Study Guide
to accompany

MOFFETT
MOFFETT
SCHAUF

Human Physiology

SECOND EDITION

Foundations & Frontiers

Ann Vernon
St. Charles County Community College

Kevin T. Patton
St. Charles County Community College

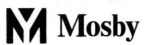 **Mosby**

St. Louis Baltimore Boston Chicago London Madrid Philadelphia Sydney Toronto

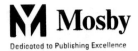

Mosby

Dedicated to Publishing Excellence

CONTENTS

STUDENT SURVIVAL GUIDE

FOR

HUMAN PHYSIOLOGY

As you begin a new course, you may feel trapped in a wilderness where the ideas are strange, the language unique, and the terrain unfamiliar. In other words, you may feel a little lost. Have no fear! This part of the *Study Guide to Accompany Human Physiology* provides a set of survival tips to help you in your trek through the strange and wondrous world of human physiology.

Look at the tips outlined in the following pages. Some you may find useful; others may not suit your style. Choose the strategies that work for you, then use them.

SURVIVAL TIP 1

Know your learning style

Learning researchers have found that each of us has a certain style of learning. This style is the way we approach new information, process that information, and then use it. Familiarity with your own learning style can be a major key to success in learning. Knowing your style lets you approach new information in a way that will enable you to learn it more efficiently.

One way to determine your own learning style is to be tested by a learning specialist. Although formal tests are available, such testing may be as informal as a chat with a staff member at your college's learning center. Another way to determine your own learning style is to use the self-quiz method. Here are a few questions you can ask yourself about your personal approach to learning:

Do I prefer a verbal explanation of a process, or a written explanation?

Do I need to see, hear, or touch a model or specimen as I learn about a process?

Do I learn better at some particular time of day than at others?

Do I learn better if I am physically active, or eating or drinking while I study?

Do I prefer to start with the "big picture" and work toward the details, or do I prefer starting with details and assembling the "big picture"?

These and other questions will help you identify your approach to learning. Once that is done, you can plan a learning strategy that will process new information in a way that works best with your learning style.

SURVIVAL TIP 2

Plan a learning strategy

Intending to learn something is a step in the right direction, but intentions only will not suffice as a learning plan. You must carefully plan a set of activities that will move you toward your goals for learning about human physiology.

You must consider two important aspects of a good learning strategy:

1. **Time management.** For any plan to work, it must account for timing. A learning strategy must be based on the careful planning of study time for your work in human physiology. If you have trouble budgeting your time, perhaps you should seek the advice of your instructor or of a learning specialist.

2. **A logical sequence of activities.** The sequence of learning activities within your budgeted study time should be determined by your learning style, any limitations you may have to live with, and a look at what has worked for others. Here is a plan that has worked for many human physiology students:

Read the appropriate chapter in the textbook.

Attend the lecture, taking careful notes.

Review and organize your notes.

Participate in related lab and demonstration activities.

Reread the textbook chapter.

Work through some learning activities, such as those in this guide.

Review the material with other students, as in a study group.

SURVIVAL TIP 3

Arrange a suitable study area

Just as the timing of study activities is important, the location in which you work can be critical to success in learning human physiology. Because none of us lives in an ideal world, you may

have to settle for less than the best. However, extra effort put
into securing a prime study site could pay big dividends at test time. Things to consider when selecting a study location:

Make sure you have good access to the site. Don't plan to study in an area that may be closed during your study time, or that is often in use by others before you get there.

Be sure that you have comfortable lighting. Some learners do best in bright lighting, others in moderately dim lighting. Also, you may find reading easier in incandescent rather than fluorescent lighting.

Ensure that the surroundings complement your learning style. In other words, make sure that your site is comfortable (without being so comfortable that you'll tend to doze).

Analyze the background noise. Few study locations are perfectly quiet. Ask yourself whether your selected site has noise that will be tolerable (loud/soft; people's voices/music/machine noises).

SURVIVAL TIP 4

Plan a reading strategy

Reading the appropriate chapters is one part of the overall learning strategy, but reading itself requires a strategy of its own. With physiology textbooks, especially, the "jump right into it" approach used for reading novels or magazines does not work very well. Instead, you must do some "prereading" and "postreading" of a new chapter if you are to understand it well.

Learning specialists have developed several reading strategies, the most popular of which are:

SQ3R (survey, question, read, recite, review)

PQRST (preview, question, read, summarize, test)

OK5R (overview, key ideas, read, record, recite, review, reflect)

You can find details of these strategies in your college or university learning center or in the school library.

A strategy that works well with this textbook is outlined here:

Read the brief chapter outline (text or study guide). This provides a framework for the chapter, enabling you to see the organization of chapter topics before you start reading.

Read the learning objectives (text or study guide). This gives you specific goals for finding meaning in the chapter.

Read the important terms aloud (study guide). Reading the words aloud will familiarize you with new terms, which in physiology can be incredibly complex. Even if you don't know what they mean yet, you'll have seen them before. As you read the chapter, you can absorb them easily, without having to stop and reread each sentence that has a new term in it.

Read the text. Try to read the chapter from beginning to end without stopping. The chapters in the textbook are designed to be brief enough that you can do this easily. If any part of the chapter is particularly troublesome, go back and reread it after you have finished the entire chapter.

Look at the illustrations while reading the text. The authors and artists who created this text spent considerable effort to balance text and illustrations. Don't miss the information in the figures referred to in the text; it is just as important as the information in the words. Some readers do well with the two-finger approach, following the text with one finger while the other traces elements of the figure.

Finish by reviewing the chapter contents by rereading the chapter objectives (to make sure that you didn't miss any important points). Although you may not have absorbed everything as well as you might like, by this point you are prepared for your professor's explanations in lecture.

SURVIVAL TIP 5

Analyze your note-taking skills. As you may know, taking notes during a lecture improves both your comprehension and your retention of information. Because note-taking requires you to organize the data you see and hear during the lecture on the spot, it improves your comprehension. Because note-taking reinforces information as you record it, it improves your retention of the material. Also, the multisensory (sight, sound, movement) character of note-taking improves your recall. Here are a few points to consider when planning your note-taking strategy:

Know the lecturer's style. Some lecturers present physiology in a well-organized manner, whereas others tend to ramble. Some speak very softly, or perhaps too loudly. Lecturers may choose to follow the textbook organization closely, or they may choose to take a completely different approach. Being aware of a lecturer's style will help you decide how you want to organize your notes; whether you may need a tape-recorder to back up your notes; and where you want to sit in the classroom.

Plan for note-taking. Decide on what style of note-taking you will rely on, what materials you need to bring, and how much lap or desk space you need.

Listen well. You cannot take effective notes without hearing what is being presented. This means making sure that you not only perceive the sound, but understand the meaning. Try to identify the speaker's personal style to determine the main points and relationships between concepts.

Structure your notes. Know ahead of time whether you will use a formal outline style or your own personal modified outline style for your notes. Be concise. Don't try to take down every word, but use phrase, abbreviations, symbols, diagrams, and so forth to summarize the points made by the lecturer. Leave space between entries so that you can fill in more information if the lecturer returns to a point. Try using highlighting pens or colored pencils to organize your notes with color. Keep your physiology notes separate form those for other classes.

Process your notes. As soon after a lecture as possible, review your notes to clarify what you have written. Fill in blank spots you may haver left and write out abbreviated terms so you'll know their meaning later. Don't completely rewrite your notes, but be sure that everything is there, and that you understand everything. If you find a gap or a muddled section, check with a classmate or the lecturer for clarification.

SURVIVAL TIP 6

Study actively.

Many students believe that studying is the same as reading, so they spend their study time only in reading and rereading their textbooks and lecture notes. Although reading is part of a study plan, additional activities are necessary is you study time is to be effective. Here are a few aggressive supplements to your study regimen:

Answer the study questions at the end of each chapter in your textbook. Write out these answers; don't just answer them mentally.

Do some or all of the many types of activities in this study guide.

Keep up with the new vocabulary by making and using flashcards, or by devising other vocabulary-strengthening activities.

Use computer-assisted tutorials, visualizations, or reviews, if they are available.

Form a study group with others in your course and discuss/review/process human physiology together. Ask each other test questions that you devise yourselves. Argue about the correct answers.

Make a "concept map" of important physiological concepts. A concept map is a graphic representation of an idea. It can take many forms. It can be a flowchart, a tree-diagram of topics and subtopics, or even a full-color sketch of a process. Your campus learning center or library will be able to help you learn how to do concept mapping.

SURVIVAL TIP 7

Use all your resources

Some learning resources are obvious: your textbook, this study guide, your notes, your instructor, the course syllabus, and so forth. Other useful resources are often less obvious; here are some:

teaching assistants, aides, and tutors

study partners (classmates)

friends who have recently taken the human physiology course

campus learning center or library

other physiology books (references, texts)

related journal or magazine articles

study skills courses, seminars, books

SURVIVAL TIP 8

Prepare for tests

Obviously, you prepare for tests by studying the appropriate course material. However, a few special tricks may help you to deal with the testing situation itself. Other students have found some of these useful:

Practice taking the test. Sometimes professors provide sample questions or old editions of physiology tests. Fortunately for you, you have a practice test in each learning module of this study guide.

Stay healthy. Don't overtax yourself in studying (especially last-minute cramming) to the point that you are sick, sleepy, or otherwise unable to work at top efficiency.

Be comfortable. Dress as comfortably as possible and find a seat in a part of the test room that suits you.

Anticipate stress. No matter how confident you may feel, the test situation is stressful. That may negatively influence your performance on a particular test. Knowing that ahead of time, you can plan for what to do if you feel pressured during the exam. Closing your eyes and calmly counting 10 slow breaths may help, as may concentrating on a relaxing image. You might even consider participating in one of the test anxiety workshops held on many campuses.

Make a final review of important physiological concepts just before the test. This review should be a refresher, not the first time you look at the material. Cramming is very seldom an effective strategy.

SURVIVAL TIP 9

Use a test-taking strategy during the examination.

Once you begin the examination, you should still be implementing a strategy. test-taking is more than just spewing forth information, It is a process that requires thought, skill, and action. Physiology students have found these hints helpful:

Know the testing style. Do what you can to find out the specifics of the test's construction (format, number of items, time to complete, wording of test items, level of complexity, and so forth).

Skim over the test before answering any questions. Read the directions for the entire test first; then briefly look at the style and content of all the questions. It only takes a few minutes, and then you'll know what you're up against.

Skip questions that stump you. If you come across a puzzling questions, save it for later (when you better know how much time you can devote to it).

Know how to evaluate objective items logically.

Understand the nature of each item (Is it fill-in, matching, or multiple-choice?) and any special instructions. (Is there more than one correct answer; can the same answer appear more than once?)

Analyze the wording. Watch for key qualifying words such as *all, every, always, never, sometimes, often, usually*. Determine whether the answer should be singular or plural, and what part of speech (noun, verb, adverb, adjective).

Eliminate choices. If several choices are offered (or occur to you) that all seem likely to be correct, try to eliminate those that are *least* likely. Such analysis may lead you to the correct choice.

If you must, guess. If blank answers are scored the same as wrong answers, and you are really stumped, guess anyway. Assuming you have studied, your answer will be an informed guess, which is certainly better than a blank.

Plan answers to short-answer and essay questions well.

Understand the directions. This is especially important for these types of items, because it will determine the approach you take in planning a response.

Understand the questions. Although key words are important, they are not the question itself. Take some time to think over the questions, to be sure that you know what it is asking.

Start with a thesis statement, which summarizes the core of your answer succinctly. Usually, a rephrasing of the question makes a suitable thesis statement.

Arrange your points logically. After stating your thesis, support it by a series of paragraphs (or sentences) that backs it up.

If possible, make a concluding statement. A restatement of the thesis (although not in exactly the same words) works well. Not only is a concluding remark good style, it allows you to emphasize your main point.

Don't dance around the central issue of the questions, Many students feel that weaving circles around an issue that they don't understand completely will fool the grader. It's more likely that the grader will not only see that critical content is missing, but also will become irritated at the student who wrote the answer. This is not a good strategy for items that are graded subjectively.

HUMAN PHYSIOLOGY STUDY MODULES

The bulk of this study guide is a series of learning activities keyed to the 26 chapters of *Human Physiology: Foundations and Frontiers*. These learning activities are based on the study strategies outlined in the "Student Survival Guide." Each module contains the following parts:

Focus The Focus section gives the learner a broad perspective of the chapter contents and organization before the study activities begin. Thus specific information is always studied within the context of the entire chapter.

Chapter outline The Chapter Outline is the first of two Focus subsections. It repeats the outline at the beginning of each textbook chapter, so it should look familiar to you.

Learning objectives The Learning Objectives is the second of the two Focus subsections. These objectives are specific goals that you must reach if you are to have a good understanding of the chapter. This word tells you what kind of goal you should have for that item. For instance, it indicates whether you should be able to *explain* a concept or merely *list* its steps. Keep these objectives in mind as you study.

Language of physiology The vocabulary of physiology can sometimes be a stumbling block to easy learning of the major concepts. The Language of Physiology section provides opportunities for you to improve your mastery of key physiological terms.

Word parts Many learners find that physiology vocabulary is easier to master if the roots, suffixes, and prefixes of the terms are recognizable. The Word Parts subsection presents common Greek and Latin word parts, which will help you in learning new terms in the chapter.

Key terms The Key Terms subsection helps you master vocabulary in two ways. First, it encourages you to read each term aloud, a multisensory approach to adding to your vocabulary. Pronunciation keys are provided for the more difficult terms. Second, this subsection helps you master the meaning of each term by grouping terms according to their meanings and by providing description/matching exercises.

The big picture This section of the study module offers a wide variety of different learning activities, each suited to the specific topic being studied. The emphasis in this section is on the relationship of separate bits of information, enabling you to appreciate the "big picture."

Learning exercises This subsection contains different learning activities, each with its own set of instructions.

Quick recall This subsection asks you to do just that: quickly recall basic information. This section serves as a review, and answers are not provided. If you get stuck here, go back over the appropriate sections in your textbook and this study guide to find the answers.

Practice test Do the Practice Test after you finish all the other study activities. This is your final preparation for taking the "real" chapter test. If you do well, you are well prepared. If you do poorly, you need to do some more studying. *Important*: Each test item has only *one* correct response.

Answers This section provides answers to all of the learning activities except for the Quick Recall items. Use this section only to verify that you have answered questions correctly, or to find the correct response if you are stumped.

Chapter 1
Human Physiology in Perspective

Focus
Review this section *first*. It will help you focus on the overall message of this chapter.

Chapter Outline
Read through the outline slowly. This activity will help your mind organize the topics of this chapter.

Human physiology—an experimental science
"How" and "why"—explanations in physiology
From single cells to organ systems
Homeostasis—a delicately balanced state

Learning Objectives
These are the learning goals for this part of the course. After reading the text, attending class, and studying this chapter, you should be able to:

♦   describe the science of physiology

♦   appreciate the history of physiology—especially in terms of its dependence upon anatomy

♦   compare and contrast different approaches to explaining life processes: vitalism, mechanism, teleology

♦   list the levels of biological organization within organisms: cell, tissue, organ, system

♦   understand the nature of the cell as the basic unit of living organisms

♦   describe the four basic tissue types found in humans

♦   recognize the major human organ systems, their component organs, and their basic functions

♦   understand the basic character of the internal environment, including its fluid nature and homeostatic balance

Language of Physiology

Physiology uses its own set of terms, many of which may be unfamiliar to you. This section will help you improve your mastery of key physiological terms.

Word Parts

Here are some combining forms often seen in physiological terms. Give an example of a term that contains each word part listed.

Word Part	Meaning	Example
cardio-	heart	1_____
extra-	outside of	2_____
homeo-	same;equal	3_____
intra-	within	4_____
mutat-	change	5_____
neuro-	nerve	6_____
physio-	nature (function) of	7_____

Key Terms

Read each of the terms in each grouping below aloud, using the pronunciation guide if necessary. This will help you to remember them better than if you read them silently. Then, write out the correct term next to each of the descriptions given.

Terms related to processes

differentiation (dif-er-en-shee-AY-shun)   natural selection
diffusion (dif-YOO-jun)   negative feedback

1. _____ process in which a variable is controlled by actions (responses) which oppose changes in that variable

2. _____ process in which the random movements of molecules result in the net movement of molecules to an area of lower concentration

3. _____ process in nature whereby only fit individuals (those with beneficial characteristics) survive

4. _____ developmental process by which relatively unspecialized cells become specialized to perform specific functions

Terms related to structures/substances

adipose tissue (AD-i-pohs)   connective tissue
blood   digestive system
bone   endocrine system (EN-doh-krin)
cardiac muscle   endocrine gland (EN-doh-krin)
cardiovascular system   epithelial tissue (ep-ih-THEE-lee-al)
    (KARD-ee-oh-VASK-yoo-ler)   exocrine gland (EKS-oh-krin)
cell   extracellular fluid (eks-trah-SEL-yoo-ler)

glial cell (GLEE-al)
immune system
integumentary system
     (in-teg-yoo-MENT-ah-ree)
interstitial fluid (in-ter-STISH-al)
intracellular fluid (in-trah-SEL-yoo-ler)
multicellular organism (muhl-tee-SEL-yoo-ler)
muscle tissue
musculoskeletal system
     (muhs-kyoo-loh-SKEL-uh-tal)
nervous system

nervous tissue
neuron (NOO-ron)
nutrient
organ system
organ
plasma
reproductive system
respiratory system
skeletal muscle
smooth muscle
tissue
urinary system (yoo-rih-NAR-ee)

1 _____ term that refers to any body fluid that surrounds the cells of multicellular organisms; includes both interstitial fluid and plasma

2 _____ loose, liquid type of connective tissue which circulates throughout the body

3 _____ type of extracellular fluid that forms the liquid portion of blood

4 _____ collection of similar cells

5 _____ group of organs that work together (that is, have a common function)

6 _____ structure composed of two or more tissue types working as a functional unit

7 _____ type of very hard connective tissue that forms most of the skeleton

8 _____ substance that serves as a molecular building block or source of energy

9 _____ organ system that transports materials throughout the body, exchanging them between organ systems

10 _____ organ system that maintains the homeostasis of extracellular fluid volume and composition—and excretes certain wastes

11 _____ organ system that functions to resist invasion from foreign materials and the growth of cancer

12 _____ organ system that protects the body from the external environment

13 _____ organ system that secretes hormones, thus regulating many body functions

14 _____ organ system that digests and absorbs nutrients

15 _____ organism composed of many cells, as is the human

16 _____ organ system that supports and moves the body, stores minerals, and produces blood cells

17 _____ organ system that sends, receives, and stores information

18 _____ organ system that takes oxygen from the atmosphere and releases carbon dioxide into the atmosphere

19 _____ organ system that functions in the reproduction and development of offspring

20 _____ cell type found in nervous tissue; specialized for supportive non-conducting functions within the nervous system

21 _____ cell type found in nervous tissue; specialized for generation and conduction of nerve impulses

22 _____ fat tissue; a type of soft connective tissue

23 _____ fluid that surrounds most tissue cells of multicellular organisms, except blood cells; a type of extracellular fluid

24 _____ fluid found inside the cells of a multicellular organism

25 _____ one of four basic tissue types; responsible for movements of body organs

26 _____ one of four basic tissue types; primarily responsible for generation and conduction of electrical impulses

27 _____ one of four basic tissue types; has large amounts of extracellular material and often contributes to the structural integrity of the body

28 _____ one of four basic tissue types; forms sheets that cover/line body parts, forms glands, forms some sensory receptors

29 _____ fundamental unit of which organisms are composed

30 _____ type of muscle tissue responsible for movement of soft internal organs

31 _____ type of muscle tissue responsible for moving the skeleton

32 _____ type of muscle tissue responsible for heart contractions

33 _____ type of gland (secreting organ) that releases material into the bloodstream

34 _____ type of gland (secreting organ) that releases material through a duct onto a surface or into a cavity

Other Key Terms

anatomy
concentration gradient (GRAY-dee-ent)
homeostasis (hoh-mee-oh-STAY-sis)
mechanism
mutation

physiology
reflex
teleology (tee-lee-AHL-o-jee)
vitalism (VIH-tahl-izm)

1 _____ chemical change in the genes of a DNA molecule (chromosome)

2 _____ response to a stimulus

3 _____ difference in the concentration of a substance over a distance

4 _____ approach to studying life processes that assumes that they are subject to physical and chemical laws

5 _____ approach to studying life processes that assumes that living organisms possess a vital life force

4

6 _____ approach to studying life processes that attempts to justify processes in terms of their value to an organism

7 _____ constancy (steady balance) of the internal environment

8 _____ science that describes how the bodies of living organisms function

9 _____ science that describes the structures of organisms

The Big Picture
Use the activities of this section to help you learn the broader concepts of this chapter.

Learning Exercises
1. Match these historically significant persons or groups with their descriptions below.

physicians of the Renaissance era   William Harvey
the physiologoi   William Beaumont

_____ American who studied the physiology of the stomach of a live patient (Alexis St. Martin) beginning in 1835

_____ correctly described the pumping action of the heart and the circulatory mechanism of the human body in 1628

_____ early scientists who attempted to understand the function of the body through anatomical studies

_____ early Greek philosophers (400 to 500 B.C.) who applied themselves to the study of all aspects of nature, rejecting supernatural explanations because they believed that everything was understandable

2. Use these terms describing different scientific approaches to label the perspective taken in each of the quotations listed below.

mechanism   vitalism
teleology

_____ "The human digestive system works like a computerized processing plant, with intricate steps and regulatory mechanisms that will someday be understood completely."

_____ "The human body is certainly composed of distinct organs and systems but is powered by the mysterious force called 'life.'"

_____ "The incredible mental processing capabilities of humans result from the need to cope in a harsh environment without the aid of great physical power or speed."

3.   Put these levels of biological organization in the correct order, beginning with the simplest level and progressing to the most comprehensive level.

biomolecule   organism
cell   organ system
organ   tissue

_____   (simplest)

_____

_____

_____

_____

_____

_____   (most comprehensive)

4.   List the four major tissue types found in humans.

_____   _____

_____   _____

5.   For each description listed, give the correct name of the major human tissue type (from No. 4 above) that applies.

1_____   responsible for movement of the body

2_____   initiates and conducts electrical impulses that regulate/control overall body functions

3_____   forms glands that secrete important substances

4_____   responsible for the heart's pumping action and the movement of food through the digestive tract

5_____   forms bones and tendons

6_____   blood is this type of tissue

7_____   stores memories

8_____   may be smooth, cardiac, or skeletal

9_____   forms sheets that line or cover body parts

6. List the major human organ systems, writing them in the correct space in the table below.

Organ System	Function
	support and movement; mineral storage; blood production
	homeostasis of extracellular fluid volume and composition
	transports nutrient, gases, metabolic end products, and hormones between organ systems
	resists infection, parasitization, and cancer
	regulation of reproduction, growth, metabolism, energy balance, extracellular fluid composition
	reproduction; sexual gratification
	digestion; absorption of nutrients
	takes up oxygen, releases carbon dioxide; produces sounds; helps regulate acidity
	protection from drying and infection; temperature regulation
	controls other systems; receives environmental information; stores memories; behavior

7. Use these terms to label Figure 1-1.

blood plasma   internal environment
external environment   interstitial fluid
extracellular fluid   intracellular fluid

Figure 1-1

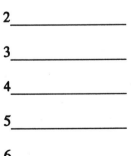

1_____

2_____

3_____

4_____

5_____

6_____

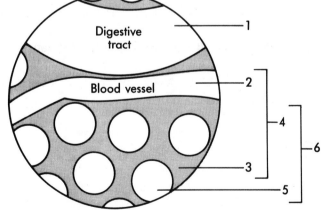

8. The graph in Figure 1-2 shows the concentration of hormone X in the blood stream over time. The line shows the normal average concentration of hormone X for 3 hours. During the fourth hour, the blood concentration of X rises significantly. Assuming that negative feedback mechanisms help regulate hormone X concentrations, predict what should happen to the hormone X concentration over the next several hours by continuing the graph line with your pencil.

Figure 1-2

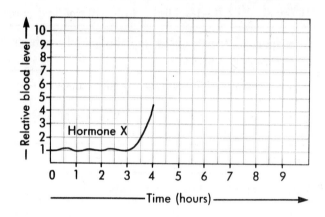

Quick Recall

Review some of the major concepts of this chapter by doing these "quick recall" activities.

1. List the two major types of glands.

2. List the three principal types of muscle tissues.

3. List the two major cell types within nervous tissue.

4. List the two functional categories of epithelium.

5. List three types of connective tissue.

6. List some major organs of each human organ system given.

   Integumentary:

   Musculoskeletal:

   Nervous:

   Endocrine:

   Cardiovascular:

   Immune:

   Urinary:

   Respiratory:

Reproductive:

Digestive:

7. List the two kinds of extracellular fluid.

8. List two evolutionary advantages of being multicellular.

Practice Test
Use this practice test to review the topics of this chapter and to prepare for your test on this material.

1. The interstitial fluid is located
   a. within cells
   b. outside the body
   c. between cells
   d. within blood vessels
   e. a and b are correct

2. The mechanistic view of physiology
   a. is no longer held by most scientists
   b. explains functions in terms of their value to the organism
   c. presupposes the existence of a "life-force"
   d. explains functions in terms of physical laws of nature

3. Initiation and conduction of electrical impulses are largely functions of which system?
   a. nervous
   b. glial
   c. brain
   d. musculoskeletal
   e. endocrine

4. Diffusion occurs
   a. across some membranes
   b. down a concentration gradient
   c. because of the random movement of molecules
   d. a and b
   e. all of the above

5. The basic unit of living organisms
   a. is the organ
   b. is the organ system
   c. is the cell
   d. has not yet been determined
   e. is called the "life force"

6. Plasma
   a. is an intracellular fluid
   b. is the interstitial fluid
   c. is a collection of functional blood cells
   d. is an extracellular fluid
   e. c and d

7. Adipose is what type of tissue?
   a. blood
   b. nervous
   c. epithelial
   d. muscle
   e. connective

8. A mechanism which returns a body function to normal (setpoint) is an example of
   a. positive feedback
   b. negative feedback
   c. motility
   d. a homeostatic muscle
   e. b and d

9. The science that deals with the study of organisms and how they function is called
   a. physiology
   b. physics
   c. teleology
   d. anatomy
   e. oncology

10. The femur bone is an organ of what system?
    a. connective
    b. musculoskeletal
    c. nervous
    d. endocrine
    e. immune

11. Human cells vary in structure and function as a result of the process of
    a. homeostasis
    b. differentiation
    c. histology
    d. negative feedback
    e. none of the above

12. A nutrient is likely to be moved from the external environment to a typical tissue cell by way of
    a. direct diffusion
    b. osmosis
    c. travel via the cardiovascular system
    d. travel via the integumentary system
    e. respiration

13. Defense against infection is a function of what system(s)?
    a. immune
    b. digestive
    c. integumentary
    d. all of the above
    e. none of the above

14. Homeostasis can be described as
    a. a dynamic steady state
    b. maintained in part by negative feedback mechanisms
    c. constancy of the internal environment
    d. constant intracellular fluid volume
    e. a, b, and c

15. A group of different tissues acting as a functional unit is usually called a(n)
    a. tissue type
    b. organ system
    c. organelle
    d. organ
    e. organism

Answers

Here are answers (or references) to some of the questions presented above.

Word Parts: (your examples may be different) 1. cardiovascular 2. extracellular 3. homeostasis 4. intracellular 5. mutation 6. neuron 7. physiology

Key Terms: Processes: 1. negative feedback 2. diffusion 3. natural selection 4. differentiation
Structures/substances: 1. extracellular fluid 2. blood 3. plasma 4. tissue 5. organ system 6. organ 7. bone 8. nutrient 9. cardiovascular system 10. urinary system 11. immune system
12. integumentary system 13. endocrine system 14. digestive system 15. multicellular organism
16. musculoskeletal system 17. nervous system 18. respiratory system 19. reproductive system
20. glial cell 21. neuron 22. adipose tissue 23. interstitial fluid 24. intracellular fluid 25. muscle tissue 26. nervous tissue 27. connective tissue 28. epithelial tissue 29. cell 30. smooth muscle
31. skeletal muscle 32. cardiac muscle 33. endocrine gland 34. exocrine gland **Other:** 1. mutation
2. reflex 3. concentration gradient 4. mechanism 5. vitalism 6. teleology 7. homeostasis
8. physiology 9. anatomy

Learning Exercises: 1. Beaumont, Harvey, Renaissance physicians, physiologoi 2. mechanism, vitalism, teleology 3. biomolecule, cell, tissue, organ, organ system, organism 4. (any order) epithelial, connective, muscle, nervous 5. 1-muscle, 2-nervous, 3-epithelial, 4-muscle, 5-connective, 6-connective, 7-nervous, 8-muscle, 9-epithelial 6. musculoskeletal, urinary, cardiovascular, immune, endocrine, reproductive, digestive, respiratory, integumentary, nervous 7. 1-external environment, 2-blood plasma, 3-interstitial fluid, 4-extracellular fluid, 5-intracellular fluid, 6-internal environment 8. The graph shows a rise from a concentration of about 1 to a level of about 4 or 5—your line should move the concentration level downward toward level 1 again, forming a bell-shaped curve.

Quick Recall: (You should be able to answer these questions easily without correction or confirmation by this point in your studies. If you cannot, review your notes, the text chapter, and the previous study activities to find the answers.)

Practice Test: 1-c, 2-d, 3-a, 4-e, 5-c, 6-d, 7-e, 8-e, 9-a, 10-b, 11-b, 12-c, 13-d, 14-e, 15-d

Chapter 2
The Chemical and Physical Foundations of Physiology

Focus
Review this section *first*. It will help you focus on the overall message of this chapter.

Chapter Outline
Read through the outline slowly. This activity will help your mind organize the topics of this chapter.

The chemical basis of physiology
     Atomic structure
     Chemical bonds
     Covalent bonds
     Ionic bonds
     Weak bonds
     Properties of water
     Aqueous solutions
     Molarity, osmolarity, and equivalency
Physiological forces and flows
     The relationship between force, resistance, and movement
     Mechanical forces
     Osmotic pressure
     Electrical forces
Thermodynamics in physiology
     The first law: energy conservation
     The second law: disorder of the universe increases
     Chemical equilibrium and the law of mass action
     The concept of dynamic steady state revisited

Learning Objectives
These are the learning goals for this part of the course. After reading the text, attending class, and studying this chapter, you should be able to:

♦   describe the structure of atoms and explain the principles of chemical bonds as they relate to the structure and behavior of biologically important compounds

- understand why water is the universal solvent for biological systems and define hydrophilic and hydrophobic

- describe solutions in terms of the molarity and osmolarity

- explain the basic chemistry of acids and bases and calculate the pH of solutions

- understand the difference between equilibrium and steady state

- describe the relationship between force, friction, and movement that will be applied in subsequent chapters to such processes as blood flow, muscle movement and the behavior of respiratory structures

- define compliance

- understand the application of thermodynamics to biological systems and define entropy and free energy

Language of Physiology

Physiology uses its own set of terms, many of which may be unfamiliar to you. This section will help you improve your mastery of key physiological terms.

Word Parts

Here are some combining forms often seen in physiological terms. Give an example of a term that contains each word part listed.

Word Part	Meaning	Example
co-	with	1_____
electro-	electrical	2_____
iso-	same	3_____
micro-	small; millionth	4_____
milli-	thousandth	5_____
neutro-	neutral	6_____
non-	not	7_____
solv-, solu-	loosen, dissolve	8_____
thermo-	heat	9_____
valen-	strength (as in bond)	10_____

Key Terms

Read each of the terms in each grouping below aloud, using the pronunciation guide if necessary. This will help you to remember them better than if you read them silently. Then, write out the correct term next to each of the descriptions given.

Descriptive terms

inorganic   organic
nonpolar   polar

1_____   describes a molecule with distinct negative and positive regions (poles) caused by unequal sharing of electrons

2_____   describes a molecule in with no distinct negative or positive region (pole)

3_____   describes a molecule that is not a complex carbon-containing molecule

4_____   describes a complex carbon-containing molecule

Terms related to measurement

acceleration   molecular weight
atomic weight   osmolarity (ahz-moh-LAYR-it-ee)
Avogadro's number (a-voh-GAD-rohz)   osmotic pressure (ahz-MAHT-ik)
compliance   pH
current   scientific notation
entropy (EN-troh-pee)   specific heat
free energy   surgace tension
friction   thermal conductivity (kahn-duk-TIV-it-ee)
heat of vaporization   valence (VAH-lents)
hydrostatic pressure (hyd-roh-STAT-ik)   velocity
molarity (mo-LAYR-it-ee)   voltage
mole

1_____   measure of hydrogen ion concentration (acidity) of a solution

2_____   manner of expressing numbers as a product of a number (between 1 and 10) and a power of 10 (such as 1.55×10^6, or 2.36×10^{-12})

3_____   electrical potential; the driving force that results from a charge imbalance

4_____   in thermodynamics, the measure of randomness (disorder)

5_____   measure of the ability of a substance to conduct heat

6_____   rate of movement; speed

7_____   rate of change of velocity over time

8_____   sum of the protons and neutrons in an atom's nucleus

9_____   sum of the atomic weights of all the atoms within a molecule

10 _____ relative density of a liquid based on the force required to break the forces holding the surface molecules together

11 _____ number of electrons an atom can donate or accept during bond formation

12 _____ gram molecular weight (6.023 x 10²³ molecules)

13 _____ amount of energy required to raise the temperature of 1 gram of a substance 1° C

14 _____ number of dissolved participles in a liter of solution

15 _____ number of moles of solute in a liter of solution

16 _____ force of pressure of fluid against a barrier (membranae)

17 _____ flow of charge (electricity)

18 _____ relationship between the degree of distortion and the force applied

19 _____ amount of a system's total energy available to do work

20 _____ amount of energy absorbed by a substance as it passes from the liquid state to the gaseous state

21 _____ mechanical resistance offered by two substances as they slide past one another

22 _____ force of pressure generated by the movement of water across a membranae into a solution (via osmosis); the potential to generate such pressure

23 _____ number of molecules in a mole of a substance (6.023 x 10²³)

Terms related to structures/substances

acid
anion (AN-i-in)
atom
base
buffer
cation (KAT-i-on)
covalent bond (koh-VAY-lent)
electrolyte (eh-LEK-troh-lyt)
electron
electron donor
electron shell (orbital)
element

hydration shell (hide-RAY-shun)
hydrogen bond
ion
ionic bond (I-ahn-ik)
isotope
neutron (NOO-trahn)
nucleus
proton
solute (SAHL-yoot)
solvent
van der Waals force (VAN-der-wahlz)

1 _____ positive ion

2 _____ weak bonding force generated by the attraction of a polar molecule to a nonpolar one in which polarity has been induced

3 _____ form of an element with the same atomic number as other forms of the element, but having a different atomic mass

4 _____ electrically charged atom or group of atoms

5 _____ positively charged particle in the nucleus of an atom

6 _____ compound that combines with a hydrogen ion

7 _____ substance that forms ions when dissolved

8 _____ negatively charged particle in the outer region of an atom

9 _____ pure substance, composed of atoms of the same atomic number

10 _____ layer of water molecules that surrounds dissolved particles

11 _____ type of chemical bond formed when electrons are shared by multiple atoms

12 _____ mixture of an acid with its conjugate base capable of minimizing changes in pH caused by the addition of strong acids or bases

13 _____ negative ion

14 _____ electrolyte that dissociates to yield hydrogen ions

15 _____ electrically neutral particle in the nucleus of an atom

16 _____ atom that tends to give up electrons during bond formation

17 _____ area (orbit) in the periphery of an atom where a certain number of electrons are likely to be found

18 _____ molecule or ion dissolved in a solution

19 _____ basic constituent of all matter; composed of a nucleus surrounded by electrons

20 _____ central structure of an atom

21 _____ liquid in which substances are dissolved—usually water

22 _____ type of chemical bond formed by the attraction of positive hydrogen (electron donor) and a negative portion of a molecule (electron acceptor)

23 _____ type of chemical bond formed when electrons are transferred between atoms and the resulting charged atoms cling together via electrical attraction

Other Key Terms

dissociation (dih-soh-see-AY-shun)   steady state
equilibrium   thermodynamics (therm-oh-dy-NAM-iks)

1_____   situation in which all system variables remain constant, without expenditure of physiological energy

2_____   situation in which some variables of a system are constant over time, usually requiring the expenditure of physiological energy

3_____   science that deals with energy transformations

4_____   splitting of chemical entities as they dissolve

The Big Picture

Use the activities of this section to help you learn the broader concepts of this chapter.

Learning Exercises

1.   Use these labels to correctly name the parts of an atom shown in the figure.

electron   nucleus
electron shell   proton
neutron

Figure 2-1

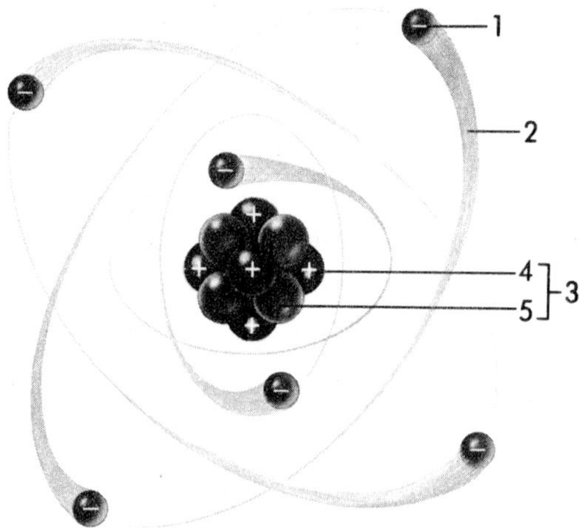

1_____

2_____

3_____

4_____

5_____

2.   Arrange these chemical bond types in order of increasing relative strength.

covalent bond   _____
hydrogen bond
ionic bond   _____

_____

3.   For Figure 2-2, fill in appropriate pH values in the spaces provided along the middle column of the graph.

Figure 2-2

H⁺ ion concentration (moles/liter)	pH value	Examples	OH⁻ ion concentration (moles/liter)

H⁺ ion concentration (moles/liter)		pH value	Examples	OH⁻ ion concentration (moles/liter)
1	▲ Increasingly acid	—	Hydrochloric acid	10^{-14}
10^{-1}		—	Stomach acid	10^{-13}
10^{-2}		—	Lemon juice	10^{-12}
10^{-3}		—	Vinegar, Coca-Cola, beer	10^{-11}
10^{-4}		—	Tomatoes	10^{-10}
10^{-5}		—	Black coffee / Normal rainwater	10^{-9}
10^{-6}		—	Urine	10^{-8}
10^{-7}	Neutral	—	Pure water / Blood, tears	10^{-7}
10^{-8}		—	Seawater	10^{-6}
10^{-9}	Increasingly basic	—	Baking soda	10^{-5}
10^{-10}		—	Great Salt Lake	10^{-4}
10^{-11}		—	Household ammonia	10^{-3}
10^{-12}		—	Bicarbonate of soda	10^{-2}
10^{-13}		—	Oven cleaner	10^{-1}
10^{-14}	▼	—	Sodium hydroxide (NaOH)	1

4.   Given these concentrations of H⁺ in solution, calculate the correct pH.

1 Molar H^+ = pH _____

.01 Molar H^+ = pH _____

.00001 Molar H^+ = pH _____

5. Match the units of measurement listed to the parameter that they measure (give the unit's abbreviation within the parentheses).

ampere   _____   ( ) length
gram   _____   ( ) mass
liter   _____   ( ) volume
millimeter of mercury _____   ( ) time
meter   _____   ( ) pressure
mole   _____   ( ) electrical resistance
ohm   _____   ( ) voltage (electrical potential)
osmole   _____   ( ) electrical current
second   _____   ( ) solute concentration
volt   _____   ( ) osmolarity

6. Use these terms to fill in the blanks in the following paragraph.

compliance   hydrostatic   resistance
elastic   osmotic   velocity
friction

        As blood moves through a vessel, it moves at a certain flow rate, or _____. The
force of _____, generated by the blood rubbing past the walls of the vessel, tends to slow
the flow rate. A force that tends to impede the flow of blood (or any material) is called
_____. The driving force of blood comes from tow sources: _____ pressure
(mechanical force of a fluid against a barrier) and _____ pressure (force generated by the
osmotic flow of water into the bloodstream). Blood vessels often exhibit an _____ restoring
force in their walls as the walls spring back into their original shape after being stretched. The relative
ability of such a membrane to spring back in this manner is termed _____.

7. Describe the relationship between these three parameters by inserting them into the blanks in the
   mathematical function given below.

                        driving force
                        flow rate
                        resistance

_____ = _____ / _____

8. Use the mathematical function in #7 above to answer these items.

    1. If the flow rate is to remain constant but the resistance increases, then the driving force
        must (increase/decrease/stay the same)
    2. If the flow rate increases but the driving force remains constant, then the resistance mist
        (increase, decrease, stay the same).
    3. If the resistance increases, the flow rate will tend to (increase, decrease, stay the same).

20

9.   Use these terms to fill in the mathematical functions describing Ohm's Law below.

current
resistance
voltage

current = _____ / _____

voltage = _____ / _____

resistance = _____ / _____

10.   Match the names of these physical principles to their descriptions below.

Newton's second law of mechanics
first law of thermodynamics
second law of thermodynamics

1_____   a process always results in an increase in the total disorder in a system
2_____   the total quantity of energy involved in a process is never lost
3_____   if increased order results from a process, an input of energy is required
4_____   if a process increases the entropy of a system, energy is released during the
                    process
5_____   a mass subject to an applied force will accelerate in the direction of the force,
                    with an acceleration that is proportional to the force

Quick Recall
Review some of the major concepts of this chapter by doing these "quick recall" activities.

1.   List the three possible particles that comprise atoms.

2.   List four types of bonds/forces that may hold atoms together.

3.   List the two forces that affect the flow rate of a fluid in a vessel.

4.   List the three electrical parameters described in Ohm's Law.

Practice Test
Use this practice test to review the topics of this chapter and to prepare for your test on this material.

1.   Steady states can be distinguished from equilibria because steady states
     a.   do not require physiological energy to maintain themselves
     b.   require physiological energy to maintain themselves
     c.   require only the random movements of molecules to maintain themselves
     d.   b and c

2. Avogadro's number
    a.   is 6.023 x 10²³
    b.   describes the number of molecules in a mole
    c.   is the number of protons in a gram of substance
    d.   all of the above
    e.   a and b

3. Of these binding forces, which is weakest?
    a.   van der Waals force
    b.   ionic bond
    c.   covalent bond

4. An acid and its conjugate base mixed in a solution
    a.   is called a buffer
    b.   tends to reduce large changes in pH
    c.   neutralize each other
    d.   cannot exist
    e.   a and b

5. The ration of the length change of an object to the applied force is termed its
    a.   compliance
    b.   conductance
    c.   resistance
    d.   capacitance
    e.   none of these

6. If a sold crystal were placed in a solution and its ions broke apart as they were surrounded by water molecules, one could say
    a.   the crystal dissolved
    b.   the ions dissociated
    c.   hydration shells were formed
    d.   electron shells were formed

7. Sodium tends to ionize and
    a.   form negative ions in solution
    b.   form positive ions in solution
    c.   form anions in solution
    d.   b and c are correct
    e.   none of the above

8. As energy is released by a process, one would expect entropy to a.   increase
    b.   decrease
    c.   stay the same
    d.   energy and entropy are unrelated

9. If tritium and deuterium are isotopes of hydrogen, one would expect that
    a.   they have the same atomic number
    b.   they have the same atomic mass
    c.   they have the same number of neutrons
    d.   they have the same gram weight

22

10. The amount of total energy available to do work in a system is called
    a. heat of friction
    b. entropy
    c. free energy
    d. acceleration
    e. conductance

11. pH
    a. is a measure of the acidity of a solution
    b. is an expression of H^+ concentration
    c. is a measure of the relative destructiveness of a substance
    d. is an expression of conjugate base concentration
    e. a and b

12. Which of these is *not* a characteristic of water?
    a. good solvent
    b. good thermal conductor
    c. low specific heat
    d. high polarity
    e. high surface tension

13. The sharing of electrons by atoms that form a molecule is termed
    a. ionic bond
    b. hydrogen bond
    c. covalent bond
    d. van der Waals force
    e. b and d

14. The difference in electrical charge between two points generates a driving force for electrical current called electrical potential or
    a. amperage
    b. voltage
    c. resistance
    d. conductance
    e. compliance

Answers

Here are answers (or references) to some of the questions presented above.

Word Parts: 1. covalent 2. electrolyte 3. isotope 4. microvolt 5. millivolt 6. neutron 7. nonpolar 8. solvent, solute 9. thermodynamics 10. covalent

Key Terms: Descriptive: 1. polar 2. nonpolar 3. inorganic **Measurement:** 1. pH 2. scientific notation 3. voltage 4. entropy 5. thermal conductivity 6. velocity 7. acceleration 8. atomic weight 9. molecular weight 10. surface tension 11. valence 12. mole 13. specific heat 14. osmolarity 15. molarity 16. hydrostatic pressure 17. current 18. compliance 19. free energy 20. heat of vaporization 21. friction 22. osmotic pressure 23. Avogadro's number
Structures/Substances: 1. cation 2. van der Waals force 3. isotope 4. ion 5. proton 6. base 7. electrolyte 9. element 10. hydration shell 11. covalent bond 12. buffer 13. anion 14. acid

15. neutron 16. electron donor 17. electron shell 18. solute 19. atom 20. nucleus 21. solvent
22. hydrogen bond 23. ionic bond **Other:** 1. equilibrium 2. steady state 3. thermodynamics
4. dissociation

Learning Exercises: 1. 1-electron, 2-electron shell, 3-nucleus, 4-proton, 5-neutron 2. hydrogen, ionic, covalent 3. (starting from top) 0, 1, 2, 3, 4, 5, 6, 7, 8, 9, 10, 11, 12 13, 14 4. 0, 2, 5 5. meter(m), gram(g), liter(l), second(s), millimeter of mercury (mm Hg), ohm(Ω), volt(v), ampere(A), molar or mole/L(M), osmole/L (Osm) 6. velocity, friction, resistance, hydrostatic, osmotic, elastic, compliance 7. flow rate, driving force, resistance 8. 1-increase, 2-decrease, 3-decrease 9. current = voltage / resistance, voltage = resistance x current, resistance = voltage / current 10. 1-second law of thermodynamics, 2-first law of thermodynamics, 3-second law of thermodynamics, 4-second law of thermodynamics, 5-Newton's second law of mechanics

Quick Recall: (You should be able to answer these questions without correction or confirmation by this point in your studies. If you cannot, review your notes, the text chapter, and the previous study activities to find the answers.)

Practice Test: 1-b, 2-e, 3-a, 4-e, 5-a, 6-e, 7-b, 8-a, 9-a, 10-c, 11-e, 12-c, 13-c, 14-b

Chapter 3
The Chemistry of Cells

Focus
Review this section *first*. It will help you focus on the overall message of this chapter.

Chapter Outline
Read through the outline slowly. This activity will help your mind organize the topics of this chapter.

Some molecular terminology
Lipids
        Types of lipids
        Fatty acids
        Acylglycerols
        Phospholipids
        Glycolipids
        Steroids
        Eicosanoids
Carbohydrates
        Monosaccharides
        Disaccharides, oligosaccharides and polysaccharides
Proteins
        Amino acids
        Protein structure and function
Enzyme catalysis
        Enzymes and the rates of biochemical reactions
        The names of enzymes
        The importance of active sites in enzymatic catalysis
        The concentration dependence of enzyme-catalyzed reactions
        The effects of temperature and pH
        Competitive inhibition
        Allosteric regulation of enzymes
Nucleic acids
        Structure of nucleic acids
        Functions of DNA and RNA
        DNA replication and base pairing
        The cell cycle and mitosis
DNA transcription and protein synthesis
        The genetic code
        DNA transcription into mRNA

mRNA translation into proteins
Selective reading of the genetic code in differentiated cells

Learning Objectives

These are the learning goals for this part of the course. After reading the text, attending class, and studying this chapter, you should be able to:

♦ describe the structure of lipids including triacylglycerols, fatty acids, steroids, and phospholipids—and state the major storage form of lipids in humans

♦ describe the structure of carbohydrates including monosaccharides, disaccharides, and the starches—and state the major storage form of carbohydrate in humans

♦ understand peptide formation

♦ compare primary, secondary, tertiary, and quaternary structure of proteins

♦ state how the sequence of amino acids in a protein is coded for by the sequence of nucleotide codons

♦ understand how enzymes catalyze chemical reactions

♦ define the terms active site, saturation, competition, and allosteric site

♦ describe DNA and how DNA replicates by complementary base-pairing

♦ understand the process of transcription of the nucleotide sequence of a gene into messenger RNA

♦ describe how messenger RNA is translated into protein

Language of Physiology
Physiology uses its own set of terms, many of which may be unfamiliar to you. This section will help you improve your mastery of key physiological terms.

Word Parts
Here are some combining forms often seen in physiological terms. Give an example of a term that contains each word part listed.

Word Part	Meaning	Example
carbo-	carbon-containing	1_____
di-	two (double)	2_____
glyco-	sugar (carbohydrate)	3_____
-hydrate	containing H, O (water)	4_____
hydro-	water	5_____
lipo-	lipid (fat)	6_____
mono-	one (single)	7_____
-philic	loving	8_____
-phobic	fearing	9_____
poly-	many	10_____

Key Terms
Read each of the terms in each grouping below aloud, using the pronunciation guide if necessary. This will help you to remember them better than if you read them silently. Then, write out the correct term next to each of the descriptions given.

Chemical substances
adenine (AD-en-een)
amino acids (ah-MEEN-oh)
carbohydrate
catalyst (KAT-ahl-ist)
cytosine (SITE-oh-seen)
deoxyribose (dee-ahks-ee-RYB-ohs)
disaccharide (dy-SAK-ah-ride)
enzyme
fatty acids
glycogen (GLY-koh-jen)
glycolipid (gly-koh-LIP-id)
guanine (GWAH-neen)
hydrocarbon (hide-roh-KAR-bon)
lipoprotein (lip-oh-PROH-teen)
messenger RNA

monosaccharide (mahn-oh-SAK-ah-ride)
nucleotide (NOO-klee-oh-tide)
phospholipid (fahs-foh-LIP-id)
polymer (PAHL-i-mer)
polysaccharide (pahl-ee-SAK-ah-ride)
proenzyme (proh-EN-zime)
prostaglandin (proh-stah-GLAND-in)
protein
ribose (RYB-ohs)
RNA
thymine (THY-meen)
transfer RNA
triglyceride (try-GLIS-er-ide)
uracil (YOO-rah-sil)

27

1_____ one of four possible bases in DNA or RNA nucleotides; combines with G

2_____ one of four possible bases in DNA nucleotides only; combines with A

3_____ one of four possible bases in DNA or RNA nucleotides; combine with T or U

4_____ one of four possible bases in DNA or RNA nucleotides; combines with C

5_____ one of four possible bases in DNA or RNA nucleotides only; combines with A

6_____ two fatty acids and one phosphoric acid/polar molecule linked to a glycerol group

7_____ 20-carbon fatty acid with 5-carbon ring; tissue regulator

8_____ a lipid-protein combination

9_____ a carbohydrate-lipid combination

10_____ animal starch; a polymer of glucose

11_____ biomolecule composed of C, H, and O in a 1:2:1 ratio

12_____ carbohydrate formed by covalent linkage of two monosaccharides

13_____ carbohydrate formed by linkage of many monosaccharides

14_____ compound consisting only of carbon and hydrogen

15_____ general term for a substance that accelerates reactions, but is not consumed in the process

16_____ hydrocarbons that have a carboxyl group at one end

17_____ inactive form in which some enzymes are first synthesized

18_____ molecule formed by the linking together of many similar subunit molecules

19_____ molecules with three fatty acid chains attached to a glycerol backbone

20_____ one of 20 small nitrogen-containing molecules commonly used by cells to make protein

21_____ organic molecule formed by the combination of many amino acids

22_____ ribonucleic acid

23_____ simple 5- or 6-carbon carbohydrate such as fructose, glucose, and galactose

24_____ substrate-specific catalysts for biochemical reactions

25_____ subunit of nucleic acids formed by a sugar, phosphate group, and nitrogen base

26 _____ sugar present in DNA nucleotides

27 _____ sugar present in RNA nucleotides

28 _____ type of RNA that carries a particular amino acid to its codon on mRNA

29 _____ type of RNA that represents a copy of a portion of a DNA molecule

Descriptive terms

allosteric effect (al-oh-STAYR-ik)   hydrophilic (hide-roh-FIL-ik)
amphipathic (am-fih-PATH-ik)   hydrophobic (hide-roh-FOHB-ik)

1 _____ describes molecules that have both polar regions and nonpolar regions

2 _____ modification of enzyme activity by binding of a modulator at a separate site

3 _____ tendency of polar molecules to attract water molecules

4 _____ tendency of nonpolar molecules to avoid interaction with water

Terms related to processes

complementary base-pairing   mitosis (my-TOH-sis)
cytokinesis (site-oh-kin-EES-is)   oxidation (ahks-id-AY-shun)
dehydration   reduction
denaturation (dee-nay-chur-AY-shun)   replication (rep-lih-KAY-shun)
enzyme competion   transcription
enzyme saturation   translation
hydrolysis (hide-RAHL-is-is)

1 _____ changes in a protein's tertiary structure caused by the breaking of some bonds

2 _____ chemical reaction in which an electron is removed from a molecule

3 _____ chemical reaction in which an electron is added to a molecule

4 _____ condensation; reaction in which molecules are joined and water is yielded

5 _____ duplication; as in duplicating the DNA molecules during interphase

6 _____ period of cell division that includes the equal and orderly distribution of DNA

7 _____ period of cell division constituted by the splitting of the cytoplasm

8 _____ principle of nucleic acid binding that states that A always bonds to T or U, and C to G

9 _____ process by which mRNA guides the synthesis of a protein

10 _____ process by which a portion of a DNA molecule is copied to form mRNA

11 _____ reaction in which subunits of a molecule are split from one another by the addition of water

12 _____ situation in which an enzyme has an affinity for two or more substrates

13 _____ situation in which increased substrate concentration does not increase the reaction rate of an enzyme

Terms related to structure

chromatid (KROHM-ah-tid)
chromosome (KROHM-o-sohm)
codon (KOH-dahn)
double helix (HEE-liks)
exon (EKS-ahn)
gene
intron (IN-trahn)

micelle (my-SEL)
mitotick spindle (my-TOT-ik)
primary sturcture
quaternary structure (kwa-TERN-ar-ee)
ribosome (RYB-oh-sohm)
secondary structure
tertiary structure (TER-shee-ar-ee)

1 _____ a portion of a DNA molecule containing the code for one polypeptide

2 _____ a DNA molecule; contains genetic codes

3 _____ alpha helix or pleated sheet conformation of a protein molecule

4 _____ complete three-dimensional conformation of a protein molecule

5 _____ intertwining of nucleotide helices forming a "twisted ladder" shape

6 _____ network of microtubules to which the chromosomes attach during mitosis

7 _____ noncoding section of an mRNA molecule

8 _____ one of two identical DNA molecules formed during replication

9 _____ relationship of constituent polypeptides within a whole protein molecule (i.e., the type of protein molecule formed by two or more tertiary molecules)

10 _____ section of mRNA molecule that contains codes for amino acids

11 _____ spherical mass of molecules that have polar and nonpolar regions

12 _____ the amino acid sequence of a protein molecule

13 _____ three-base code for a particular amino acid (within a gene sequence)

14 _____ tiny cell organelle that serves as the site for protein synthesis

Other Key Terms

activation energy   metaphase (MET-ah-fayz)
affinity (a-FIN-it-ee)   peptide bond
anaphase (AN-ah-fayz)   prophase (PROH-fayz)
interphase (IN-ter-fayz)   telophase (TEE-loh-fayz)

1 _____ chemical bond between amino acids formed by dehydration

2 _____ energy required to "start" a chemical reaction

3 _____ expression of the relative binding of various substrates to an enzyme

4 _____ last step in mitosis; new nuclear membranes appear around two daughter nuclei

5 _____ step in mitosis in which separated chromosomes are drawn to opposite poles

6 _____ step in cell's life cycle between mitotic divisions

7 _____ step in mitosis during which the nucleus disintegrates and chromosomes condense

8 _____ step in mitosis during which chromosomes attach to spindle and line up

The Big Picture

Use the activities of this section to help you learn the broader concepts of this chapter.

Learning Exercises

1.   Put these chemical types into the correct category in the table below.

disaccharides   monosaccharides   RNA
DNA   polysaccharides   steroids
enzymes   prostaglandins   structural proteins

Lipids	Carbohydrates	Proteins	Nucleic Acids

2. Put these chemical subunits into the correct category of macromolecule given in the table below.

adenine	fatty acids	ribose
amino acids	glycerol	saccharides
cytosine	guanine	thymine
deoxyribose	nucleotides	uracil

Lipids	Carbohydrates	Proteins	Nucleic acids

3. Identify these molecules by matching them with the figures below.

amino acid	polypeptide	steroid
monosaccharide	polysaccharide	triglyceride
nucleotide		

1_____

2_____

3_____

4_____

5_____

6_____

7_____

Figure 3-1

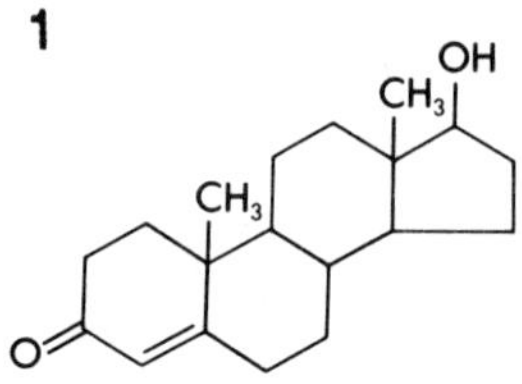

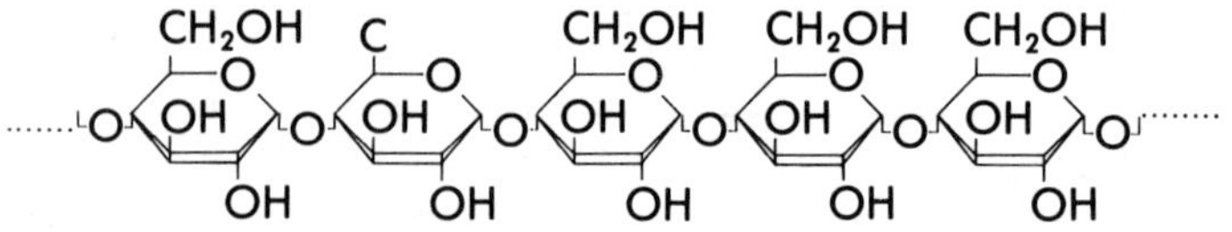

Figure 3-1, continued

3

$$H_2N-\underset{\underset{H}{|}}{\overset{\overset{CH_3}{|}}{C}}-\underset{\underset{O}{||}}{C}-OH$$

4

Phosphate group, 5-carbon sugar, Nitrogen base

6

5

7

4. Put these events of the cell life cycle in the order in which they occur.

1 <u>interphase - G1</u>   prophase
                                          interphase - S
2 _____   anaphase
                                          telophase
3 _____   interphase - G1
                                          metaphase
4 _____   interphase - G2

5 _____

6 _____

7 _____

5.   Put these events of protein synthesis in the order in which they occur.

mRNA combines with a ribosome in the cytoplasm
Two strands of a DNA molecule separate locally
Amino acids are joined together in proper sequence
mRNA strand is formed on the DNA template (transcription)
Introns are removed from mRNA in the nucleus
The ribosome accepts transfer RNAs (tRNAs) according to the mRNA codons (translation)

1_____

2_____

3_____

4_____

5_____

6_____

6.   Use the terms given to fill in the blanks of the paragraph that follows.

alpha   quaternary   tertiary
primary   secondary

        Protein molecules are long chains of amino acids that are often twisted into complicated, three-dimensional shapes. The linear sequence of amino acids in a protein molecule is called the
_____ structure. Hydrogen bonds can form between the carboxyl portion of a peptide bond and the amino group of a peptide bond farther down the chain. Such interactions result in a twisted
_____ helix or a pleated sheet shape, both of which are termed the _____
structure of the protein molecule. The complete three-dimensional shape of a protein, its
_____ structure, is stabilized by hydrophobic interactions and disulfide bonds. Two or more polypeptides may be assemble to form a protein molecule. In such a case, the relationship of the constituent polypeptides within the whole molecule constitutes the _____ structure of the protein.

Quick Recall
Review some of the major concepts of this chapter by doing these "quick recall" activities.

1.   List the chemical groups that form each of these lipids:

Triglycerides:

Fatty acids:

Steroids:

Phospholipids:

2.   In a word or two describe the major distinguishing characteristic of each carbohydrate.

Monosaccharide:

Disaccharide:

Polysaccharide:

3.   State the major storage form of lipids in the human body.

4.   List important functions of proteins in the human body.

5.   List factors that can influence the activity of enzymes.

6.   List the purine and pyridimine bases that can be found in

RNA nucleotides:

DNA nucleotides:

Practice Test
Use this practice test to review the topics of this chapter and to prepare for your test on this material.

1.   Lipids
    a.   are water soluble
    b.   are present in biological cell membranes
    c.   may be amphipathic
    d.   include steroids
    e.   b, c, d are all correct

2.   The sequence of amino acids making up a protein is termed its
    a.   primary structure
    b.   secondary structure
    c.   tertiary structure
    d.   quaternary structure
    e.   none of the above

3.   Enzymes
      a.   are proteins
      b.   act as catalysts
      c.   reduce activation energies
      d.   may act on more than one substrate
      e.   all of these

4.   The process of forming protein molecules from a messenger RNA template is termed
      a.   transcription
      b.   replication
      c.   translation
      d.   allosteric regulation
      e.   none of these

5.   Which of the following serve(s) as the primary site(s) of protein syntheses?
      a.   plasma membrane
      b.   ribosomes
      c.   nucleus
      d.   smooth endoplasmic reticulum
      e.   lysosomes

6.   Carbohydrates contain
      a.   carbon
      b.   oxygen
      c.   hydrogen
      d.   a and b only
      e.   a, b, and c

7.   Proteins are composed of a combination of a possible __ different types of amino acid.
      a.   24
      b.   20
      c.   23
      d.   15
      e.   4

8.   When one substrate is more likely to react with an enzyme than a second substrate, we say that the first enzyme has a greater __ for the enzyme.
      a.   allosteric effect
      b.   activation energy
      c.   affinity
      d.   molarity
      e.   amphipathism

9.   Lipid molecules with both polar and nonpolar regions may be termed
      a.   allosteric
      b.   hydrostatic
      c.   denatured
      d.   amphipathic
      e.   none of these

10. During mitosis, the nucleus reforms during
    a. prophase
    b. telophase
    c. metaphase
    d. anaphase
    e. interphase

11. A chemical reaction in which water is used in breaking chemical bonds is called
    a. hydrolysis
    b. anabolism
    c. cytokinesis
    d. dehydration
    e. a and d only

12. The primary stored form of carbohydrates in humans is
    a. adipose tissue
    b. glucose
    c. maltose
    d. steroids
    e. glycogen

13. A situation in which an increased amount of substrate does not increase the reaction rate is called
    a. enzyme competition
    b. enzyme saturation
    c. affinity
    d. allosteric effect
    e. none of these

14. The tendency of nucleotides to pair up in certain combinations can be called
    a. competition
    b. complementary base-pairing
    c. hydrolysis
    d. translation
    e. cytokinesis

15. Enzymes may first be formed as inactive
    a. introns
    b. extrons
    c. proenzymes
    d. exons
    e. genes

Answers

Here are answers (or references) to some of the questions presented above.

Word Parts: (your examples may be different) 1. carbohydrate 2. disaccharide 3. glycolipid 4. carbohydrate 5. hydrolysis 6. lipoprotein 7. monosaccharide 8. hydrophilic 9. hydrophobic 10. polypeptide

Key Terms: Chemicals: 1. cytosine 2. thymine 3. adenine 4. guanine 5. uracil 6. phospholipid 7. prostaglandin 8. lipoprotein 9. glycolipid 10. glycogen 11. carbohydrate 12. disaccharide 13. polysaccharide 14. hydrocarbon 15. catalyst 16. fatty acids 17. proenzyme 18. polymer 19. triglyceride 20. amino acid 21. protein 22. RNA 23. monosaccharide 24. enzyme 25. nucleotide 26. deoxyribose 27. ribose 28. transfer RNA 29. messenger RNA

Descriptive: 1. amphipathic 2. allosteric effect 3. hydrophilic 4. hydrophobic

Processes: 1. denaturation 2. oxidation 3. reduction 4. dehydration 5. replication 6. mitosis 7. cytokinesis 8. complementary base-pairing 9. translation 10. transcription 11. hydrolysis 12. enzyme competition 13. enzyme saturation

Structures: 1. gene 2. chromosome 3. secondary structure 4. tertiary structure 5. double helix 6. mitotic spindle 7. intron 8. chromatid 9. quaternary structure 10. exon 11. micelle 12. primary structure 13. codon 14. ribosome

Other: 1. peptide bond 2. activation energy 3. affinity 4. telophase 5. anaphase 6. interphase 7. prophase 8. metaphase

Learning Exercises: 1. **Lipids:** phospholipids, prostaglandins, steroids, triglycerides **Carbohydrates:** disaccharides, monosaccharides, polysaccharides **Proteins:** enzymes, structural proteins **Nucleic acids:** DNA, RNA 2. **Lipids:** fatty acids, glycerol **Carbohydrates:** saccharides **Proteins:** amino acids **Nucleic acids:** adenine, cytosine, deoxyribose, guanine, nucleotides, ribose, thymine, uracil 3. 1-steroid, 2-polysaccharide, 3-amino acid, 4-nucleotide, 5-triglyceride, 6-polypeptide, 7-monosaccharide 4. interphase G1, interphase S, interphase G2, prophase, metaphase, anaphase, telophase 5. Two strands of a DNA molecule separate locally; mRNA strand is formed on the DNA template (transcription); Introns are removed from mRNA in the nucleus; mRNA combines with a ribosome in the cytoplasm; the ribosome accepts tRNAs according to the mRNA codons (translation); Amino acids are joined together in proper sequence 6. primary, alpha, secondary, tertiary, quaternary

Quick Recall: (You should be able to answer these questions easily without correction or confirmation by this point in your studies. If you cannot, review your notes, the text chapter, and the previous study activities to find the answers.)

Practice Test: 1-e, 2-a, 3-e, 4-c, 5-b, 6-e, 7-b, 8-c, 9-d, 10-b, 11-a, 12-e, 13-b, 14-b, 15-c

Chapter 4
The Structure and Energy Metabolism of Cells

Focus
Review this section *first*. It will help you focus on the overall message of this chapter.

Chapter Outline
Read through the outline slowly. This activity will help your mind organize the topics of this chapter.

Basic cell structure
>	The cell membrane
>	Endocytosis and exocytosis
>	Nucleus

Cytoplasmic organelles
>	Endoplasmic reticulum
>	Golgi apparatus
>	Lysosomes
>	Mitochondria
>	Cytoskeleton

Junctions between cells
>	Desmosomes
>	Gap junctions
>	Tight junctions

Energy metabolism
>	High energy phosphates: the energy currency of cells
>	Electron carriers: NADH and $FADH_2$
>	Glycolysis
>	Intermediary oxidative metabolism: the Krebs cycle
>	Terminal oxidative metabolism and oxidative phosphorylation
>	The yield of ATP from complete oxidation of glucose
>	Energy metabolism of fatty acids, amino acids, and nucleic acids

Control of energy metabolism
>	Respiratory control of ADP
>	Control of enzymes by ADP, ATP, and metabolic intermediates

Learning Objectives
These are the learning goals for this part of the course. After reading the text, attending class, and studying this chapter, you should be able to:

♦	identify the major organelles of cells and provide a brief description of their physiological roles

- describe the structure and function of desmosomes, tight junctions and gap junctions

- outline the biochemical pathways by which carbohydrates are metabolized, distinguishing between the processes that occur under anaerobic and aerobic conditions

- distinguish between substrate-level phosphorylation and oxidative phosphorylation

- describe the ways amino acids and fatty acids can enter the metabolic pathways of the cell and thus be used as energy sources

- describe the mechanism of oxidation—phosphorylation coupling according to the chemiosmotic hypothesis

- summarize the net yields of ATP obtained under anaerobic and aerobic conditions

- describe the mechanisms of respiratory control and control of glycolysis by phosphofructokinase

Language of Physiology

Physiology uses its own set of terms, many of which may be unfamiliar to you. This section will help you improve your mastery of key physiological terms.

Word Parts

Here are some combining forms often seen in physiological terms. Give an example of a term that contains each word part listed.

Word Part	Meaning	Example
crist-	crest, fold	1_____
cyt-	cell	2_____
lys-	break apart	3_____
nucl-	pertaining to nucleus	4_____
phago-	eat	5_____
pino-	drink	6_____
-plasm	fluid	7_____
reticul-	network, netlike	8_____
-some	body	9_____

Plural Forms

In regular English, plurals are often formed by adding an "s" or "es." Because many physiological terms are really borrowed from Latin or Greek, they are pluralized according to Latin or Greek, not English, rules. Here are few hints at pluralization:

1. If the singular form ends with "-us," the plural form drops the "-us" and adds "-i." (e.g. villus, villi)

2. If the singular form ends in "-is," the plural form drops the "-is" and adds "-es." (e.g. arthrosis, arthroses).

3. If the singular form ends in "-a," the plural form adds "-e" (to make "-ae"). (e.g. ampulla, ampullae).

4. If the singular form ends in "-on," the plural form drops the "-on" and adds "-a." (e.g. mitochondrion, mitochondria).

5. If the singular from ends in "-um," the plural form drops the "-um" and adds "-a." (e.g. datum, data).

(NOTE: As luck would have it, not all foreign-based terms are pluralized with the foreign rules. Some are pluralized with English rules. Science dictionaries are good sources for determining the correct plural form in new words that you encounter.)

Take this opportunity to try your hand at making these terms plural. Check the answer list if you are stumped by an item.

Singular Form	Plural Form
crista	1 _____
endocytosis	2 _____
mitochondrion	3 _____
nucleolus	4 _____
nucleus	5 _____
equilibrium	6 _____

Key Terms

Read each of the terms in each grouping below aloud, using the pronunciation guide if necessary. This will help you to remember them better than if you read them silently. Then, write out the correct term next to each of the descriptions given.

Descriptive Terms

aerobic (er-OH-bik)   receptor-mediated
anaerobic (an-er-OH-bik)   (ree-SEPT-or MEE-dee-ayt-ed)

1_____   descriptive term meaning "not requiring oxygen"

2_____   descriptive term referring to a process that requires the presence of a
                           receptor molecule
3_____   descriptive term meaning "requiring oxygen"

Terms related to processes

chemiosmotic hypothesis   glycolysis (gly-KAHL-i-is)
  (kem-ee-ahz-MAH-tik)   Krebs cycle
anabolism (an-AB-ohl-izm)   oxidation-reduction reaction
catabolism (kat-AB-ohl-izm)   oxidative phosphorylation
decarboxylation   (ahks-ih-DAY-tiv fahs-for-ih-LAY-shun)
  (dee-karb-ahks-il-AY-shun)   phagocytosis (FAY-goh-site-oh-sis)
endocytosis (en-doh-site-OH-sis)   pinocytosis (PEE-noh-site-oh-sis)
exocytosis (eks-oh-site-OH-sis)

1_____   explanation of the process by which energy is transferred from a reduced
                           coenzyme to form ATP (in the mitochondrion)
2_____   cyclic sequence of metabolic reactions that occurs in the mitochondria;
                           also known as the citric acid cycle
3_____   metabolic process in which glucose is catabolized to yield pyruvate

4_____   receptor-mediated cell process in which molecules in solution (a bit of
                           extracellular fluid) is brought into the cell by means of inward bulging of
                           the membrane; type of endocytosis
5_____   receptor-mediated cell process in which a solid particle is brought into the
                           cell by means of inward bulging of the membrane; a type of endocytosis
6_____   cell process in which a vesicle of intracellular material fuses with the cell
                           membrane, then opens to the extracellular environment
7_____   cell process in which the membrane bulges inwardly, forming a vesicle of
                           substances trapped from the extracellular environment
8_____   chemical process in which a carboxyl (COOH) group is removed from a
                           molecule
9_____   breakdown of organic compounds to yield energy; a type of metabolism

10_____   metabolic process in which protons (H^+ ions) and electrons, carried by
                           coenzymes, are transferred to O_2 during ATP synthesis

11 _____ synthesis of complex molecules from simpler ones; a type of metabolism

12 _____ type of chemical reaction in which some reactants donate electrons (oxidation) and some gain those electrons (reduction)

Terms related to structures/substances

acetyl CoA (ah-SEET-al KO-en-zime A)
adenosine diphosphate [ADP]
  (ad-EEN-oh-sin dy-FAHS-fayt)
adenosine triphosphate [ATP]
  (ad-EEN-oh-sin try-FAHS-fayt)
crista (KRIS-tah)
cytochrome (SYT-oh-krohm)
cytoskeleton (SYT-oh-skel-et-on)
desmosome (DES-moh-sohm)
electrochemical gradient
endoplasmic reticulum [ER]
  (en-doh-PLAZM-ik ret-IK-yoo-lum)
FAD$^+$, FADH
gap junction
Golgi apparatus (GOHL-jee)
intermediate filaments

lactate (LAK-tayt)
lysosome (LY-soh-sohm)
microfilament (my-kroh-FIL-ah-ment)
microtubule (my-kroh-TOOB-yool)
mitochondrion (my-toh-KON-dree-ahn)
NAD$^+$, NADH
neurotransmitter (noo-roh-TRANS-mit-er)
nuclear membrane (NOO-klee-er)
nuclear pore (NOO-klee-er)
nucleolus (noo-klee-OH-lus)
nucleus
plasma (cell) membrane
pyruvate (py-ROO-vayt)
ribosome (RYB-oh-sohm)
tight junction
vesicle (VES-ih-kal)

1 _____ bilayer of phospholipids with imbedded proteins forming a boundary around the cell

2 _____ cell organelle consisting of a vesicle filled with digestive (lysing) enzymes

3 _____ chemical released from neurons that reacts with receptors in the next neuron or in a muscle or gland cell

4 _____ difference in the distribution of electrical charges over distance

5 _____ double membrane that forms the outer boundary of the cell nucleus

6 _____ double-membraned organelle that contains the principal complement of the cell's DNA molecules

7 _____ fold of the inner membrane of a mitochondrion

8 _____ membranous organelle formed by a serious of flattened membranous sacs containing molecules that migrated there from the ER

9 _____ molecule that results from the hydrolysis of ATP, in which the terminal (end) phosphate group is removed to release its energy

10 _____ molecule that is the end result of anaerobic metabolism of glucose; lactic acid

11 _____ simple molecule resulting from the catabolism of glucose (during glycolysis)

12 _____ tiny hole in the nuclear membrane formed by fusion of its two layers

13 _____ tiny bladder within a cell, formed by a spherical piece of cellular membrane

14 _____ acetyl group bound to coenzyme A; the form in which glucose, amino acids, and fatty acids can enter the Krebs cycle

15 _____ organelle formed by a membranous network of flattened sacs and canals; the ER

16 _____ organelle within the cell nucleus composed largely of ribosomal RNA (rRNA); site of ribosome construction

17 _____ cell organelle bounded by a double membrane; contains enzymes for extracting energy from carbohydrates

18 _____ flavine adenine dinucleotide; a coenzyme that transfers protons and electrons (and therefore energy) in certain metabolic pathways

19 _____ interlacing network of proteins within the cell that supports its shape and the position of certain organelles and molecules

20 _____ iron-containing enzyme in the mitochondrion that transports electrons from one molecule to another (electron transport chain)

21 _____ nicotinamide adenine dinucleotide; a coenzyme that transfers protons and electrons (and therefore energy) in certain metabolic pathways

22 _____ organelle that serves as the site of protein synthesis; found free in the cytoplasm, or on rough ER

23 _____ protein strands (larger than microfilaments) that provide most of the stability of the cytoskeleton

24 _____ small, hollow tube formed by tubulin (protein) molecules; forms part of the cytoskeleton

25 _____ solid, double strand of protein (largely actin) that forms part of the cytoskeleton

26 _____ "energy currency" of cells; a molecule with high-energy phosphate bonds that break to release energy used in cell processes

27 _____ type of "loose" cell junction that binds cells mechanically by means of connecting filaments

28 _____ type of cell junction in which the membranes of connected cells seem to be fused — often preventing molecules from diffusing easily through a sheet of cells

29 _____ type of cell junction, composed of paired connexons, that allows molecules to pass from one cell to the other, thus forming a continuous pathway for electrical transmission

The Big Picture

Use the activities of this section to help you learn the broader concepts of this chapter.

Learning Exercises

1.   Use these terms to identify the major cell organelles labeled in the figure.

Golgi apparatus   nucleolus   rough ER
lysosome   nucleus   smooth ER
microtubule   plasma (cell) membrane   vesicle
mitochondrion   ribosomes

Figure 4-1

1 _____

2 _____

3 _____

4 _____

5 _____

6 _____

7 _____

8 _____

9 _____

10 _____

11 _____

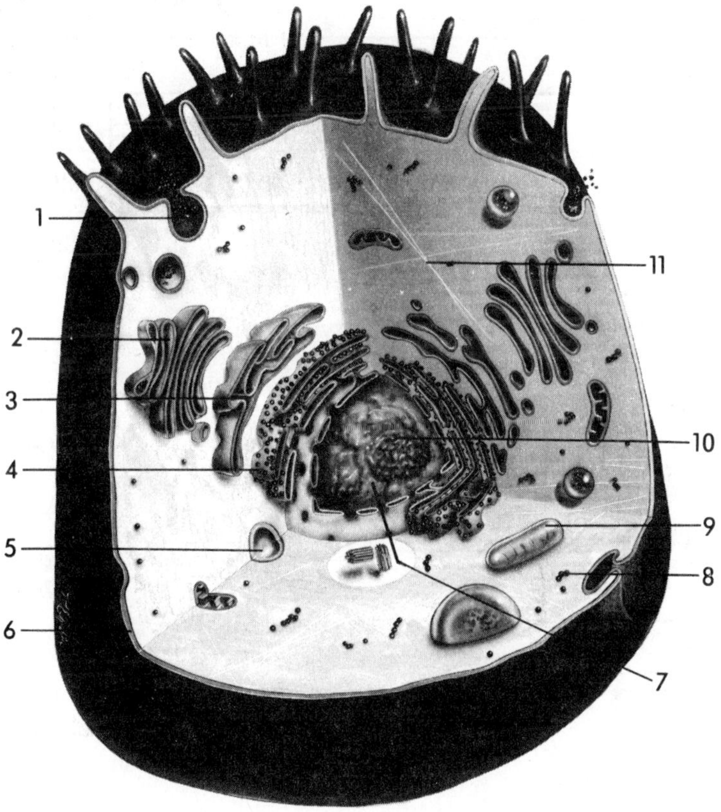

2.   Use the organelles listed in No. 1 to fill in the table below.

Organelle	Functional role
	defines limit of cell; solute transport
	pinocytosis; phagocytosis; exocytosis
	controls all cell processes; stores DNA
	synthesis and transport of proteins to be excreted
	synthesis site for proteins/polypeptides
	membrane synthesis; fatty acid/steroid synthesis
	incorporation of materials into secretory vesicles
	intracellular digestion
	oxidative phosphorylation
	cell shape; positioning of some organelles

3. Identify these cell junction types in Figure 4-2.

desmosome   gap junction   tight junction

Figure 4-2

1_____

2_____

3_____

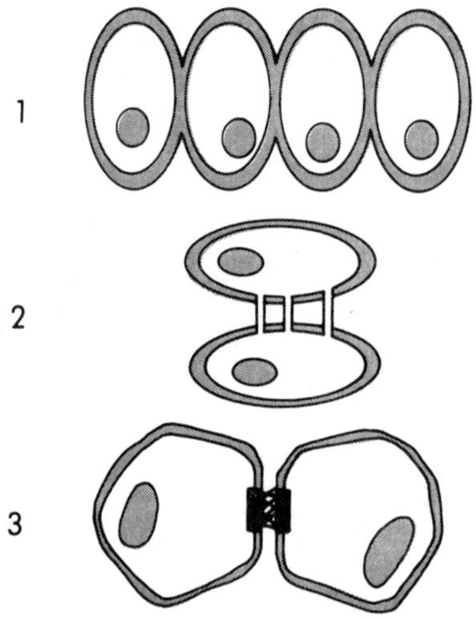

4.　Identify the following components of the cytoskeleton by matching them with the correct descriptions below.

intermediate filament　　　　　　microfilament　　　　　　microtubule

_____ hollow; composed of tubulin

_____ most stable component of the cytoskeleton

_____ composed mostly of actin

5.　Arrange these molecules, or groups of molecules, in the order in which they appear during the first portion of glucose catabolism.

acetyl-CoA　　　　　　　　　　　　glucose-6-phosphate
glucose　　　　　　　　　　　　　　pyruvate

1_____

2_____

3_____

4_____

6.　Arrange these Krebs cycle intermediates in the order in which they appear (see text, Figure 4-23, if you need help).

α-ketoglutaric acid　　　　　fumaric acid　　　　　　oxaloacetic acid
cis-aconitic acid　　　　　　　　isocitric acid　　　　　succinic acid
citric acid　　　　　　　　　　　malic acid

Preparation stage　　　　　　1__citric acid_____　　< ─┐
　　　　　　　　　　　　　　　　　　　　　　　　　　　│
　　　　　　　　　　　　　　2_____　│
　　　　　　　　　　　　　　　　　　　　　　　　　　　│
　　　　　　　　　　　　　　3_____　│
　　　　　　　　　　　　　　　　　　　　　　　　　　　│
Energy extraction stage　　　4_____　│
　　　　　　　　　　　　　　　　　　　　　　　　　　　│
　　　　　　　　　　　　　　5_____　│
　　　　　　　　　　　　　　　　　　　　　　　　　　　│
　　　　　　　　　　　　　　6_____　│
　　　　　　　　　　　　　　　　　　　　　　　　　　　│
Regeneration stage　　　　　7_____　│
　　　　　　　　　　　　　　　　　　　　　　　　　　　│
　　　　　　　　　　　　　　8_____　─┘

7.   Use these terms to fill in the blanks found in the paragraphs that follow.

ADP   mitochondrion
aerobic   oxidative
anacrobic   substrate-level
ATP

There are two mechanisms for the regeneration of _____. The first

is referred to as _____ phosphorylation because a phosphate group is

transferred to _____ from an intermediate compound to form ATP.

Sometimes this type of phosphorylation occurs in the absence of oxygen, a situation termed

_____ metabolism. The second means of ATP production is

_____ phosphorylation, that occurs in the inner membrane of the

_____. It requires oxygen and produces most of the ATP used by the

body. This type of phosphorylation and the metabolic pathways that serve it are referred to collectively as

_____ metabolism.

8. Use these terms to identify the numbered labels in Figure 4-3.

acetyl-CoA   anaerobic metabolism   Kreb's cycle
ADP   glycolysis   lactate
ATP   H₂O   NADH
aerobic metabolism

Figure 4-3

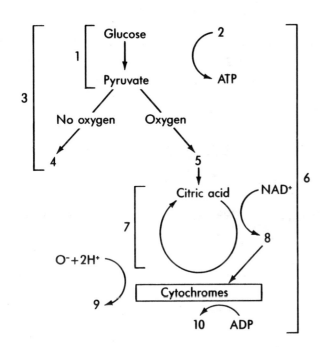

1 _____

2 _____

3 _____

4 _____

5 _____

6 _____

7 _____

8 _____

9 _____

10 _____

9. Fill in the blank portions of the catabolism flowchart below (Figure 4-4).

Figure 4-4

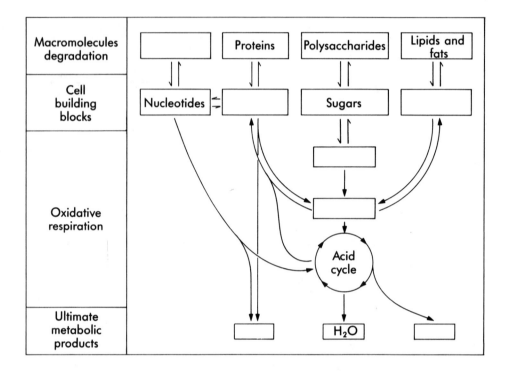

Quick Recall

Review some of the major concepts of this chapter by doing these "quick recall" activities.

1. List three components of the cytoskeleton.

2. List three functions of the plasma membrane.

3. List three types of cell junctions.

4. List two types of endocytosis.

5. Name two types of endoplasmic reticulum.

6. List two nucleotides that transfer electrons from one molecule to another during glucose catabolism.

7. Name two type of phosphorylation (ATP synthesis) typical of human cell metabolism.

Practice Test
Use this practice test to review the topics of this chapter and to prepare for your test on this material.

1.   The cell membrane functions to
    a.   help provide shape to the cell
    b.   transport materials into the cell
    c.   keep the cell intact
    d.   transport materials out of the cell
    e.   all are correct

2.   If the cell membrane pinches inward, trapping a bacterium within the vesicle thus formed, the process could be identified as
    a.   pinocytosis
    b.   exocytosis
    c.   phagocytosis
    d.   endocytosis
    e.   c and d are correct

3.   The nuclear pores
    a.   allow material to pass into and out of the cell
    b.   provide a pathway for the movement of mRNA molecules
    c.   provide a pathway for the movement of DNA molecules
    d.   are too small to allow organic molecules to pass
    e.   a and b are correct

4.   Rough ER can synthesize proteins because of the presence of
    a.   ribosomes
    b.   Golgi apparatus
    c.   membrane
    d.   DNA
    e.   lysosomes

5.   The cell organelle that processes and packages proteins transported by the ER for eventual export from the cell is called the
     a.   ribosome
     b.   Golgi apparatus
     c.   seminal vesicle
     d.   nucleolus
     e.   mitochondrion

6.   Which of these is a membranous organelle?
     a.   mitochondrion
     b.   chromosome
     c.   cytoskeleton
     d.   lysosome
     e.   a and d are correct

7.   A cell junction that allows relatively free movement of cytoplasmic materials between the joined cells is termed a
     a.   gap junction
     b.   desmosome
     c.   synapse
     d.   tight junction
     e.   a and c are correct

8.   Oxidative phosphorylation is the formation of new
     a.   cells
     b.   ADPs
     c.   ATPs
     d.   cyclic adenosine monophosphates (cAMPs)
     e.   glucose molecules

9.   Which of these processes always requires oxygen?
     a.   glycolysis
     b.   Krebs cycle
     c.   lactate formation
     d.   anaerobic metabolism
     e.   all of the above

10. Protein molecules can be converted to __, which can enter the Krebs cycle directly.
     a.   glucose
     b.   acetyl-CoA
     c.   pyruvate
     d.   lactate
     e.   a and c are correct

11. The primary goal of the Krebs cycle is to
     a.   produce citric acid
     b.   use oxygen
     c.   produce carbon dioxide
     d.   extract energy from food molecules
     e.   extract energy from ATP molecules

12. The nature of ATP synthesis in human cells is best explained by
   a. natural selection
   b. photosynthetic theory
   c. chemosmotic hypothesis
   d. endocytosis
   e. c and d are correct

13. The function of FADH and NADH in energy metabolism is to
   a. carry electrons
   b. act as a coenzyme
   c. transfer energy
   d. a and c are correct
   e. all are correct

14. Aerobic respiration produces more ATP than anaerobic respiration.
   a. true
   b. false

15. Under anaerobic conditions, pyruvate is converted to
   a. citric acid
   b. glucose
   c. NADH
   d. lactate
   e. glucose-6-phosphate

Answers

Here are answers (or references) to some of the questions presented above.

Word Parts: (your examples may be different) 1. crista 2. cytoplasm 3. lysosome 4. nuclear membrane 5. phagocytosis 6. pinocytosis 7. endoplasmic 8. reticulum 9. ribosome

Plural Forms: 1. cristae 2. endocytoses 3. mitochondria 4. nucleoli 5. nuclei 6. equilibria

Key Terms: Descriptive: 1. anaerobic 2. receptor-mediated 3. aerobic
Processes: 1. chemosmotic hypothesis 2. Krebs cycle 3. glycolysis 4. pinocytosis 5. phagocytosis 6. exocytosis 7. endocytosis 8. decarboxylation 9. catabolism 10. oxidative phosphorylation 11. anabolism 12. oxidation-reduction reaction
Structures/Substances: 1.plasma (cell) membrane 2.lysosome 3. neurotransmitter 4. electrochemical gradient 5. nuclear membrane 6. nucleus 7. crista 8. Golgi apparatus 9. adenosine diphosphate [ADP] 10. lactate 11. pyruvate 12.nuclear pore 13. vesicle 14. acetyl-CoA 15.endoplasmic reticulum 16. nucleolus 17. mitochondrion 18. FAD^+, FADH 19. cytoskeleton 20. cytochrome 21. NAD^+, NADH 22.ribosome 23. intermediate filaments 24.microtubule 25. microfilament 26. adenosine triphosphate [ATP] 27. desmosome 28. tight junction 29. gap junction

Learning Exercises: 1. 1-vesicle, 2-Golgi apparatus, 3-smooth ER, 4-rough ER, 5-lysosome, 6-plasma membrane, 7-nucleus, 8-ribosomes, 9-mitochondrion, 10-nucleolus, 11-microtubule 2. plasma membrane, vesicle, nucleus, rough ER, ribosome, smooth ER, Golgi apparatus, lysosome, mitochondrion, microtubule 3. tight, gap, desmosome 4. microtubule, intermediate filament, microfilament 5. glucose, glucose-6-phosphate, pyruvate, acetyl-CoA 6. citric acid, cis-aconitic acid, isocitric acid, α-ketoglutaric acid, succinic acid, fumaric acid, malic acid, oxaloacetic acid 7.ATP, substrate-level, ADP, anaerobic, oxidative, mitochondrion, aerobic 8. 1-glycolysis, 2-ADP, 3-

anaerobic metabolism, 4-lactate, 5-acetyl-CoA, 6-aerobic metabolism, 7-Krebs cycle, 8-NADH, 9-H_2O, 10-ATP 9. see text, Figure 4-28

Quick Recall: (You should be able to answer these questions easily without correction or confirmation by this point in your studies. If you cannot, review your notes, the text chapter, and the previous study activities to find the answers.)

Practice Test: 1-e, 2-e, 3-b, 4-a, 5-b, 6-e, 7-a, 8-c, 9-b, 10-b, 11-d, 12-c, 13-e, 14-a, 15-d

Chapter 5
Homeostatic Controls:
Neural and Endocrine Control Mechanisms

Focus
Review this section first. It will help you focus on the overall message of this chapter.

Chapter Outline
Read through the outline slowly. This activity will help your mind organize the topics of this chapter.

Control Theory
        Feedback
        Negative feedback loops
        A practical example: driving
        Gain and time lag in negative feedback systems
        Matching of feedback response to physiological role
        Positive feedback in disease and normal function
        Open loop systems
        Levels of physiological regulation
Mechanisms of intrinsic regulation
        Cellular self-regulation
        Tissue coordination by gap junctions
        Chemical regulation at the tissue level: paracrine and autocrine agents
        An example: blood flow autoregulation in tissues
Extrinsic regulation: reflex categories
        Reflex arcs
        Neural and endocrine reflexes
        Somatic motor control
        Autonomic reflexes
Endocrine reflexes
        Mechanisms of chemical communication between cells
        Chemical classes of hormones
        Hormonal signal amplification
        Action of steroid hormones and thyroid hormones
        Hormones with membrane-bound receptors
        Second messenger regulation of protein kinases
        Duration of hormone effects

Hormone receptor regulation
Functional classes of hormones
The posterior pituitary and its hormones
The anterior pituitary and its hormones
Regulation of blood glucose: an example of the principles of endocrine control
Failure of glucose regulation in endocrine diseases

Learning Objectives

These are the learning goals for this part of the course. After reading the text, attending class, and studying this chapter, you should be able to:

♦ describe the elements of a negative feedback control system and show how such systems stabilize physiological variables

♦ understand how positive feedback leads to instability

♦ provide examples of intracellular, local, and extrinsic control processes in the body

♦ recognize several common mechanisms of intrinsic regulation

♦ appreciate the variety and importance of paracrine and autocrine agents

♦ distinguish between somatic, autonomic, and hormonal reflexes

♦ state the characteristics of hormones and describe the three major chemical classes of hormones

♦ understand what is meant by down-regulation and up-regulation

♦ describe the factors controlling hormone release from the posterior pituitary

♦ describe the role of releasing and release-inhibiting hormones in control of anterior pituitary hormone secretion

♦ provide examples of several second messenger systems

♦ compare the intracellular mechanisms of action of steroid and peptide/protein hormones

Language of Physiology

Physiology uses its own set of terms, many of which may be unfamiliar to you. This section will help you improve your mastery of key physiological terms.

Word Parts

Here are some combining forms often seen in physiological terms. Give an example of a term that contains each word part listed.

Word Part	Meaning	Example
af-	toward	1 _____
auto-	self	2 _____
baro-	pressure	3 _____
cortico-	pertaining to cortex	4 _____
-crine	release; secrete	5 _____
ef-	away from	6 _____
endo-	within	7 _____
inter-	between	8 _____
lact-	milk; milk production	9 _____
pro-	first; promoting	10 _____
troph-	grow; nourish	11 _____

Key Terms

Read each of the terms in each grouping below aloud, using the pronunciation guide if necessary. This will help you to remember them better than if you read them silently. Then, write out the correct term next to each of the descriptions given.

Chemical substances

adenylate cyclase
(ad-EEN-il-ayt SY-klayz)
adrenocorticotropic hormone [ACTH]
(ad-ree-noh-kort-ih-koh-TROH-pik)
antidiuretic hormone [ADH]
(an-tee-dy-yoo-RET-ik)
calmodulin (kal-MOD-yoo-lin)
cyclic AMP (SIK-lik A-M-P)
epinephrine (ep-ih-NEF-rin)
follicle-stimulating hormone [FSH]
(FAH-lih-kal)
gastrin (GAS-trin)
growth hormone [somatotropin]

hormone
insulin (IN-soo-lin)
luteinizing hormone [LH]
(LOO-ten-ize-ing)
melanocyte-stimulating hormone [MSH]
(mel-AN-oh-site)
neurohormone (noo-roh-HOHR-mohn)
oxytocin (ahks-ih-TOH-sin)
parahormone (pair-ah-HOHR-mohn)
prolactin (proh-LAK-tin)
protein kinase (KIN-ayz)
release-inhibiting hormone
releasing hormone

second messenger
thyroid hormone [T$_3$, T$_4$]

thyroid-stimulating hormone [TSH]
   (THY-royd)
vitamin D

1_____   calcium-receptor molecule within cells that may help regulate metabolism within the cell

2_____   category of hormones or factors that includes chemical messengers from the brain that stop or slow the anterior pituitary's secretion of one or more of its hormones

3_____   category of hormones or factors that includes chemical messengers from the brain that cause the anterior pituitary to secrete one of its hormones

4_____   molecule that is formed by interaction of a ligand with a membrane-bound receptor that subsequently acts to modify intracellular metabolic processes

5_____   also called adrenaline; a hormone secreted by the adrenal medulla

6_____   enzyme on the inner surface of the cell membrane that catalyzes the conversion of ATP to cyclic AMP

7_____   any of several hormones secreted from the thyroid that are derived from the amino acid tyrosine

8_____   cell enzymes that control enzyme phosphorylation; these enzymes are controlled themselves by second messengers

9_____   chemical messenger such as oxytocin that acts like a regular hormone but is secreted by neurosecretory (rather than endocrine) cells

10_____   chemical messenger secreted by endocrine glands into the blood to affect the metabolism of distant target cells

11_____   cyclic adenosine monophosphate, one of the cyclic nucleotides; an important "second messenger" in the chemical processes triggered by some hormones

12_____   hormone produced by the anterior pituitary that stimulates growth of ovarian follicles

13_____   hormone produced by the anterior pituitary that stimulates the thyroid gland

14_____   hormone produced by stomach cells that is required for normal growth and repair of the stomach lining and also stimulates acid secretion by the stomach lining

15_____   hormone produced by the anterior pituitary that promotes lactation in the mammary glands

16_____   hormone produced by the pancreas that helps regulate blood glucose levels by stimulating glucose uptake by tissue cells

17_____   hormone produced by the anterior pituitary that stimulates development of the corpus luteum of the ovary

18_____   hormone produced by the anterior pituitary that stimulates melanin-producing cells and may have other effects yet to be determined

19_____   hormone produced by the anterior pituitary that stimulates the adrenal cortex

20_____   hormone released by the posterior pituitary that is important in stimulating labor and regulating lactation

21_____   hormone released by the posterior pituitary that helps regulate fluid balance by causing the kidney to conserve water; also called vasopressin

22_____ type of hormone secreted by the anterior pituitary that promotes growth of body tissues such as muscle and bone, known to be secreted in a pulse just after the onset of deep sleep

23_____ substance derived from cholesterol that is considered by endocrinologists to be a steroid hormone

Descriptive Terms

afferent (AF-er-ent)
agonistic (a-gahn-IST-ik)
efferent (EF-er-ent)
half-life
nuclear
paracrine (payr-ah-KRIN)

permissiveness
postsynaptic (pohst-sin-AP-tik)
presynaptic (pree-sin-AP-tik)
stereotyped
synergistic (sin-erj-IST-ik)
trophic (TROH-fik)

1_____ characteristic of some hormone combinations, it describes two or more hormones that have an effect equal to the sum of their individual effects

2_____ characteristic of some hormones, it is the ability of one hormone to affect a target cell in a way that allows a second hormone to have its full effect

3_____ characteristic of some hormone combinations, it describes the effects of two hormones together that is greater than the sum of their effects individually

4_____ characteristic of hormones, it is the time required for half of a given amount of hormone in the plasma to be metabolized or excreted

5_____ describes a reflex that is constant in its response pattern (always repeating exactly the same response)

6_____ descriptive term meaning "within, or of, the (cell) nucleus"

7_____ descriptive term applied to agents or glands that have only local effects

8_____ descriptive term meaning "toward" something; applied to nerves, means toward the central nervous system (sensory information)

9_____ descriptive term meaning "away from" something; applied to nerves, means away from the central nervous system (motor information)

10_____ term that means "after the synapse," referring to a cell that receives a signal from a neuron

11_____ term that means "before the synapse," referring to a neuron that transmits a signal across a synapse to another cell

12_____ term that describes hormones that have a growth-stimulating, or developmental, effect (but may also have a secretion-stimulating effect on target glands)

Terms related to processes

down-regulation
enzyme phosphorylation
  (fahs-for-ih-LAY-shun)
extrinsic regulation (eks-TRIN-zik)

intrinsic regulation
positive feedback
reflex arc
up-regulation

1_____ negative feedback process within target cells that results in a decrease in the number of receptor molecules caused by overexposure to a hormone or other chemical messenger

2_____ positive feedback process within target cells that results in an increase in the number of receptor molecules caused by initial exposure to a hormone or other chemical messengers; also called the priming effect

3_____ type of feedback in which the response is an increase in the deviation of a variable rather than a decrease in deviation back toward normal

4_____ negative feedback system in which a sensory stimulus leads to a motor response that diminishes the magnitude of the eliciting stimulus

5_____ process of activating or inhibiting cell enzymes by the binding of phosphate groups to allosteric control sites on the enzymes themselves; regulated by protein kinases

6_____ regulation (control) that occurs outside the tissues or organs being regulated; nervous or endocrine regulation is this type of regulation

7_____ regulation (control) that occurs within tissues or organs (small groups of cells

Terms related to structures

adrenal gland (ad-REEN-al)
antagonistic muscles
autonomic nervous system [ANS]
  (aw-toh-NAHM-ik)
baroreceptor (BA-roh-ree-sep-tor)
central nervous system [CNS]
chemoreceptor (KEEM-oh-ree-sep-tor)
effector
hypothalamus (hy-poh-THAL-ah-mus)
integration center
interneuron (IN-ter-noo-ron)

islets of Langerhans (LAHN-ger-hahnz)
motor neuron
neurosecretory cell
  (noo-roh-SEEK-reh-toh-ree)
open-loop system
osmoreceptor (AHZ-moh-ree-sep-tor)
pituitary gland (pih-TOO-it-ayr-ee)
portal circulatory systems
synapse (SIN-aps)
target cell
thermoreceptor (THERM-oh-ree-sep-tor)

1_____ junction of a neuron with another cell (another neuron or an effector cell)

2_____ structure that responds to stimuli of the nervous or endocrine system; a muscle or gland

3_____ also called an association neuron; this nerve cell type forms the integration center of a reflex arc, connecting incoming to outgoing signals

4_____ uncontrolled system with no feedback regulation; disease can disrupt closed feedback systems to make them uncontrolled

5_____ cell that is a neuron specialized to secrete hormonelike substances into the bloodstream

6_____ cell with receptor molecules for a particular chemical messenger

7_____ collection of neurons in the spinal cord that connects incoming sensory signals to the proper outgoing motor signals, integrating them to form a reflex arc

8_____ efferent nerve cell — one that conducts impulses away from the brain or cord and toward an effector

9_____ endocrine gland located on the superior aspect of each kidney; also called suprarenal gland

10_____ gland along the ventral surface of the brain, divided into anterior and posterior lobes; secretes at least eight different hormones

11_____ isolated masses of endocrine cells within the pancreas; also called pancreatic islets

12_____ main portion of the nervous system; includes the brain and spinal cord

13_____ muscles that oppose one another's actions (one pulls one way, the other in the opposite direction)

14_____ portion of the central nervous system (brain and cord) that regulates internal organs (autonomic, or visceral, effectors)

15_____ region of the brain ventral to the cerebrum that serves as a control center of homeostatic feedback mechanisms

16_____ sensory receptor specialized to detect osmolarity of a solution (such as blood or other extracellular fluid)

17_____ sensory receptor specialized to detect changes in temperature

18_____ sensory receptor specialized to detect chemical components of a substance (e.g., O_2, CO_2 in the blood)

19_____ sensory receptor that detects changes in pressure, especially blood pressure

20_____ system of blood vessels that directly connects the capillary networks of two different tissues or organs

Other Key Terms
endocrinology (en-doh-krin-AHL-oh-jee)
gain

1_____ measure of the sensitivity of a negative feedback system

2_____ science that deals with endocrine structure and function

The Big Picture

Use the activities of this section to help you learn the broader concepts of this chapter.

Learning Exercises

1. Figure 5-1 shows a flowchart that describes a closed-loop negative feedback system. Insert these labels into the proper location within the flowchart.

effector   perturbing factors
integrator   sensor

Figure 5-1

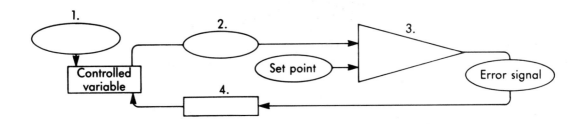

2. The graph in Figure 5-2 shows the concentration of hormone X in the bloodstream over time. The graph shows the normal average concentration of hormone X for 3 hours. During the fourth hour, the blood concentration of X rises significantly. Assuming that positive feedback mechanisms respond to this increase, predict what should happen to the hormone X concentration level over the next several hours by continuing the graph line with your pencil.

Figure 5-2

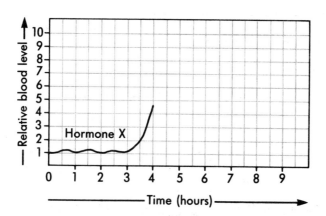

3. Use these terms describing different types of control processes to identify each situation outlined below.

extrinsic control   intrinsic control

_____   the heart rate increases during a stress situation, as a result of the effects
                            of epinephrine
_____   prostaglandin E_2 increases acid secretion in the stomach
_____   arm muscle cells contract in response to the hand touching a hot flask
_____   flow autoregulation

63

4. Put these different reflexes into the correct categories in the table below.

hand pulled away from a hot flask
increased blood flow to skin as a result of high internal temperature
increased heart activity as a result of decreased blood pressure
skeletal muscle stretch reflex
uterine lining thickens in response to high estrogen levels

Somatic motor reflexes	Autonomic reflexes	Endocrine reflexes

5. Put these hormones into the correct categories, based on their chemical characteristics.

adrenocorticotropic hormone
antidiuretic hormone
calcitonin
cortisol
epinephrine
estrogen
follicle-stimulating hormone

growth hormone
hypothalamic hormones
insulin
luteinizing hormone
melanocyte-stimulating
hormone
melatonin
oxytocin

parathyroid hormone
progesterone
prolactin
somatostatin
testosterone
thyroid-stimulating hormone
thyroxine

Proteins	Glycoproteins	Polypeptides	Amino acid derivatives	Steroids

6. Put these terms into the correct location in the flowchart shown in Figure 5-3.

anterior pituitary   hypothalamus   target gland

Figure 5-3

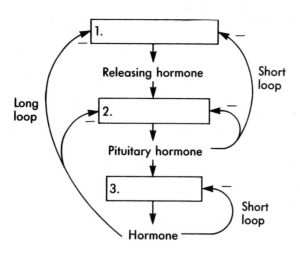

7. Use these terms to fill in the blanks found in the paragraph below.

calmodulin   inositol triphosphate   second
cyclic AMP   nonsteroid   steroid
cyclic guanosine   nuclear   target
  monophosphate (cGMP)   protein molecules

_____ hormones are recognized by mobile cytoplasmic receptors.

Once in the nucleus, the hormone-receptor complex reacts with a _____

receptor that is associated with the DNA. This triggers the production of specific mRNA molecules, that

in turn triggers the production of thousands of specific _____ within the cell.

_____ hormones, on the other hand, are recognized by fixed receptors on the surface of _____ cells. Most of the effects of this type of hormone-receptor

complex are mediated by _____ messengers. A common example of such a

messenger is a form of adenosine monophosphate called _____. This

molecule then acts to influence cell metabolism. Other chemicals that may act in this way include

_____, 1-2 diacylglycerol, and _____. Ca^{++}

may also act as a messenger molecule, binding to the intracellular receptor

_____, that may be a regulatory subunit attached to an enzyme.

Quick Recall

Review some of the major concepts of this chapter by doing these "quick recall" activities.

1. List two types of feedback mechanisms possible in the human body.

2. List three kinds of reflexes observed in human physiology.

3. State the major classes of hormones (according to chemical structure).

4. Name six hormones secreted by the anterior pituitary.

5. Name two hormones released by the posterior pituitary.

6. Name two releasing hormones and the endocrine hormone each regulates.

7. Name five molecules known to act as second messengers.

Practice Test

Use this practice test to review the topics of this chapter and to prepare for your test on this material.

1.   Negative feedback mechanisms
    a.   may involve motor reflexes
    b.   may involve glandular secretion
    c.   are inherently stable
    d.   have an error signal
    e.   all of the above

2.   Positive feedback
      a.   is stable
      b.   is unstable
      c.   occurs only in the nervous system
      d.   all of the above
      e.   b and c only

3.   Hormones
      a.   may be steroids
      b.   are released directly into the blood
      c.   affect only target cells
      d.   a and b are correct
      e.   all are correct

4.   Protein and peptide hormones
      a.   do not exist
      b.   bind to fixed receptors
      c.   bind to mobile cytoplasmic receptors
      d.   usually trigger synthesis of mRNA
      e.   c and d are correct

5.   Prostaglandins are
      a.   involved in local control mechanisms
      b.   chemical messengers
      c.   only secreted by the stomach lining
      d.   considered proteins
      e.   a and b are correct

6.   Releasing hormones
      a.   are secreted by the anterior pituitary
      b.   are manufactured in the hypothalamus
      c.   are manufactured in the posterior pituitary
      d.   affect the thyroid directly
      e.   a and c are correct

7.   Muscles can
      a.   only be somatic effectors
      b.   only be autonomic effectors
      c.   only be endocrine effectors
      d.   be somatic, autonomic, or endocrine effectors
      e.   none of the above

8.   Two hormones that have a greater effect in combination than the sum of each acting alone are
      called
      a.   agonists
      b.   antagonists
      c.   synergists
      d.   nonsteroids
      e.   a and b are correct

9. A reflex
   a.   can involve nerve cells
   b.   requires an integrating center
   c.   can involve endocrine responses
   d.   always decreases stability
   e.   a, b, and c are correct

10. _____ is an example of a second messenger.
    a.   cyclic GMP
    b.   cATP
    c.   acetyl-CoA
    d.   epinephrine
    e.   a and b

11. Oxytocin
    a.   is released by the anterior pituitary
    b.   affects the mammary glands only
    c.   affects the mammary glands and the uterus
    d.   is released by the ovary
    e.   a and c are correct

12. Calmodulin
    a.   may regulate certain enzymes
    b.   has a receptor site for Ca^{++}
    c.   is a nonsteroid hormone
    d.   a and b are correct
    e.   all are correct

13. Down-regulation
    a.   involves a decrease in hormone receptors
    b.   involves an increase in hormone receptors
    c.   is an example of positive feedback
    d.   occurs only in afferent neurons
    e.   a and c are correct

14. Osmoreceptors detect changes in
    a.   blood O_2 levels
    b.   pH
    c.   water concentration
    d.   temperature
    e.   none of the above

15. Paracrine agents
    a.   act locally
    b.   act intracellularly
    c.   act globally (throughout the body)
    d.   do not affect human cells
    e.   none of the above

Answers

Here are answers (or references) to some of the questions presented above.

Word Parts: (your examples may be different) 1. afferent 2. autoregulation 3. baroreceptor 4. adrenocorticotropin 5. endocrine 6. efferent 7. endocrine 8. interneuron 9. prolactin 10. prolactin 11. trophic hormone

Key Terms: Chemicals: 1. calmodulin 2. release-inhibiting hormone 3. releasing hormone 4. second messenger 5. epinephrine 6. adenylate cyclase 7. thyroid hormone (T_3, T_4) 8. protein kinase 9. neurohormone 10. hormone 11. cyclic AMP 12. follicle-stimulating hormone (FSH) 13. thyroid-stimulating hormone (TSH) 14. gastrin 15. prolactin 16. insulin 17. luteinizing hormone (LH) 18. melanocyte-stimulating hormone (MSH) 19. adrenocorticotrophic hormone (ACTH) 20. oxytocin 21. antidiuretic hormone (ADH) 22. growth hormone (somatotrophin) 23. vitamin D
Descriptive: 1. agonistic 2. permissiveness 3. synergistic 4. half-life 5. stereotyped 6. nuclear 7. paracrine 8. afferent 9. efferent 10. postsynaptic 11. presynaptic 12. trophic
Processes: 1. down-regulation 2. up-regulation 3. positive feedback 4. reflex arc 5. enzyme phosphorylation 6. extrinsic regulation 7. intrinsic regulation
Structures: 1. synapse 2. effector 3. interneuron 4. open-loop system 5. neurosecretory cell 6. target cell 7. integration center 8. motor neuron 9. adrenal gland 10. pituitary gland 11. islets of Langerhans 12. central nervous system (CNS) 13. antagonistic muscles 14. autonomic nervous system (ANS) 15. hypothalamus 16. osmoreceptor 17. thermoreceptor 18. chemoreceptor 19. baroreceptor 20. portal circulatory systems
Other: 1. gain 2. endocrinology

Learning Exercises: 1. 1-perturbing factors, 2-sensor, 3-integrator, 4-effector 2. The graph shows a rise from a level of about 1 to a level about 4 or 5 — your line should continue the upward trend by moving into the 6, 7, 8 range or higher. 3. extrinsic, local, extrinsic, intrinsic 4. Somatic: hand pulled away from a hot flask, stretch reflex; Autonomic: increased heart activity as a result of decreased blood pressure, increased blood flow to skin as a result of high internal temperature; Hormonal: uterine lining thickens in response to high estrogen levels 5. Proteins: growth hormone, prolactin, insulin, parathyroid hormone; Glycoproteins: follicle-stimulating hormone, luteinizing hormone, thyroid-stimulating hormone; Polypeptides: oxytocin, antidiuretic hormone, calcitonin, melanocyte-stimulating hormone, adrenocorticotrophic hormone, hypothalamic hormones, somatostatin; Amino acid derivatives: epinephrine, thyroxine, melatonin; Steroids: estrogen, progesterone, testosterone, cortisol 6. 1-hypothalamus, 2-anterior pituitary, 3-target gland 7. steroid, nuclear, protein molecules, nonsteroid, target, second, cyclic AMP, cyclic guanosine monophosphate (cGMP), inositol triphosphate, calmodulin

Quick Recall: (You should be able to answer these questions easily without correction or confirmation by this point in your studies. If you cannot, review your notes, the text chapter, and the previous study activities to find the answers.)

Practice Test: 1-e, 2-b, 3-e, 4-b, 5-e, 6-b, 7-d, 8-c, 9-e, 10-a, 11-c, 12-d, 13-a, 14-c, 15-a

Chapter 6
Transport Across Cell Membranes

Focus
Review this section *first*. It will help you focus on the overall message of this chapter.

Chapter Outline
Read through the outline slowly. This activity will help your mind organize the topics of this chapter.

The molecular structure of cell membranes
      Properties of phospholipids in membranes
      The fluid mosaic model of proteins and phospholipids in the membranes
      Functions of membrane proteins
Diffusion
      Random motion and diffusional equilibrium
      Determinants of the rate of diffusion
      Diffusion through cell membranes
      Osmosis
      Determinants of cell volume
Membrane transport proteins
      Mediated transport
      Active versus passive transport
      Channels
      Carriers
The membrane potential
      Electrical gradients across cell membranes
      Ionic gradients and diffusion potentials
      Determinants of the resting potential of a cell

Learning Objectives
These are the learning goals for this part of the course. After reading the text, attending class, and studying this chapter, you should be able to:

♦   describe the bilayer structure of cell membranes, identifying intrinsic and extrinsic proteins

♦   understand why pure lipid bilayers are impermeable to polar solutes and ions

♦   understand the factors that determine the rate of diffusion

- define the terms isotonic, hypotonic, and hypertonic and be able to apply them to determine how cells will change their volumes in these solutions

- understand why cell volume regulation requires that Na^+ be effectively impermeant

- describe the characteristics of mediated transport systems

- distinguish among facilitated diffusion, primary active transport, and secondary or gradient-driven active transport

- describe the origin of the membrane potential and be able to determine the magnitude and sign of the resting potential knowing the permeabilities and concentration gradients of Na^+ and K^+

Language of Physiology

Physiology uses its own set of terms, many of which may be unfamiliar to you. This section will help you improve your mastery of key physiological terms.

Word Parts

Here are some combining forms often seen in physiological terms. Give an example of a term that contains each word part listed.

Word Parts	Meaning	Example
-ase	(signifies an enzyme)	1_____
bi-	two; double	2_____
counter-	against	3_____
hyper-	over; above	4_____
hypo-	under; below	5_____
permea-	passage of fluids (or solutes)	6_____
-tonic	pressure	7_____

Key Terms

Read each of the terms in each grouping below aloud, using the pronunciation guide if necessary. This will help you to remember them better than if you read them silently. Then, write out the correct term next to each of the descriptions given.

Descriptive Terms

hyperosmotic (hy-per-ahz-MAH-tik)
hypertonic (hy-per-TAHN-ik)
hypoosmotic (hy-poh-ahz-MAH-tik)
hypotonic (hy-poh-TAHN-ik)
impermeant (im-PERM-ee-ant)

isosmotic (ice-ahz-MAH-tik)
isotonic (ice-oh-TAHN-ik)
permeant (PERM-ee-ant)
tonicity (tahn-IS-it-ee)

1_____ descriptive term that describes a solute that cannot cross a membrane

2_____ descriptive term that describes a solute that can cross a membrane

3_____ term that describes a solution with a lower concentration of solute particles than another

4_____ term referring to the tendency of a solution to cause an increase or decrease in the volume of a cell

5_____ term that describes a solution that will cause a decrease in the volume of a cell bathed in that solution

6_____ term that describes a solution that will cause an increase in the volume of a cell bathed in that solution

7_____ term that describes solutions with the same osmotic pressure (even though the types of solute particles may differ)

8_____ term that describes a solution with a higher concentration of solute particles than another

9_____ term that describes a solution that will not cause a cell to change volume when the cell is bathed in that solution

Terms related to measurement

diffusion coefficient
equilibrium potential
membrane potential

Nernst equation
permeability coefficient
  (perm-ee-ah-BIL-ih-tee)
resting potential

1_____ equation describing the equilibrium potential for a particular ion; for K^+, $E_K = C \log_{10} ([K^+]_{right}/[K^+]_{left})$

2_____ numerical expression that describes the ease with which substances cross membranes

3_____ imbalance in electrical charge across the membranes of all living cells, expressed in volts (V) or millivolts (mV)

4_____ measure of the rate of a solute's thermal motion at a standard temperature (expressed as cm^2/sec)

5_____ membrane potential of a living cell at rest (not actively conducting an impulse); typically between 40 mV and 80 mV in most cells

6_____ voltage that would exist across a membrane if it were exclusively permeable to one ion

Terms related to processes

active transport
countertransport
facilitated diffusion
  (fah-SIL-ih-tayt-ed)
gradient-driven cotransport

gradient-driven countertransport
mediated transport
osmosis (ahz-MOH-sis)
permeation (perm-ee-AY-shun)

1_____ general name for any membrane transport process that involves the concurrent movement of two particles but in opposite directions (the same or different carriers or other mechanisms may be involved)

2_____ general term referring to any cell membrane transport process that requires physiological energy from the cell

3_____ general term referring to the act of passing through (a membrane)

4_____ general term referring to any cell membrane transport process requiring mediation by a transport protein

5_____ diffusion of water across a membrane that is permeable to water

6_____ type of transport in which two particles are transported together (in different directions) but the movement is powered by the tendency of one of the particles to move down its concentration gradient

7_____ type of transport in which two particles are transported together (in the same direction) but the movement is powered by the tendency of one of the particles to move down its concentration gradient

8_____ type of diffusion that is mediated by a transport protein that allows solute particles to move down their concentration gradient more rapidly than they would by dissolving through the lipid bilayer

Terms related to structures/substances

bilayer (BY-lay-er)
carrier protein
channel protein
gated channel
glycoprotein (gly-koh-PROH-teen)
Na^+-K^+ ATPase (A-T-P-ayz)

Na^+-K^+ pump
receptor protein
recognition protein
selectivity filter
transport protein

1_____ double sheet of molecules that forms most cellular membranes; the double sheet formation results from the interaction of the polar ends of the molecules (causing them to face each other, leaving the nonpolar ends to face outward)

2_____ region in a membrane transport channel that determines which solutes may enter the channel

3_____ enzyme that hydrolyzes ATP to provide energy for the active transport accomplished by the Na^+-K^+ pump

4_____ intrinsic membrane protein that returns Na^+ to the extracellular fluid in exchange for K^+, against their concentration gradients

5_____ molecule formed by a protein with an attached carbohydrate chain

6_____ type of membrane transport channel whose opening is regulated by an external factor (that acts to open or close a biochemical "gate")

7_____ type of receptor protein with sites for the binding of immune system cells, allowing those cells to recognize foreign cells

8_____ type of transport protein that forms a passageway for the movement of molecules across the membrane

9_____ type of membrane transport protein that must undergo a cycle of solute binding and conformational change, carrying one or more particles across the membrane as it does so

10_____ type of membrane protein that acts to transport substances across the membrane

11_____ type of membrane protein with one or more binding sites specific to certain extrinsic proteins such as hormones or immune system cells

Other Key Terms

fluid mosaic model   net flux
flux

1 _____   figurative representation of the nature of the cell membrane as a mosaic of
                     molecules that are often free to flow in a two-dimensional plane
2 _____   general term meaning "flow"

3 _____   difference between two unidirectional fluxes; for any process at equilibrium, it is
                     equal to 0

The Big Picture

Use the activities of this section to help you learn the broader concepts of this chapter.

Learning Exercises

1.   Use these labels to identify the portions of cell membrane indicated in Figure 6-1.

carbohydrate chains   nonpolar region of phospholipid
channel protein   polar region of phospholipid
lipid bilayer   receptor protein

Figure 6-1

1 _____

2 _____

3 _____

4 _____

5 _____

6 _____

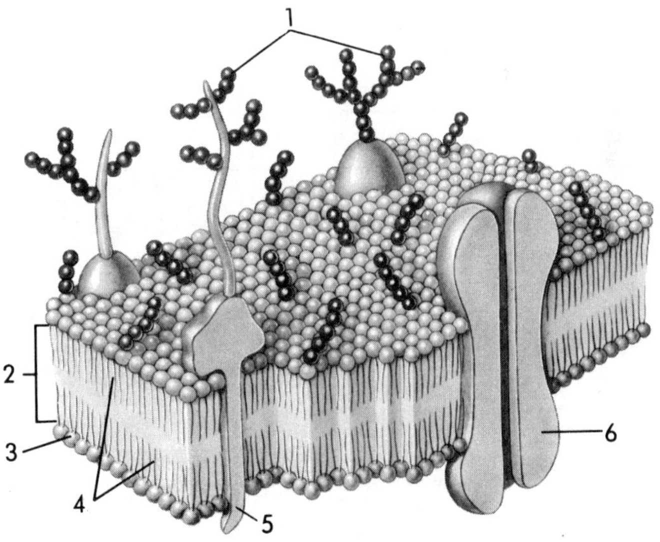

2.   Figure 6-2 shows a side view of a phospholipid bilayer. Use your pencil to label the polar and
        nonpolar portions of the phospholipid molecules in both sections. Label where you would likely
        find water molecules in relation to the bilayer.

Figure 6-2

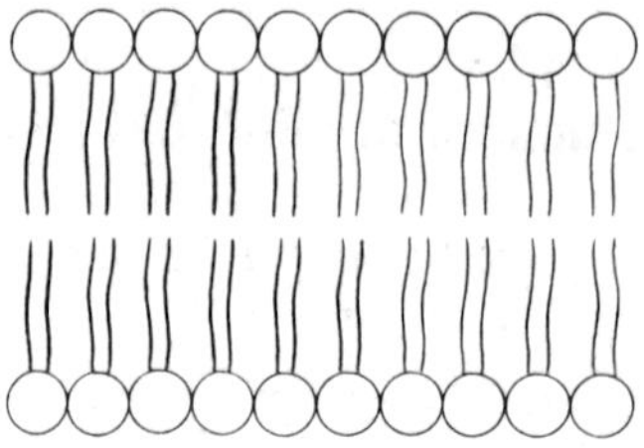

3.   With Figure 6-2 (above) in mind, tell which of these types of molecules may or may not pass
        through a pure phospholipid membrane. In each case explain why the molecule may or may not
        pass.

Molecule	May pass	May not pass	Explanation
steroid (nonpolar)	[]	[]	
amino acid (polar)	[]	[]	
Na^+	[]	[]	
sugar (polar)	[]	[]	
Cl^-	[]	[]	
water	[]	[]	

4. Polar molecules can pass through living cell membranes because of the presence of proteins in these
membranes, not represented in Figure 6-2. Use these terms to fill in the blanks found in the paragraph
on solute transport.

active   countertransport   polar
carrier   facilitated   saturated
channel   gated   selectivity
cotransport   mediated

_____ solute molecules are able to cross cell membranes by means of

a process called _____ transport, referring to protein molecules that actively

or passively enable passage. If cell energy is required for transport, the mechanism is called

_____ transport; if no cell energy is required, the process is termed

_____ diffusion, a type of passive transport. Transport proteins can become

_____ because there is a limit to how many solute particles they can handle at

any one time. Certain transport proteins called _____ proteins allow polar

molecules to pass through a water-filled tube to the other side of the membrane. They may have a region

called a _____ filter, which permits only certain molecules to pass, or may be

_____ , which means that their openings are regulated by external factors.

_____ proteins, on the other hand, change their structural conformations,

carrying the solute particles across the membrane as they do so. Sometimes two different types of

particles are moved at the same time. If they move in the same direction, the process is called

_____ ; if they move in opposite directions across the membrane, the process

is called _____ .

5.   The rate of solute movement by means of diffusion is determined by a variety of factors, some of
       which are listed here. Match the terms listed to their descriptions below.

diffusion coefficient
geometry of the path
magnitude of concentration gradient

_____   provides the driving force for net flux

_____   incorporates the factors of temperature and
                                                         the size of the solute molecule (this factor
                                                         is greater if the particles are small and the
                                                         temperature high)

_____   the greater the area available to the
                                                         diffusion solute (and the shorter the travel
                                                         distance) the greater the rate of diffusion

6.   Figure 6-3 shows a giant cell in a tiny beaker. Of course, the fluid inside the cell is intracellular fluid (A) and the fluid in the beaker is extracellular fluid (B). Use this figure to answer the questions below.

1 - If B is hypotonic to A, what would happen to the cell over time?

2 - If B is hypertonic to A, what would happen to the cell over time?

Figure 6-3

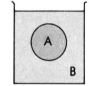

3 - If B is isotonic to A, what would happen to the cell over time?

7.   Assume that the fluids in Figure 6-3 have these characteristics (you may want to label Figure 6-3, in erasable pencil, accordingly). Remember, a living cell is represented.

A: contains K^+ (permeant), Cl^- (permeant), and Pr^- (impermeant) in water

B: contains K^+ (permeant) and Cl^- (permeant) in water

1 - Describe the equilibrium that would eventually develop across the membrane.

2 - If Na^+ were added to B and was impermeant, how would the situation change?

3 - The cell usually does create and maintain the situation described in the preceding question. How is this accomplished?

8.   Using Figure 6-3 as a visual aid, use the Nernst equation to determine the approximate equilibrium potentials asked for below. The first is done for you.

1 - A: 1 mM/L Na^+ What is the Na^+ equilibrium potential?
    B: 100 mM/L Na^+

[Answer: Plug the values given into the Nernst equation and you have $E_{Na}+ = C \log_{10} ([Na^+]_B/[Na^+]_A)$ = $(60) \log_{10} (100/1) = (60) (2) = 120$ mV. NOTE: C = 60 mV for monovalent ion at body temperature — $\log_{10}$ can be determined easily for multiples of 10 without much calculation; for example: $\log_{10} (10) = 1$, $\log_{10} (100) = 2$, and so on; $\log_{10} (.1) = -1$, $\log_{10} (.01) = -2$, and so on]

2 - A: 1 mM/L K^+ What is the K^+ equilibrium potential?
    B: 100 mM/L K^+

3 - A: 100 mM/L Na^+ What is the Na^+ equilibrium potential?
    B: 1 mM/L Na^+

4 - A: 10 mM/L K^+ What is the K^+ equilibrium potential?
    B: 100 mM/L K^+

Quick Recall
Review some of the major concepts of this chapter by doing these "quick recall" activities.

1.   List three molecule types found in cell membranes.

2.   List five possible functions of membrane proteins.

3.   List three factors that affect the rate of diffusion of a substance in aqueous solution.

4. List three characteristics of mediated transport systems.

5. List two cations whose permeabilities and gradients are important in determining cell membrane potential.

Practice Test
Use this practice test to review the topics of this chapter and to prepare for your test on this material.

1. Phospholipid bilayers
    a. tend to prevent passage of polar molecules
    b. tend to prevent passage of nonpolar molecules
    c. tend to form micelles
    d. require concentration gradients to remain stable
    e. a and c are correct

2. Membrane proteins
    a. may be glycoproteins
    b. may be involved in countertransport
    c. may form channels
    d. a and c are correct
    e. a, b, and c are correct

3. The net flux of water across a membrane
    a. is determined, in part, by the osmolarity on each side
    b. is determined, in part, by the presence of glycoproteins
    c. is termed permeability
    d. usually results from active transport

4. Diffusion rate becomes greater when
    a. temperature decreases
    b. temperature increases
    c. carriers become saturated
    d. concentration gradient decreases
    e. a and d

5. Constant cell volume requires that
    a. there is no net flux of water
    b. there is no net osmosis
    c. Na^+ is relatively impermeant
    d. all of the above
    e. a and b are correct

6. Polar molecules
   a. cannot pass through cell membranes
   b. can always pass through cell membranes
   c. can pass through cell membranes under certain circumstances
   d. are seldom observed in cells
   e. none of the above

7. Na^+-K^+ ATPase
   a. provides energy for passive diffusion
   b. helps provide energy for some ion pumps
   c. hydrolyzes Na^+-K^+
   d. renders K^+ impermeant
   e. b, c, and d are correct

8. A cell placed in a hypertonic solution will
   a. swell
   b. remain stable
   c. shrivel
   d. lyse
   e. a and d are correct

9. Carrier proteins
   a. work by changing shape
   b. work by providing water-filled passageways for ions
   c. allow only certain molecules to cross the membrane
   d. a and c are correct
   e. none of the above

10. Facilitated diffusion is
    a. a form of active transport
    b. a form of passive transport
    c. gradient driven
    d. a and b are correct
    e. b and c are correct

11. 100 mM/L of NaCl is isotonic to
    a. 100 mM/L glucose
    b. 200 mM/L glucose
    c. 100 mM/L $CaCl_2$
    d. 150 mM/L KCl
    e. none of the above

12. If extracellular $[K^+] = 10$ and intracellular $[K^+] = 100$, then the potassium equilibrium potential is about
    a. -60 mV
    b. -70 mV
    c. 60 mV
    d. 100 mV
    e. 10 mV

13. The equilibrium potential for Na$^+$ is 60 mV and for K$^+$ is -90 mV, with an observed resting potential of -65 mV. Which ion is more permeable in this case?
    a. they are the same
    b. K$^+$
    c. Na$^+$
    d. insufficient data is given

14. If $E_{Na}+$ = 60 mV and E_K+ = -60 mV, then the resting potential across a membrane permeable only to K$^+$ would most likely be
    a. 60 mV
    b. 30 mV
    c. 0 mV
    d. -30 mV
    e. -60 mV

15. If $E_{Na}+$ = 60 mV and E_K+ = -60 mV, then the resting potential across a membrane permeable only to Na$^+$ would most likely be
    a. 60 mV
    b. 30 mV
    c. 0 mV
    d. -30 mV
    e. -60 mV

Answers

Here are answers (or references) to some of the questions presented above.

Word Parts: (your examples may be different) 1. ATPase 2. bilayer 3. countertransport 4. hypertonic 5. hypotonic 6. permeability 7. isotonic

Key Terms: Descriptive: 1. impermeant 2. permeant 3. hypoosmotic 4. tonicity 5. hypertonic 6. hypotonic 7. isosmotic 8. hyperosmotic 9. isotonic
Measurement: 1. Nernst equation 2. diffusion equation 3. permeability coefficient 4. membrane potential 5. diffusion coefficient 6. resting potential 7. equilibrium potential
Processes: 1. countertransport 2. active transport 3. permeation 4. mediated transport 5. osmosis 6. gradient-driven countertransport 7. gradient-driven cotransport 8. facilitated diffusion
Structures/substances: 1. bilayer 2. selectivity filter 3. Na$^+$-K$^+$ ATPase 4. Na$^+$-K$^+$ pump 5. glycoprotein 6. gated channel 7. recognition protein 8. channel protein 9. carrier protein 10. transport protein 11. receptor protein
Other: 1. fluid mosaic model 2. flux 3. net flux

Learning Exercises: 1. 1-carbohydrate chains, 2-lipid bilayer, 3-polar region of phospholipid, 4-nonpolar region of phospholipid, 5-receptor protein, 6-channel protein 2. the polar portions of the molecules are the spherical "heads," the nonpolar portions are the wavy "tails," water would be above and below the bilayer 3. steroid (may pass), amino acid (not pass), Na$^+$ (not pass), sugar (not pass), Cl$^-$ (not pass), water (not pass), nonpolar molecules may pass because they are soluble in the nonpolar lipid molecules forming the bilayer — polar molecules can't dissolve through the lipid bilayer 4. polar, mediated, active, facilitated, saturated, channel, selectivity, gated, carrier, cotransport, countertransport 5. magnitude of concentration gradient, diffusion coefficient, geometry of the path 6. 1-the cell would swell and possibly burst (lyse) because of the influx of water by means of osmosis, 2-the cell would shrivel because of the outflux of water by means of osmosis, 3-the cell should remain stable, since water is already at an equilibrium 7. 1-This is a tricky question, because no equilibrium could develop. Since the total number of negative and positive charges on each side of the membrane must balance, and Pr is confined to A, there will always be more K^+ than Cl^- in A (to balance the Pr). The K^+/Cl^- ratio in B is balanced. Given this situation, the osmotic imbalance (too may particles in A, making it hypertonic to B) would cause the cell to eventually burst. 2-Na^+ on the outside of the cell would balance the excess of K^+ on the inside (described in No. 1). A would then be both electrically and osmotically balanced with B. 3-Na^+-K^+ ATPase catalyzes the hydrolysis of ATP, yielding energy that is used by Na^+-K^+ pumps to push Na^+ out of the cell in exchange for K^+. 8. 1-(120mV), 2-(120mV), 3-(-120mV), 4-(60mV)

Quick Recall: (You should be able to answer these questions easily without correction or confirmation by this point in your studies. If you cannot, review your notes, the text chapter, and the previous study activities to find the answers.)

Practice Test: 1-a, 2-e, 3-a, 4-b, 5-d, 6-c, 7-b, 8-c, 9-d, 10-e, 11-b, 12-a, 13-b, 14-e, 15-a

Chapter 7
Action Potentials

Focus
Review this section first. It will help you focus on the overall message of this chapter.

Chapter Outline
Read through the outline slowly. This activity will help your mind organize the topics of this chapter.

Electrical events in membranes
       Categories of electrical events
       Resting potential
       Receptor and synaptic potentials
       Action potentials
Molecular basis of electrical events in membranes
       Membrane repolarization
       Action potential threshold
Voltage clamp studies
       Voltage clamp of giant axons
       Measuring membrane conductances
Voltage-gated channels
       Channels in electrically excitable membranes
       Properties of Na^+ and K^+ channels
       Changes in permeability during action potentials
       Role of Na^+-K^+ pump in excitability
Refractory period and firing frequency
       Absolute and relative refractory period
       Repetitive firing during prolonged depolarization
       Extracellular Ca^{++} and excitability
Propagation of action potentials
       Spread of excitation
       Differences in propagation velocity
       Effect of diameter and myelin on propagation velocity
       Propagation in myelinated nerve fibers
       Comparison of nonmyelinated and myelinated nerves
       The compound action potential in nerve trunks

Learning Objectives
These are the learning goals for this part of the course. After reading the text, attending class, and studying this chapter, you should be able to:

- compare action potentials, receptor potentials, and synaptic potentials

- describe the behavior of voltage-gated Na^+ and K^+ channels in excitable membranes as a function of voltage and time

- understand how an action potential is initiated, using the concept of threshold

- understand how inactivation of Na^+ channels and opening of K^+ channels combine to terminate the action potential

- state the factors governing the velocity of conduction of action potentials in an axon or muscle cell

- understand the role of myelin as an insulator and characterize saltatory conduction

- understand the origin of the compound action potential of a nerve trunk and account for the origin of its various components

Language of Physiology

Physiology uses its own set of terms, many of which may be unfamiliar to you. This section will help you improve your mastery of key physiological terms.

Word Parts

Here are some combining forms often seen in physiological terms. Give an example of a term that contains each word part listed.

Word Part	Meaning	Example
calc-	calcium	1_____
de-	down from, undoing	2_____
-emia	(refers to blood condition)	3_____
pol-	axis, having poles	4_____
saltat-	to dance, leap	5_____
sub-	under	6_____

Key Terms

Read each of the terms in each grouping below aloud, using the pronunciation guide if necessary. This will help you to remember them better than if you read them silently. Then, write the correct term next to each of the descriptions given.

Descriptive Terms

depolarized (de-POH-ler-ized)
excitable

graded
hyperexcitable (hy-per-ek-SITE-ih-bil)

hyperpolarized (hy-per-POH-ler-ized)   nonmyelinated (nahn-my-el-in-AYT-ed)
inexcitable (in-ek-SITE-ih-bil)   polarized (POH-ler-ized)
myelinated (my-el-in-AYT-ed)

1_____   descriptive term meaning "having myelin"

2_____   descriptive term meaning "not having myelin"

3_____   refers to a membrane incapable of experiencing an action potential,
                             although it may exhibit a graded potential

4_____   refers to a membrane that has a potential across it; that is, one side is
                             positive with respect to the other

5_____   refers to a nerve or muscle cell with a membrane that may discharge
                             action potentials continuously, without stimulation (as when extracellular
                             Ca^{++} is low)

6_____   refers to a membrane that can experience an action potential, not just a
                             graded potential

7_____   refers to a membrane that has a potential more negative than the resting
                             potential

8_____   refers to a membrane that had been significantly polarized (having distinct
                             negative and positive poles) but has been rendered less polar or nonpolar

9_____   term that means "having gradations"; refers to processes that occur at
                             different intensities

10_____   all-or-none membrane depolarization that is propagated along nerve fibers
                             without any decrease in amplitude

Terms related to processes

decremental conduction   repetitive firing
  (dee-kre-MENT-al)   repolarization (ree-POH-ler-iz-ay-shun)
demyelination (dee-my-el-in-AY-shun)   saltatory conduction (SALT-ah-toh-ree)
Na^+ activation   summation (sum-AY-shun)
Na^+ inactivation
nondecremental conduction
  (non-dee-kre-MENT-al)

1_____   loss or removal of all or part of the myelin coating (sheath) of affected
                             neurons; a symptom or result of certain disease conditions such as
                             diabetes, alcoholism, and multiple sclerosis

2_____   process in which several receptor/synaptic potentials add together to create
                             a greater membrane potential

3_____   process in which the voltage-gated Na^+-selective ion channels close
                             spontaneously, after having opened briefly

4_____   process in which a membrane returns to a polarized state after having been
                             briefly depolarized

5_____   process in which the voltage-gated Na^+-selective ion channels open,
                             allowing Na^+ to pass through the membrane

6_____   series of action potentials resulting from prolonged depolarization

7_____ type of spreading action of a membrane potential where the intensity of the potential drops as it travels across the membrane

8_____ type of action potential conduction in which the action potential seems to "leap" from one node of Ranvier to the next, increasing the overall speed of conduction

9_____ type of spreading action of a membrane potential in which the intensity of the potential does not decrease as it travels, as in an action potential

Terms related to structures/substances

axon
axon hillock
giant axon
leak channel
myelin (MY-el-in)
nerve trunk

node of Ranvier (RAHN-vee-ay)
oligodendrocyte
   (ahl-ih-goh-DEN-droh-site)
Schwann cell (shwahn)
stimulus-gated channel
voltage clamp
voltage-gated channel

1_____ apparatus (and the technique involved in using it) that controls the voltage of a cell membrane and indirectly measures the movement of ions across the membrane

2_____ bundle of axons supported by glial cells; same as a "nerve" in the terminology of gross anatomy

3_____ gap in a myelin sheath (1 to 2 μm wide) that allows for saltatory conduction of action potentials

4_____ gated membrane channel that opens and closes in response to physical and chemical stimuli; it is involved in creating receptor and synaptic potentials

5_____ gated membrane channel that opens and closes in response to changes in the membrane potential; it is involved in creating action potentials

6_____ long cell process projecting from the neuron cell body which bears synaptic terminals on its distal end

7_____ membrane channel that lets most ions through the cell membrane and is not sensitive to changes in membrane potential

8_____ nerve fibers, efferent with respect to the neuron cell body, of a particularly large diameter that are useful in voltage clamp studies

9_____ portion of the neuron where the cell body (soma) extends to become the axon; also called the "initial segment"

10_____ type of glial cell that produces a myelin sheath around peripheral nerve fibers

11_____ type of glial cell that produces myelin in the central nervous system

12_____ whitish lipid substance produced by some glial cells

Other Key Terms

action potential
all-or-none principle
compound action potential
hypocalcemia (hy-poh-kal-SEEM-ee-ah)

potential
receptor potential
refractory period (ree-FRAKT-oh-ree)
safety factor

squid
subthreshold potential

synaptic potential
threshold potential

1_____ composite response of many (or all) axons in the nerve trunk that are stimulated simultaneously to produce action potentials

2_____ condition of relatively low blood concentration of Ca^{++}, usually resulting in low Ca^{++} levels in interstitial fluid surrounding nerve and muscle cells

3_____ difference in electric charge, measured in volts or millivolts (mV)

4_____ generator potential; the change in voltage that occurs when a sensory receptor is activated by a stimulus

5_____ graded, decremental potential that results from physical or chemical events at the synapse, and may be summed; similar to a receptor potential

6_____ interval after an action potential in which another action potential cannot be generated (absolute) or has an increased threshold (relative)

7_____ membrane potential of a magnitude less than that required to produce an action potential

8_____ minimum magnitude (mV) of the membrane potential at which an action potential can be produced

9_____ principle applied to a variety of different processes, it states that the process happens completely or not at all — that is, the event or process is not graded

10_____ ratio of the current flowing along a nerve fiber to the minimum amount needed to sustain conduction

11_____ saltwater invertebrate animal (specifically, a cephalopod) possessing anatomical features that make it desirable for neuron research and as an appetizer

The Big Picture

Use the activities of this section to help you learn the broader concepts of this chapter.

Learning Exercises

1.   Use these terms to fill in the blanks in the following paragraph (some terms are used more than once).

action K^+ channels   repolarization
depolarization Na^+ conductance   voltage-gated
K^+ conductance Na^+ channels

_____ potentials are explained on the basis of the behavior of

_____ protein channels in the excitable membranes:

_____ are activated rapidly by _____ and then

inactive spontaneously; _____ are activated more slowly by depolarization

and do not inactivate, but rather close in response to _____ . An

_____ potential is initiated when a depolarizing stimulus opens enough

voltage-gated Na^+ channels so that the _____ exceeds the

_____ , setting up a positive feedback cycle in which

_____ rapidly opens the remaining _____ .

2.   Fill in this table, which compares electrical events in membranes as indicated. Some portions
     have already been done for you.

Characteristic	Receptor/synaptic potentials	Action potentials
Location	sensory endings _____ junctions between nerve and muscle	_____ muscle cells
Stimulus type	_____ chemical stimuli	_____
Nature of event	_____	all-or-none
Magnitude (mV)	less than 10mV	_____
Propagation	no	_____
Conduction type	_____	nondecremental
Threshold	no	_____
Summation	yes	_____
Direction	_____ hyperpolarizing	_____
Electrically excitable?	_____	yes
Ion channel type	_____	voltage-gated

90

3. Use these terms to label Figure 7-1 below. Label the abscissa and ordinate (including probable approximate values).

action potential   absolute refractory   hyperpolarization
depolarization   period   threshold
repolarization   relative refractory
                             period

Figure 7-1

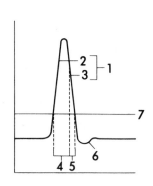

1 _____

2 _____

3 _____

4 _____

5 _____

6 _____

7 _____

4. Use Figure 7-1 to answer these questions:

____ At what point are most of the Na$^+$ channels inactivated, while K$^+$ permeability decreases?

____ At what point is the membrane's permeability to Na$^+$ increasing dramatically?

____ At what point is the membrane's permeability to K$^+$ increasing, while permeability to Na$^+$ is decreasing?

5.   Use these terms to label the neuron pictured in Figure 7-2.

axon   dendrite   Schwann cell
axon hillock   node of Ranvier   synaptic end of axon
cell body (soma)

Figure 7-2

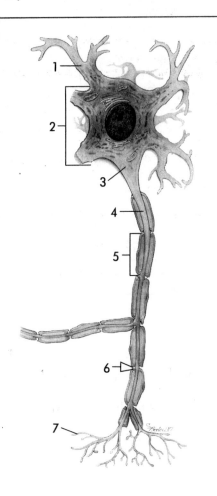

1_____

2_____

3_____

4_____

5_____

6_____

7_____

6.   Arrange this list of nerve fibers in order of conduction velocity, beginning with the fastest
conductor and ending with the slowest.

motor neuron - diameter 20 μm   sensory neuron - diameter 10 μm
sensory neuron - diameter 1 μm   sensory neuron - diameter 5 μm

_____

_____

_____

_____

92

7. Group these characteristics according to the action potential types shown in the table.

continuous spread of depolarization
regenerative action potentials at nodes
relatively fast velocity
relatively slow velocity

requires no myelinization of fibers
requires myelinization of fibers
velocity increases as fiber diameter
increases

Saltatory conduction	Nonsaltatory conduction

8. The graphs in Figure 7-3 show action potentials in three different situations, listed here. Match these situations to the appropriate graphs (A, B, C) which represent them.

Hypercalcemia
Hypocalcemia
Normal Ca^{++} level (in extracellular fluid)

Figure 7-3

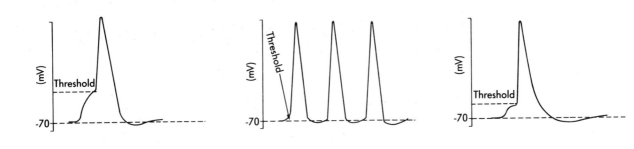

A:_____   B:_____
C:_____

Quick Recall
Review some of the major concepts of this chapter by doing these "quick recall" activities.

1. Name four differences between action potentials and receptor/synaptic potentials.

2. List two kinds of voltage-gated channels important in determining membrane potential.

3.   List the events leading to the initiation of an action potential.

4.   Repolarization is the result of what two factors?

5.   Name three factors that determine conduction velocity in a nerve fiber.

6.   Name two cell types that produce myelin.

Practice Test

Use this practice test to review the topics of this chapter and to prepare for your test on this material.

1.   An action potential
    a.   is propagated
    b.   has a refractory period
    c.   has a threshold
    d.   a and b are correct
    e.   all are correct

2.   Receptor and synaptic potentials
    a.   are propagated
    b.   have thresholds
    c.   are graded
    d.   a and b are correct
    e.   none are correct

3.   During an action potential, which open first?
    a.   voltage-gated Na^+ channels
    b.   voltage-gated K^+ channels
    c.   both open at the same time
    d.   neither opens at all during an action potential

4. A direct result of the opening of voltage-gated Na^+ channels is that
   a. the membrane potential becomes more negative
   b. the membrane potential becomes more positive
   c. the membrane potential stabilizes
   d. neurotransmitters are always released
   e. none of the above

5. As the membrane potential reaches the threshold level
   a. most Na^+ channels become inactivated
   b. there is a net flux of Na^+ inward
   c. all the Na^+ channels have opened
   d. there is a net flux of K^+ inward
   e. all are correct

6. As an action potential begins, the membrane
   a. depolarizes
   b. repolarizes
   c. hyperpolarizes
   d. a and c are correct
   e. all are correct

7. The action potential repolarizes as the
   a. voltage-gated K^+ channels open
   b. voltage-gated K^+ channels close
   c. voltage-gated Na^+ channels close
   d. voltage-gated Na^+ channels open
   e. a and c are correct

8. As a membrane repolarizes after an action potential peak
   a. Na^+ channels inactivate
   b. Na^+ channels activate
   c. the RMP becomes more negative
   d. a and c are correct
   e. none are correct

9. During the absolute refractory period
   a. action potentials can occur but have a high threshold
   b. action potentials cannot occur
   c. most Na^+ channels are inactivated
   d. a and b are correct
   e. b and c are correct

10. During the relative refractory period
    a. action potentials can occur but have a high threshold
    b. action potentials cannot occur
    c. most K^+ channels are inactivated
    d. a and b are correct
    e. b and c are correct

11. Myelin
    a. is a carbohydrate
    b. has an electrically insulating characteristic
    c. tends to allow an increase in conduction velocity
    d. b and c are correct
    e. all are correct

12. Nerve fibers may have relatively high conduction velocities if
    a. they are partially coated with carbohydrate
    b. they are of large diameter
    c. they are of small diameter
    d. a and b are correct
    e. none are correct

13. Saltatory conduction
    a. requires the presence of certain glial cells
    b. requires the presence of myelin
    c. has a relatively high velocity
    d. b and c are correct
    e. all are correct

14. Hypercalcemia can affect conducting cells by
    a. decreasing the threshold for action potentials
    b. increasing the threshold for action potentials
    c. causing spontaneous action potentials
    d. encasing them in crystalline calcium
    e. a and c are correct

15. In a compound action potential, one would expect
    a. involvement of multiple axons
    b. one large action potential peak at each point a change is observed
    c. one small action potential peak at each point a change is observed
    d. a and c are correct
    e. a and b are correct

Answers

Here are answers (or references) to some of the questions presented above.

Word Parts: (your examples may be different) 1-hypercalcemia, 2-depolarization, 3-hypocalcemia, 4-polarization, 5-saltatory, 6-subthreshold

Key Terms: Descriptive: 1. myelinated 2. nonmyelinated 3. inexcitable 4. polarized 5. hyperexcitable 6. excitable 7. hyperpolarized 8. depolarized 9. graded 10. action potential **Processes:** 1. demyelination 2. summation 3. Na^+ inactivation 4. repolarization 5. Na^+ activation 6. repetitive firing 7. overshoot 8. decremental conduction 9. saltatory conduction 10. nondecremental conduction

Structures/Substances: 1. voltage clamp 2. nerve trunk 3. node of Ranvier 4. stimulus-gated channel 5. voltage-gated channel 6. axon 7. leak channel 8. giant axon 9. axon hillock 10. Schwann cell 11. oligodendrocyte 12. myelin

Other: 1. compound action potential 2. hypocalcemia 3. potential 4. receptor potential 5. synaptic potential 6. refractory period 7. subthreshold potential 8. threshold potential 9. all-or-none principle 10. safety factor 11. squid

Learning Exercises: 1. action, voltage-gated, Na^+ channels, depolarization, K^+ channels, repolarization, action, Na^+ conductance, K^+ conductance, depolarization, Na^+ channels 2. (see Table 7-1 in text for answers) 3. 1-action potential, 2-depolarization, 3-repolarization, 4-absolute refractory period, 5-relative refractory period, 6-hyperpolarization, 7-threshold, ordinate-potential(mV), abscissa-time(msec) (check text, Figure 7-5, for numerical values) 4. 6, 2, 3
5. 1-dendrite, 2-cell body (soma), 3-axon hillock, 4-axon, 5-Schwann cell, 6-node of Ranvier, 7-synaptic end of axon 6. motor neuron - diameter 20 μm, sensory neuron - diameter 10 μm, sensory neuron - diameter 5 μm, sensory neuron - diameter 1 μm 7. Saltatory: requires myelinization of fibers, relatively fast velocity, regenerative action potentials at nodes, velocity increases as fiber diameter increases; Nonsaltatory: requires no myelinization of fibers, relatively slow velocity, continuous spread of depolarization, velocity increases as fiber diameter increases 8. A-hypercalcemia, B-hypocalcemia, C-normal

Quick Recall: (You should be able to answer these easily without correction or confirmation by this point in your studies. If not, review your notes, the text chapter, and the previous study activities to find the answers.)

Practice Test: 1-e, 2-c, 3-a, 4-b, 5-b, 6-a, 7-e, 8-d, 9-e, 10-a, 11-d, 12-b, 13-e, 14-b, 15-a

Chapter 8
Initiation, Transmission, and Integration of Neural Signals

Focus
Review this section *first*. It will help you focus on the overall message of this chapter.

Chapter Outline
Read through the outline slowly. This activity will help your mind organize the topics of this chapter.

Neuron structure and information transfer
      Input and output segments of neurons
      Axoplasmic transport
Overview of sensory system organization
      How sensory cells receive information
      Sensory modalities
      Receptive fields and their central representations
Physiological properties of sensory receptors
      Sensory receptors as transducers
      Receptor potentials
      Intensity coding by the receptor potential
      Linear and logarithmic coding
      Sensory adaptation
Synaptic transmission
      Electrical and chemical synapses
      Anatomical specializations of chemical synapses
      Neurotransmitters
      Control of neurotransmitter release by calcium
      Synaptic efficacy
      Fates of released neurotransmitter
      Neurotransmitter receptor families
Principles of information processing in the nervous system
      Categorizing postsynaptic potentials
      Integration of postsynaptic potentials
      Processing of pain signals

Learning Objectives

These are the learning goals for this part of the course. After reading the text, attending class, and studying this chapter, you should be able to:

- understand the functions of the input and output segments of neurons.

- explain how intensity of a stimulus is coded by the receptor potential and how this is translated into action potentials in the afferent neuron.

- describe the two types of specialized cells that transduce the energy provided by stimuli into membrane potential changes.

- define a modality and discuss categories of sensory information that are not included in modalities because they are not consciously experienced.

- summarize the types of receptor adaptation.

- understand the functional differences between electrical and chemical synapses.

- know major classes into which neurotransmitters can be categorized.

- distinguish between excitatory postsynaptic potentials and inhibitory postsynaptic potentials.

- understand the role of Ca^{++} in transmitter release and how synaptic efficacy can be modulated.

- understand how painful sensations can be modulated in the periphery and in the central nervous system (CNS).

Language of Physiology

Physiology uses its own set of terms, many of which may be unfamiliar to you. This section will help you improve your mastery of key physiological terms.

Word Parts

Here are some combining forms often seen in physiological terms. Give an example of a term that contains each word part listed.

Word Part	Meaning	Example
-aps, -apt	fit; fasten	1 _____
con-	with; together	2 _____
corp-	body	3 _____
dendr-	tree; branched structure	4 _____
-icle	(diminutive)	5 _____
karyo-	nucleus	6 _____
post-	after	7 _____
pre-	before	8 _____
quant-	amount	9 _____
syn-	together	10 _____
tempo-	time	11 _____
trans-	across; through	12 _____
vesic-	bladder; blister	13 _____

Key Terms

Read each of the terms in each grouping below aloud, using the pronunciation guide if necessary. This will help you to remember them better than if you read them silently. Then, write out the correct term next to each of the descriptions given.

Descriptive Terms

modality (moh-DAL-it-ee)
postsynaptic (post-sin-APT-ik)
presynaptic (pree-sin-APT-ik)

quantal content (KWAN-tal)
synaptic efficacy
(sin-APT-ik EF-ih-kah-see)

1 _____   degree to which any single synapse can affect the activity of the postsynaptic cell

2 _____   descriptive term meaning "before the synapse," referring to the sending cell at a chemical synapse

3_____	descriptive term meaning "after the synapse," referring to the receiving cell at a chemical synapse
4_____	number of quanta of neurotransmitter released by a presynaptic neuron as the result of a single action potential
5_____	refers to the nature of a sensory stimulus — touch, smell, sound, visual, kinesthetic, heat, cold, pain, and so on

Terms related to processes

adaptation	presynaptic inhibition
axoplasmic transport (aks-oh-PLAZ-mik)	(pree-sin-APT-ik)
linear response (LIN-ee-er)	silent inhibition
logarithmic response (log-ah-RITH-mik)	spatial summation (SPAY-shahl)
presynaptic excitation	synaptic delay (sin-APT-ik)
(pree-sin-APT-ik)	synaptic transmission (sin-APT-ik)
	temporal summation

1_____	ATP-dependent process involving neurofilaments and neurotubules that moves materials away from (anterograde) or toward (retrograde) the soma of the neuron
2_____	decrease in the quanta of transmitter released from a presynaptic neuron resulting from stimulation of the presynaptic axon at an axoaxonic synapse
3_____	delay of about 0.5 msec between the arrival of the action potential at the presynaptic axon terminal and the beginning of the response of the postsynaptic cell
4_____	general term for any decrease in the responsiveness of a receptor cell during continued use
5_____	increase in the quanta of transmitter released from a presynaptic neuron resulting from stimulation of the presynaptic axon at an axoaxonic synapse
6_____	inhibition of an action potential produced by increased membrane permeability to Cl⁻, which stabilizes the membrane potential at the Cl⁻ equilibrium potential (also the resting potential), thus opposing depolarization
7_____	transmission across a synapse (neuron-to-neuron or neuron-to-effector junction)
8_____	type of summation of membrane potentials that occurs when simultaneous inputs at different sites combine to produce a larger potential change
9_____	type of summation of membrane potentials that occurs when serial inputs to a single region repeat rapidly enough to have a combining effect
10_____	type of neuron response to a sensory stimulus in which the receptor potential is directly proportional to the intensity of the stimulus
11_____	type of neuron response to a sensory stimulus in which the receptor potential is not directly proportional to the intensity of the stimulus; in this case, the neuron is quite sensitive to changes in weak stimuli but not so sensitive as the stimuli become stronger

Terms related to structures/substances

acetylcholine (ah-seet-al-KOH-leen)
axoaxonic synapse (aks-oh-aks-AHN-ik)
axon varicosity (var-ih-KAHS-ih-tee)
chemical synapse (SIN-aps)
dendrite (DEN-drite)
dorsal root ganglion (GANG-lee-ahn)
electrical synapse (SIN-aps)
G protein
labeled line
mixed receptor
neuromodulator (noo-roh-MAHD-yoo-lay-tor)

neuropeptide (noo-roh-PEP-tide)
pacinian corpuscle
  (pah-CHIN-ee-an KOHR-pus-il)
phasic receptor (FAYZ-ik)
receptive field
sensory neuron
soma
stimulus-sensitive receptor proteins
synaptic cleft (sin-APT-ik)
synaptic vesicle (sin-APT-ik VES-ih-kal)
tonic receptor
transducer (tranz-DOOS-er)

1_____ 30 to 50 nm space between the presynaptic and postsynaptic cells forming a chemical synapse

2_____ branched extension of the neuron cell body that typically receives input from other cells or receptors; a portion of the input segment of neurons

3_____ group of afferent neuron cell bodies located within the dorsal root of a spinal nerve

4_____ in sensory physiology, this term identifies an afferent nerve as being ordered — that is, specific sensory data travel via particular afferent fibers to appropriate sensory receiving areas

5_____ membrane proteins that are ion channels (or coupled to ion channels) that open or close in response to appropriate stimuli

6_____ neuron that typically receives sensory input and relays it toward the CNS; an afferent neuron

7_____ one of a family of intrinsic membrane proteins that act as second messengers within membranes

8_____ one of a series of enlargements along efferent autonomic nerve fibers from which neurotransmitters are released into the organs innervated by these fibers

9_____ peptide released from a neuron that acts as a hormone, such as oxytocin or somatostatin

10_____ perikaryon, or cell body, of a neuron

11_____ portion of an afferent neuron in which an appropriate stimulus of adequate intensity can result in a change in the permeability of that neuron's membrane; determined by the location of the input segment

12_____ small membranous sphere containing neurotransmitter molecules; found within presynaptic neurons

13_____ specific transmitter substance associated particularly with neuromuscular junctions and certain autonomic pathway synapses

14_____ structure capable of transforming energy from one type to another; for example, a receptor can transform light energy into a neural code

15_____ substance that acts to alter the effect of a neurotransmitter, usually by activating an intracellular second messenger, which then modifies an ion channel

16_____ type of sensory receptor that continues to discharge at the same rate no matter how long a stimulus lasts; equivalent to "nonadapting receptor"

17_____ type of synapse formed when one axon ends on another axon

18_____ type of neuronal junction involving a 30 to 50 nm space between the cells that is traversed by small amounts of neurotransmitter, which affect the potential of the receiving cell; allows transmission in only one direction (from presynaptic toward postsynaptic)

19_____ type of sensory receptor that displays an initial transient response (proportional to the rate of change of the stimulus) followed by a steady state response of smaller magnitude (proportional to the intensity of the stimulus)

20_____ type of neuronal junction formed by gap junctions between the cells, allowing depolarizing current to flow directly from one cell to another (in either direction)

21_____ type of sensory receptor that gives a burst of action potentials at the onset of stimulation, but as the stimulus continues, the rate diminishes (ultimately to zero); equivalent to "rapidly adapting receptor"

22_____ vibration-sensitive receptor found in the deeper skin layers, composed of multiple layers of connective tissues that slip past one another

Other Key Terms

convergence
divergence
excitatory postsynaptic potential
  (ek-SITE-ah-toh-ree post-sin-APT-ik)
inhibitory postsynaptic potential
  (in-HIB-ih-toh-ree post-sin-APT-ik)

local current
postsynaptic potential
  (post-sin-APT-ik)
quantum (KWAN-tum)

1_____ EPSP; a postsynaptic potential that is more positive than the resting potential — that is, a depolarizing potential (making it more likely to reach the threshold)

2_____ flow of electricity (current) at a specific site of a cell membrane (local)

3_____ IPSP; a postsynaptic potential that is more negative than the resting potential (reducing the likelihood that the threshold will be reached)

4_____ Latin for "how much"; in neurophysiology, the amount of neurotransmitter contained in a single synaptic vesicle

5_____ property of neural pathways that involves the formation of synapses of several presynaptic neurons with a single postsynaptic cell

6_____ property of neural pathways that involves the signaling of multiple postsynaptic cells by a single presynaptic neuron

7_____ transient change in the postsynaptic membrane's potential (in either direction) that results from neurotransmitter-receptor interactions

The Big Picture

Use the activities of this section to help you learn the broader concepts of this chapter.

Learning Exercises

1. Review the characteristics of membrane potentials by putting these descriptive phrases into the correct column in the table below.

Begins with opening of both Na^+ and K^+ channels
Begins with an opening of only Na^+ channels
Is always a depolarization
May result from opening of channels coupled to receptor proteins
May be a depolarization or hyperpolarization
Often results from opening of stimulus-gated channels
Propagates
Propagates decrementally
Results from opening of voltage-gated channels

Action potential	Receptor (generator) potential

2. Figure 8-1 represents different ways that receptors may process sensory information. Fill in the blank labels indicated in the diagram with the choices given here (may be used more than once). Then answer the questions given below.

action   linear   receptor
CNS   logarithmic   stimulus
labeled line

Figure 8-1

1 _____

2 _____

3 _____

4 _____

5 _____

6 _____

7 _____

8 _____

9 ___ Which letter (A,B,C) represents lowest intensity stimuli?

10 ___ Which letter represents highest intensity stimuli?

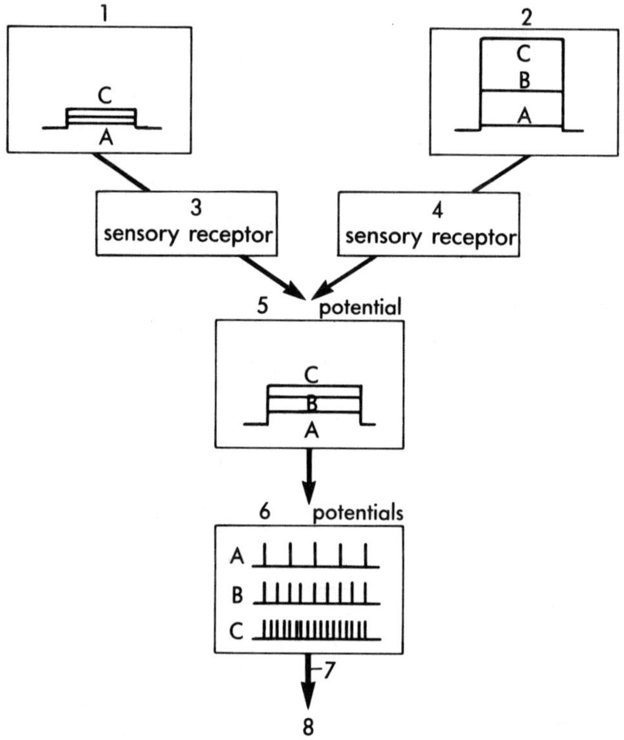

3.   The graph lines in Figure 8-2 show receptor potentials during three different kinds of adaptation exhibited by receptor cells. Identify them by labeling each graph line in blanks A, B, and C.

Figure 8-2

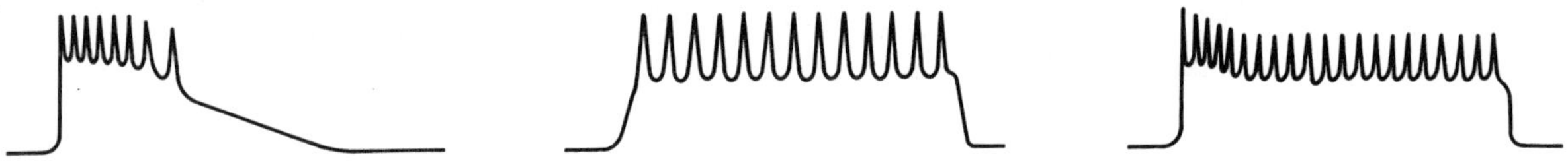

A:_____   B:_____   C:_____

4.   Use the sensory adaptation types that you labeled in No. 3 above to identify these examples.

_____   discharge of potentials at the same rate, no matter how long the stimulus lasts

_____   exhibits a burst of potentials at the onset of stimulation but gradually diminishes to zero

_____   exhibits a burst of potentials but soon decreases to a steady series of lower potentials until the stimulation stops

_____   rapidly adapting type

_____   nonadapting type

_____   for example, the painful sensation associated with a splinter continues for hours, until the splinter is removed

_____   for example, the touch sensations felt when a wristwatch is first put on diminish over time so that eventually the wristwatch is not felt

5.   Arrange these events of synaptic transmission in the order in which they occur.

voltage-gated Na^+ channels in axon fiber open, propagating action potential
action potential invades the presynaptic terminal
depolarization at terminal triggers opening of voltage-gated Ca^{++} channels
Ca^{++} influx facilitates exocytosis of transmitters from terminal vesicles
transmitters diffuse across synaptic cleft
transmitters bind to receptor proteins in postsynaptic membrane
postsynaptic membrane potential deviates from the resting potential
reuptake of some of the transmitters by the presynaptic neuron

1 _____

2 _____

3 _____

4 _____

5 _____

6 _____

7 _____

8 _____

6.   Put these characteristics of membrane potentials into the categories given in the following table.
      (They may be used more than once.)

a move toward 0 mV (from RMP)
a move away from 0 mV (from RMP)
are graded
can be summated
makes an action potential more likely
reduces the possibility of an action potential
results from an increased K^+ permeability
results from an increased Na^+ permeability
tends to be a hyperpolarization

IPSP	EPSP

7.   Refer to Figure 8-3 and write these terms in the correct spaces in the paragraph below.

Figure 8-3

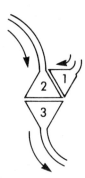

axoaxonal
chemical
EPSP
IPSP
neuromodulator
neurotransmitter
presynaptic inhibition
presynaptic
   facilitation

The junction between 2 and 3 is a regular _____ synapse, whereas

the synapse between 1 and 2 is a special type called _____. A change in 2

resulting from stimulation from 1 may be _____ if the amount of

transmitter sent to 3 is decreased, or it may be _____ if the amount of

transmitter sent to 3 is increased. If the transmitter sent to 3 tends to hyperpolarize that cell, an

_____ is created. On the other hand, if 3 becomes less polarized, an

_____ is created. Short-term effects observed in 3 result from regular

_____ released from 2. Long-term effects in 3, such as subtle changes in

ion permeability, may result from peptides called _____, also released from 2.

8.   Use the space on the next page to draw a logical circuit of neurons that meets the specifications
      given. Do not attempt to draw realistic cell sketches; instead, use this as a neuron symbol:
      ¤——<, where ¤ is the receptive field or dendritic endings, —— (curved, shortened, or
      lengthened as needed), is the axon fiber, and < is the axon terminal. Thus a simple two neuron
      series would be rendered ¤——<¤——<. The direction of this neuron figure represents the
      direction of conduction, so be careful of your placement. Be sure to label areas of convergence
      and divergence and any special synapse or neuron types.

Specifications
This circuit is a reflex arc that begins with a set of six receptors and ends with four effector cells. One
interneuron mediates the reflex. Sensory impulses travel through a series of two neurons before reaching
the interneuron, and motor impulses travel through a series of three neurons after leaving the interneuron.
As the sensory input is integrated by the interneuron, it is also sent to conscious sensing centers in the
brain. Also, at some point before entering the CNS, sensory information may be enhanced through
presynaptic facilitation.

Quick Recall
Review some of the major concepts of this chapter by doing these "quick recall" activities.

1.   Name two ways in which the intensity of a sensory stimulus may be coded.

2.   Name three different types of adaptation in sensory receptor cells.

3.   List two different types of postsynaptic potential.

4.   List two different types of synapse (based on structure).

5. Name three (chemical) categories of neurotransmitters.

6. Name three different substances secreted by neurons.

7. Name two different types of summation.

Practice Test
Use this practice test to review the topics of this chapter and to prepare for your test on this material.

1. Sensory information reaches the CNS
    a. by way of labeled lines
    b. by way of neurons
    c. where it may be integrated by interneurons
    d. where it is always translated into efferent signals
    e. a, b, and c are correct

2. Phasic receptors
    a. tend to have rapidly decreasing generator potentials
    b. tend to have continuous generator potentials
    c. have decreasing generator potentials that eventually even out and continue
    d. are seldom found in the human body
    e. none of the above

3. A receptor that is sensitive to stimuli by orders of magnitude, such as sound, would most likely be
    a. linear
    b. logarithmic
    c. sensitive to only low-magnitude stimuli
    d. sensitive to only high-magnitude stimuli
    e. a and c are correct

4. A receptor that does not adapt to a stimulus is
    a. phasic
    b. tonic
    c. not found in the human organism
    d. hyperpolarized
    e. a and d are correct

5. The receptor potential
    a. is a generator potential
    b. propagates well along the membrane
    c. travels faster along myelinated fibers
    d. has no refractory period
    e. a and d are correct

6.   Receptor adaptation
    a.   has no survival value
    b.   prevents certain stimuli from becoming overly distracting
    c.   is common among many touch receptors in the skin
    d.   b and c are correct
    e.   all are correct

7.   Calcium ions
    a.   have no effect on neuron function
    b.   tend to trigger endocytosis of transmitter molecules
    c.   tend to trigger exocytosis of transmitter molecules
    d.   trigger voltage-gated chloride channels responsible for the action potential
    e.   none of the above

8.   An IPSP
    a.   is more negative than the resting potential
    b.   is less negative than the resting potential
    c.   results mainly from an increase in K^+ permeability
    d.   results mainly from an increase in Na^+ permeability
    e.   a and c are correct

9.   Presynaptic inhibition results
    a.   from signals sent by means of axoaxonic synapses
    b.   from signals sent by means of dendrodendritic synapses
    c.   in the release of more transmitters than usual
    d.   in a greater postsynaptic potential
    e.   a and d are correct

10. Postsynaptic excitation
    a.   results in greater depolarization in the postsynaptic membrane
    b.   results in hyperpolarization in the postsynaptic membrane
    c.   results in increased K^+ permeability in the postsynaptic membrane
    d.   results in decreased Na^+ permeability in the postsynaptic membrane
    e.   a and c are correct

11. Spatial summation is most likely to occur in a case of
    a.   convergence
    b.   rapidly repeating stimuli
    c.   divergence
    d.   a postsynaptic neuron with multiple dendrites
    e.   a and d are correct

12. After being released from the binding sites on postsynaptic receptors, neurotransmitters
    a.   are metabolized by enzymes
    b.   are transported back into the presynaptic neuron
    c.   are transported into the postsynaptic neuron
    d.   act as hormones
    e.   a and b are possible

13. Acetylcholine is a
    a.   hormone
    b.   transmitter found at neuromuscular junctions
    c.   transmitter found at some autonomic synapses
    d.   substrate of the Krebs cycle
    e.   b and c are correct

14. Long-term changes in synaptic efficacy can be accomplished through the action of
    a. classical neurotransmitters
    b. acetylcholine
    c. neuromodulators
    d. steroids
    e. none of the above

Answers
Here are answers (or references) to some of the questions presented above.

Word Parts: (your examples may be different) 1-synapse, 2-convergence, 3-pacinian corpuscle, 4-dendrite, 5-vesicle, 6-perikaryon, 7-postsynaptic, 8-presynaptic, 9-quantum, 10-synapse, 11-temporal summation, 12-transducer, 13-vesicle

Key Terms: Descriptive: 1. synaptic efficacy 2. presynaptic 3. postsynaptic 4. quantal content 5. modality
Processes: 1. axoplasmic transport 2. presynaptic inhibition 3. synaptic delay 4. adaptation 5. presynaptic excitation 6. silent inhibition 7. synaptic transmission 8. spatial summation 9. temporal summation 10. linear response 11. logarithmic response
Structures/Substances: 1. synaptic cleft 2. dendrite 3. dorsal root ganglion 4. labeled line 5. stimulus-sensitive receptor proteins 6. sensory neuron 7. G protein 8. axon varicosity 9. neuropeptide 10. soma 11. receptive field 12. synaptic vesicle 13. acetylcholine 14. transducer 15. neuromodulator 16. tonic receptor 17. axoaxonic synapse 18. chemical synapse 19. mixed receptor 20. electrical synapse 21. phasic receptor 22. pacinian corpuscle
Other: 1. excitatory postsynaptic potential 2. local current 3. inhibitory postsynaptic potential 4. quantum 5. convergence 6. divergence 7. postsynaptic potential

Learning Exercises: 1. ACTION POTENTIAL: Results from opening of voltage-gated channels, Begins with an opening of only Na^+ channels, Is always depolarization, Propagates RECEPTOR POTENTIAL: Often results from opening of stimulus-gated channels, May result from opening of channels coupled to receptor proteins, Begins with opening of both Na^+ and K^+ channels, May be depolarization or hyperpolarization, Propagates decrementally 2. 1-stimulus, 2-stimulus, 3-linear, 4-logarithmic, 5-receptor, 6-action, 7-labeled line, 8-CNS, 9-A, 10-C 3. A:phasic, B:tonic, C:mixed (phasic/tonic) 4. tonic, phasic, mixed, phasic, tonic, tonic, phasic 5. 1-voltage-gated Na^+ channels in axon fiber open, propagating action potential, 2-action potential invades the presynaptic terminal, 3-depolarization at terminal triggers opening of voltage-gated Ca^{++} channels, 4-Ca^{++} influx facilitates exocytosis of transmitters from terminal vesicles, 5-transmitters diffuse across synaptic cleft, 6-transmitters bind to receptor proteins in postsynaptic membrane, 7-postsynaptic membrane potential deviates from the resting potential, 8-reuptake of some of the transmitters by the presynaptic neuron 6. INHIBITORY POSTSYNAPTIC POTENTIAL: a move away from 0 mV, results from an increased K^+ permeability, reduces the possibility of an action potential, can be summated, are graded, tends to be a hyperpolarization; EXCITATORY POSTSYNAPTIC POTENTIAL: a move toward 0 mV, results from an increased Na^+ permeability, makes an action potential more likely can be summed, are graded 7. chemical, axo-axonal, presynaptic inhibition, presynaptic facilitation, IPSP, EPSP, neurotransmitter, neuromodulator 8. (Figures may vary. Check text, Figures 8-3, 8-20, and 8-23 for ideas. If uncertain, check with your instructor or teaching assistant)

Quick Recall: (You should be able to answer these easily without correction or confirmation by this point in your studies. If not, review your notes, the text chapter, and the previous study activities to find the answers.)

Practice Test: 1-e, 2-a, 3-b, 4-b, 5-e, 6-d, 7-c, 8-e, 9-a, 10-a, 11-a, 12-e, 13-e, 14-e, 15-c

Chapter 9
The Somatosensory System and an Introduction to Brain Function

Focus
Review this section *first*. It will help you focus on the overall message of this chapter.

Chapter Outline
Read through the outline slowly. This activity will help your mind organize the topics of this chapter.

Anatomy of the nervous system
      Segregation of axons and cell bodies
      Central and peripheral components of the nervous system
      Subdivisions of the central nervous system
      The cortex of the cerebral hemispheres
      Cortical organization
Sensory Processing
      Projection of sensory inputs
The somatosensory system
      Overview of somatosensory receptors
      Touch receptors
      Temperature receptors
      Pain perception
Integration in the somatosensory system
      Somatosensory projections to the thalamus
      Somatosensory maps
      Two-point discrimination
      The reticular activating system
Learning and memory
      Distinctions between learning and memory
      Short-term and long-term memory
Specializations of the human brain
      Hemispheric specializations
      Evidence for language specialization
      Split-brain individuals
      Specializations of the right hemisphere
      Cortical regions involved in memory, emotion, and self-image
Sleep and the wakeful state
      Sleep as an active function
      Sleep states and waking states
      The sleep cycle

Learning Objectives

These are the learning goals for this part of the course. After reading the text, attending class, and studying this chapter, you should be able to:

◆ distinguish between the peripheral and central nervous systems, and describe the location of the major subdivisions of the brain: the brainstem, cerebellum, thalamus, hypothalamus, and cerebral hemispheres

◆ understand what is meant by a topographic representation and why it is important in the central processing of sensory information

◆ outline the elements of the somatosensory afferent pathways, identifying the different routes taken by the submodalities of touch, vibration, temperature and pain

◆ state the function of the reticular activating system

◆ understand the difference between short-term memory and long-term memory

◆ appreciate the significance of the term "dominant hemisphere" and identify the location of the language areas

◆ identify the characteristics of the stages of sleep

Language of Physiology

Physiology uses its own set of terms, many of which may be unfamiliar to you. This section will help you improve your mastery of key physiological terms.

Word Parts

Here are some combining forms often seen in physiological terms. Give an example of a term that contains each word part listed.

Word Part	Meaning	Example
cephalo-	head	1_____
derm-	skin	2_____
-gram*	something written, drawn	3_____
-graph*	to write, draw	4_____
hemi-	half	5_____
peri-	around; surrounding	6_____
tom-	a cutting; a segment	7_____
top-	place; region	8_____

* in current physiological usage, a term ending in "-graph" refers to an apparatus or technique that results in a visual image or record of biological phenomena, whereas a term ending in "-gram" is the record itself. For instance, an electrocardio*graph* is used in producing an electrocardio*gram*.

Key Terms

Read each of the terms in each grouping below aloud, using the pronunciation guide if necessary. This will help you to remember them better than if you read them silently. Then, write out the correct term next to each of the descriptions given.

Terms related to processes

fast pain
feature extraction
lateral inhibition
learning
memory
memory consolidation

rapid eye movement [REM] sleep
referred pain
segmental reflex
slow pain
slow wave sleep [SWS]

1 _____ nerve reflex process in which the reflex arc is completed within a single spinal segment

2 _____ process of pain sensation in which the perception of pain seems localized at a cutaneous site when it is actually coming from a visceral site (as in the surface chest pain experienced during a heart attack)

3 _____ process whereby experience (memory) modifies centrally controlled behavior

4 _____ process of pain sensation in which the perception is diffuse (rather than well localized) and persists after removal of the stimulus (as in prolonged contact with a hot object)

5 _____ process of pain sensation in which the perception is well localized but rapidly disappears without residual effects (as in a needle jab)

6 _____ process in which the brain emphasizes important aspects of a particular modality at the expense of less important aspects; for example, in detecting the boundary outlines of an object or in detecting the feature of motion in a visual field

7 _____ process in which inputs to adjacent regions of a sensory area of the cortex tend to inhibit one another (the stronger inhibits the weaker), magnifying the difference in sensations

8 _____ general term referring to the process of storage and retrieval of data regarding experience

9 _____ stage of deep sleep observed on an electroencephalogram (EEG) as a period of slow (delta) waves

10 _____ stage of sleep in which the brain is relatively active, seen outwardly as rapid movement of the eyes under the closed lids; the "dream" stage of sleep

11 _____ process of shifting stored memory data from the short-term memory form to the long-term memory form

Terms related to structure

association neuron
brainstem
cerebellum (sair-eh-BEL-um)
cerebral lobe (ser-EE-bral)
cerebral hemisphere
cerebral cortex (ser-EE-bral KOHR-tex)
corpus callosum (KORP-us kal-OH-sum)
corpus striatum (KORP-us stry-AYT-um)
cranial nerve (KRAYN-ee-al)
dermatome (DERM-ah-tohm)
diencephalon (dy-en-SEF-ah-lahn)
dorsal column pathway
ganglion (GANG-lee-ahn)
gray matter
limbic system (LIM-bik)
medulla (meh-DOO-lah)
midbrain

mixed nerves
motor tract
nucleus (NOO-klee-us)
peripheral nervous system [PNS]
    (per-IH-fer-al)
pons (pahnz)
reticular formation (ret-IK-yoo-ler)
sensory tract
spinal cord
spinal nerve (SPY-nal)
spinothalamic tract
    (spy-noh-THAL-ah-mik)
telencephalon (tel-en-SEF-ah-lahn)
thalamus (THAL-ah-mus)
white matter

1_____ region of the body surface innervated by a particular spinal nerve

2_____ loosely packed network of neurons in the brainstem that serves as the anatomical component of the reticular activating system, a system responsible for conscious arousal of higher brain divisions

3_____ general term referring to a bundle of sensory (afferent, or ascending) fibers within the CNS

4_____ thick bundle of fibers that connects the left and right cerebral hemispheres

5_____ nerve (bundle of nerve fibers outside the CNS) that contains a mix of sensory and motor fibers

6_____ portion of the brain responsible for emotional responses; includes the hippocampus and olfactory cortex

7_____ general term referring to a bundle of motor (efferent, or descending) fibers within the CNS

8_____ 3 cm thick wrinkled sheet of gray matter forming the outer section of each cerebral hemisphere; composed of three subdivisions: neocortex, hippocampus, and olfactory lobes

9_____ interneuron; a neuron that is involved in linking sensory inputs to motor outputs (a function called integration)

10_____ any of 62 (31 pairs) nerves that exit directly from the spinal cord; have dorsal and ventral roots at their exit from the cord

11_____ any association of neuronal cell bodies within the PNS

12_____ any of 24 (12 pairs) nerves that exit directly from the brain

13_____ any of several principal regions of the cerebral cortex (frontal, temporal, occipital, parietal) defined by sulci or fissures formed between the raised gyri of the cortex

14_____ cylindrical portion of the brain that connects the superior brain divisions

15 _____	to the spinal cord below; composed of the midbrain, pons, and medulla
	division of the brain composed mainly of the thalamus and hypothalamus
16 _____	in the context of neurohistology, any association of neuronal cell bodies within the CNS
17 _____	inferior portion of the CNS, in the shape of a long cylinder composed of ascending and descending nerve tracts and a core of interneurons
18 _____	inferior portion of the brainstem, where it meets the spinal cord
19 _____	middle portion of the brainstem, between the medulla and midbrain
20 _____	nervous tissue composed largely of myelinated axons, giving it a lighter appearance than tissue composed of nonmyelinated structures
21 _____	nervous tissue composed largely of cell bodies and nonmyelinated fibers; since the cell bodies are nonmyelinated, this tissue normally appears darker than the whitish myelinated axons
22 _____	one of two half-spherical portions of the cerebrum (telencephalon) — left and right
23 _____	portion of the diencephalon superior to the hypothalamus; acts as a relay point for ascending and descending fibers
24 _____	portion of the overall nervous system outside the brain and spinal cord (CNS)
25 _____	region deep within each cerebral hemisphere that contains several nuclei; the basal ganglia
26 _____	spherical division of the brain dorsal to the brainstem; acts as a coordinator of muscle movements
27 _____	superior portion of the brainstem, above the pons, containing the red nucleus; mesencephalon
28 _____	lemniscal system; the ascending somatosensory tract (of the CNS) that carries signals from specialized cutaneous receptors and proprioceptors, forming the most "direct" sensory pathway
29 _____	anterolateral system; a pathway for sensory nerve fibers carrying kinesthetic and fine touch information to the higher brain centers via the thalamus
30 _____	the most superior division of the brain; the cerebrum

Other Key Terms

alpha [α] wave (AL-fah)
aphasia (a-FAY-jah)
beta [β] wave (BAY-tah)
decussate (dee-KUS-ayt)
delta [δ] wave
dominant hemisphere

electroencephalogram [EEG]
    (el-ek-troh-en-SEF-ah-loh-gram)
principle of parallel processing
theta [θ] wave (THAY-tah)

1 _____	principle of neurophysiology that states that information arising from a single population of receptors can follow divergent pathways and be mapped in several regions of the brain, so that different relevant features can be extracted and integrated
2 _____	deficit in expressing or understanding language

119

3 _____ visual representation of the electrical activity of the cortex (voltage versus time)

4 _____ on an EEG, a wave of moderately low frequency observed at the onset of sleep

5 _____ on an EEG, a wave of high frequency (18 to 20 Hz) observed during attentive waking states

6 _____ on an EEG, a wave of very low frequency (high amplitude) observed during deep (slow wave) sleep

7 _____ on an EEG, a wave of moderately high frequency (8 to 13 Hz) observed in relaxed individuals (eyes shut)

8 _____ cerebral hemisphere in which a person's language ability resides, often the left hemisphere

9 _____ cross over from one side to another (as do some nerve fibers in the CNS)

The Big Picture

Use the activities of this section to help you learn the broader concepts of this chapter.

Learning Exercises

1. Place these terms in their proper place in the table that follows.

autonomic ganglia   midbrain
brain   motor cortex
brainstem   pons
cerebrum   sensory receptor
cranial nerve   sensory cortex
dorsal root ganglia   spinal nerve
hypothalamus   spinal cord
medulla   thalamus

Central nervous system	Peripheral nervous system

2. Shade in and/or label Figure 9-1 to include these features. The use of color pencils or pens to completely shade in areas is recommended, since it will help you to remember shapes and spatial relationships better than just labeling parts.

Figure 9-1

Broca's area
cerebellum
frontal cerebral lobe
medulla
motor cortex
occipital cerebral lobe
parietal cerebral lobe
pons
primary auditory cortex
spinal cord
temporal cerebral lobe
visual cortex
Wernicke's area

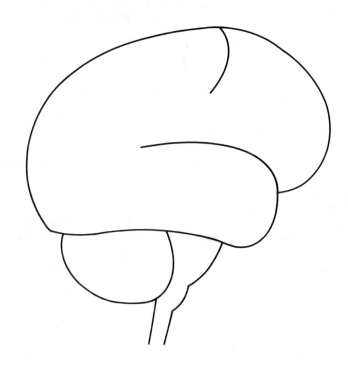

3. Match these divisions of the CNS with their functions. (Some terms may be used more than once.)

cerebellum   spinal cord
hypothalamus   telencephalon
medulla   thalamus
pons/midbrain

1_____   relay sensory information; spinal reflexes

2_____   sensory afferent nuclei; reticular activating system; visceral control centers

3_____   reticular activating system; visceral control centers

4_____   basal ganglia and red nucleus for motor control

5_____   visceral function; neuroendocrine control

6_____   coordination of movements; balance

7_____   hippocampus: memory, emotion

8_____   relay station for ascending and descending fibers; control of visceral function (diencephalon)

9_____   neocortex: higher integrative functions

4.   Put each of these characteristics of the different somatosensory afferent pathways into the correct column of the table below. (May be used more than once.)

also called the lemniscal system
also called anterolateral system
crosses over in the spinal segment it enters
decussate in the medulla
is relayed through the thalamus
mediates proprioception and fine touch

mediates crude touch, fast pain, cold
one neuron from receptor to thalamus
this tract has somatotopic representation
this tract tends to be nonsomatotopic
two neurons from the receptor to thalamus

Dorsal column pathway	Spinothalamic tract

5.   Put these terms into the correct blanks in the paragraph below.

diverge
extracting
filter

parallel
topically

    Sensory pathways commonly _____ to carry signals to more than one

brain region for _____ processing. Central processing areas

_____ the incoming signals, _____ novel or important

features for further analysis. Central processing areas are usually organized

_____ (somatotopic, etc.), so that receptors from a spot on the body surface

project to a corresponding spot in the relevant brain area.

6. Use the terms given to label the types of EEG waves shown in Figure 9-2. Then fill in the blanks below.

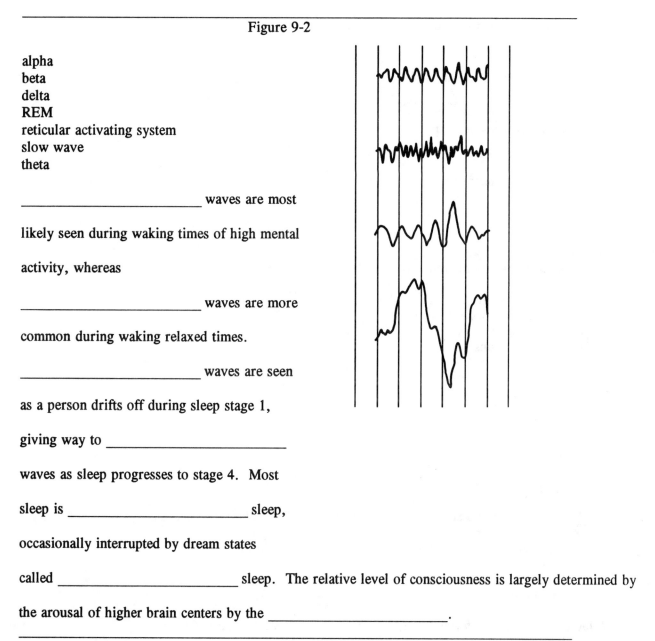

Figure 9-2

alpha
beta
delta
REM
reticular activating system
slow wave
theta

_____ waves are most likely seen during waking times of high mental activity, whereas

_____ waves are more common during waking relaxed times.

_____ waves are seen as a person drifts off during sleep stage 1,

giving way to _____ waves as sleep progresses to stage 4. Most

sleep is _____ sleep, occasionally interrupted by dream states

called _____ sleep. The relative level of consciousness is largely determined by

the arousal of higher brain centers by the _____.

Quick Recall

Review some of the major concepts of this chapter by doing these "quick recall" activities.

1. List the two main divisions of the nervous system and their primary organs.

2.   List the main subdivisions of the brain.

3.   List two different routes of somatosensory pathways.

4.   Describe four types of brain waves.

5.   Name two main types of sleep.

6.   List two forms of memory stored in the brain.

Practice Test
Use this practice test to review the topics of this chapter and to prepare for your test on this material.

1.   The peripheral nervous system includes
   a.   somatic sensory receptors
   b.   spinal nerve roots
   c.   dorsal columns
   d.   spinal cord
   e.   a and b are correct

2.   The portion of the brain that coordinates muscle movement is the
   a.   cerebrum
   b.   medulla
   c.   cerebellum
   d.   pons
   e.   corpus callosum

3.   The portion of the brain serving as the major center of the autonomic nervous system is the
   a.   pons
   b.   hypothalamus
   c.   thalamus
   d.   medulla
   e.   cerebrum

4.   A layer of gray matter forming the outer part of the telencephalon is the
   a.   cortex
   b.   medulla
   c.   ganglion
   d.   nucleus
   e.   a and d are correct

5.   The brain can precisely locate a pinprick on the finger by means of the characteristic of
   a.   tonotopism
   b.   habituation
   c.   somatotopism
   d.   thalamic relay
   e.   associative learning

6. A relay station for somatosensory nerves, before they are projected into the cortex, is the
    a. brainstem
    b. hypothalamus
    c. cerebellum
    d. thalamus
    e. lateral ventricle

7. The reticular activating system is responsible for
    a. level of consciousness
    b. sleep
    c. attentiveness
    d. stimulation of the cortex
    e. all of the above

8. Crude sensations of touch travel via the
    a. dorsal column pathway
    b. ventral column pathway
    c. spinothalamic pathway
    d. efferent fibers
    e. cerebellum

9. The spinothalamic pathway involves
    a. decussation in the brainstem
    b. cross-over in the spinal segment
    c. intervention of the cerebellum
    d. precise mapping of sensations
    e. all of the above

10. Learning
    a. is the same as memory
    b. involves memory storage
    c. always involves association of neutral and nonneutral stimuli
    d. often requires sensory processing
    e. b and d are correct

11. Short-term memory
    a. is often consolidated into long-term memory
    b. involves electrical activity in neuronal   circuits
    c. involves changes in synaptic responsiveness
    d. requires sensory input
    e. a, b and d are correct

12. Dominance of a hemisphere
    a. involves the language centers
    b. is related to "handedness"
    c. is determined by size
    d. is no longer accepted
    e. is not seen in normal individuals

13. Alpha waves are likely to be seen during
    a. SWS sleep
    b. REM sleep
    c. waking, attentive states
    d. waking, nonattentive states
    e. b and d are correct

14.	Delta waves are likely to be seen
  a.	during SWS sleep
  b.	during REM sleep
  c.	as drowsiness turns to sleep
  d.	during waking, nonattentive states
  e.	during waking, attentive states

15.	Aphasia refers specifically to a problem in
  a.	levels of consciousness
  b.	ability to learn
  c.	language ability
  d.	memory retention

Answers

Here are answers (or references) to some of the questions presented above.

Word Parts (your examples may be different) 1-electroencephalogram, 2-dermatome, 3-electroencephalogram, 4-electroencephalograph, 5-cerebral hemisphere, 6-peripheral nervous system, 7-dermatome, 8-tonotopic

Key Terms: Processes: 1. segmental reflex 2. referred pain 3. learning 4. slow pain 5. fast pain 6. feature extraction 7. lateral inhibition 8. memory 9. slow wave sleep [SWS] 10. rapid eye movement [REM] sleep 11. memory consolidation
Structure: 1. dermatome 2. reticular formation 3. sensory tract 4. corpus callosum 5. mixed nerves 6. limbic system 7. motor tract 8. cerebral cortex 9. association neuron 10. spinal nerve 11. ganglion 12. cranial nerve 13. cerebral lobe 14. brainstem 15. diencephalon 16. nucleus 17. spinal cord 18. medulla 19. pons 20. white matter 21. gray matter 22. cerebral hemisphere 23. thalamus 24. peripheral nervous system [PNS] 25. corpus striatum 26. cerebellum 27. midbrain 28. dorsal column pathway 29. spinothalamic tract 30. telencephalon
Other: 1. principle of parallel processing 2. aphasia 3. electroencephalogram [EEG] 4. theta [θ] wave 5. beta [β] wave 6. delta [δ] wave 7. alpha [α] wave 8. dominant hemisphere 9. decussate

Learning Exercises: 1. CNS:brain, brainstem, cerebrum, hypothalamus, medulla, midbrain, motor cortex, pons, sensory cortex, spinal cord, thalamus; PNS:autonomic ganglia, cranial nerve, dorsal root, ganglia, sensory receptor, spinal nerve 2. (compare your sketch to the brain figures in Chapter 9) 3. 1-spinal cord, 2-medulla, 3-pons/midbrain, 4-telencephalon, 5-hypothalamus, 6-cerebellum, 7-telencephalon, 8-thalamus, 9-telencephalon 4. DORSAL COLUMN PATHWAY:one neuron from receptor to thalamus, also called the lemniscal system, decussate in the medulla, mediates proprioception and fine touch, this tract has somatotopic representation, is relayed through the thalamus; SPINOTHALAMIC TRACT: two neurons from the receptor to thalamus, also called anterolateral system, crosses over in the spinal segment it enters, mediates crude touch, fast pain, cold, this tract tends to be nonsomatopic, is relayed through the thalamus 5. diverge, parallel, filter, extracting, topically, 6. learning, nonassociative, sensitization, habituation, associative, short-term, long-term, consolidation 7. Figure: alpha, beta, theta, delta; Paragraph: beta, alpha, theta, delta, slow wave, REM, reticular activating system

Quick Recall: (You should be able to answer these questions easily without correction or confirmation by this point in your studies. If you cannot, review your notes, the text chapter, and the previous study activities to find the answers.)

Practice Test: 1-e, 2-c, 3-b, 4-a, 5-c, 6-d, 7-e, 8-c, 9-b, 10-e, 11-e, 12-a, 13-e, 14-a, 15-c

Chapter 10
The Special Senses

Focus
Review this section *first*. It will help you focus on the overall message of this chapter.

Chapter Outline
Read through the outline slowly. This activity will help your mind organize the topics of this chapter.

The auditory system
     Physics of sound
     The outer ear and tympanic membrane
     Sound transmission through the middle ear
     Structure of the cochlea
     Sympathetic resonance and frequency coding in the cochlea
     Hair cells—the auditory receptors
     Auditory afferent pathways
     Tonotopic organization of the auditory system
     Localization of sounds in space
The vestibular system
     Functions of the vestibular system
     Vestibular receptors
     Detection of head position and linear acceleration
     Detection of head rotations
     Rotational nystagmus
The visual system
     Structure of the eye
     The eye as an image-generating device
     Accommodation for distance
     Disorders of image formation
     The retina
     The rod and cone photoreceptors
     Photopigment bleaching—the first step in photoreception
     Maintenance of photoreceptor sensitivity and dark adaptation
     From photopigment bleaching to photoreceptor potentials
     ON and OFF pathways from photoreceptors to ganglion cells
     Lateral inhibition in the retina
     What the retina tells the brain
     Central visual pathways

Detection of shape and movement
The chemical senses: taste and smell
Submodalities of taste
Mechanisms of transduction in taste buds
Olfactory receptors
Central olfactory pathways

Learning Objectives

These are the learning goals for this part of the course. After reading the text, attending class, and studying this chapter, you should be able to:

◆ describe how the tympanic membrane and auditory ossicles transmit sound energy to the cochlea

◆ understand how the resonance properties of the cochlea translate sound energy into displacements of hair cells on the basilar membrane

◆ understand how sound sources are localized in space

◆ appreciate how the structure of the vestibular system translates gravitational or inertial forces into hair cell displacement

◆ understand the process of image formation in the eye and describe accommodation

◆ appreciate how lateral inhibition makes retinal ganglion cells respond to spots on contrasting backgrounds—distinguish between ON center/OFF surround and OFF center/ON surround cells in terms of the synaptic connections in the retina

◆ summarize the principles of feature extraction in the visual system

◆ describe the organization of cortical columns in the visual cortex

◆ describe the modalities of taste and olfaction

Language of Physiology

Physiology uses its own set of terms, many of which may be unfamiliar to you. This section will help you improve your mastery of key physiological terms.

Word Parts

Here are some combining forms often seen in physiological terms. Give an example of a term that contains each word part listed.

Word Part	Meaning	Example
bas-	base	1 _____
chromo-	color	2 _____
-itis	(signifies "inflammation of")	3 _____
kin-	to move	4 _____
-lith	stone; rock	5 _____
oto-	ear	6 _____
photo-	light	7 _____
semi-	half	8 _____
son(o)-	sound	9 _____
tect-	to cover	10 _____
tympan-	drum	11 _____

Key Terms

Read each of the terms in each grouping below aloud, using the pronunciation guide if necessary. This will help you to remember them better than if you read them silently. Then, write out the correct term next to each of the descriptions given.

Descriptive Terms

binaural (byn-AWR-al)
dark-adapted
decibel (DES-ih-bel)
Hertz [Hz]
intensity difference
intensity

olfactory (ohl-FAK-tor-ee)
phase difference
pitch
pure tone
resonant frequency (REZ-oh-nant)

1 _____   characteristic of binaural interpretation of high-frequency sound, when the difference in the decibel levels of the sounds reaching each ear is used to determine the location of the sound

2 _____   characteristic of binaural interpretation of low-frequency sound, when a certain point of the sound wave reaches each ear at a slightly different time, allowing the brain to compute the location of the sound

3 _____   descriptive term referring to the sense of smell

4 _____   descriptive term referring to the ability to hear with two, rather than one or more than two, ears

5 _____   descriptive term for a rod cell with all or most of its rhodopsin in the unbleached form

6 _____   quality of sound exhibited when there is a distinctly dominant frequency

7 _____   sound with only one frequency, rather than the mix of frequencies exhibited by voice and most other environmental sources

8 _____   quality of sound that is determined by the amount of pressure in a sound wave; loudness

9 _____   unit expressing intensity (loudness) of a sound on a logarithmic scale

10 _____   measure of frequency of an energy wave in cycles/second

11 _____   frequency at which external forces applied to harmonic oscillators — objects such as pendulums or springs — cause a progressive increase in the amplitude of the resulting oscillations (sympathetic resonance)

Terms related to processes

accommodation

bleaching

impedance matching system (im-PEED-ans)

photopic vision (foh-TOP-ik)

place coding

rotational nystagmus (nis-TAG-mus)

scotopic vision (skoh-TOP-ik)

spatial analysis (SPAY-shahl)

temporal analysis (TEM-poh-rel)

visual acuity (ak-YOO-it-ee)

1 _____   process of visual interpretation that determines the locations of images within the visual field

2 _____   process in which the resonant frequency of the cochlear tissue differs from place to place, resulting in certain frequencies stimulating only certain places, thus coding for frequency

3 _____   process of visual interpretation that determines relative movement of images within the visual field

4 _____   process in photoreception in which the retinal molecule changes conformation when exposed to the proper wavelength of light; it leads to a change in membrane potential of the photoreceptor cell

5 _____   process in which the shape of the lens is altered to allow images at various (near) distances to be focused sharply on the retina

6 _____   combination of factors that results in an increase in sound wave pressure from the middle to inner ear, required for the transition from low-resistance air to high-resistance fluid

7 _____   daytime (bright-light) vision, mediated by cones

8 _____   low-light vision, mediated by the rods

9 _____   relative ability to distinguish images at a distance

10 _____   unusual back-and-forth movement of the eyes after prolonged rotation of the head, caused by a reflex associated with the continued movement of semicircular endolymph shortly after rotation has stopped

Terms related to structures/substances of the ear

ampulla (amp-YOO-lah)
auditory canal
auditory ossicle (AHS-ik-il)
basal body (BAY-zal)
basilar membrane (BAZ-ih-lar)
cochlea (KOH-klee-ah)
cupula (CYOO-pyoo-lah)
endolymph (EN-doh-limf)
eustachian tube (yoo-STAY-shun)
hair cell
kinocilium (kin-oh-SIL-ee-um)
organ of Corti (KOR-tee)
otolith (OH-toh-lith)

otolithic membrane (oh-toh-LITH-ik)
oval window
perilymph (PAIR-ih-limf)
pinna (PIN-ah)
scala tympani (SKAL-ah TIM-pan-ee)
scala media (SKAL-ah MEE-dee-ah)
scala vestibuli (SKAL-ah vest-IB-yoo-lee)
semicircular canal
stereocilia (stayr-ee-oh-SIL-ee-ah)
tectorial membrane (tek-TOR-ee-al)
tympanic membrane (tim-PAN-ik)
vestibular membrane (vest-IB-yoo-ler)
vestibule (VEST-ib-yool)

1_____ gelatinous membrane in the utricle and in the saccule embedded with calcium carbonate crystals and covering the hair cells

2_____ ball of gelatinous material covering the hair cells of the ampulla that occludes the movement of fluid within the semicircular canal

3_____ portion of the inner ear resembling a coiled snail or turban

4_____ calcium carbonate crystal found embedded in the gelatinous membrane covering the hair cells of the utricle and saccule

5_____ membrane that forms a "roof" over the basilar membrane of the cochlea

6_____ bubblelike enlargement at the base of each semicircular canal

7_____ drumlike covering of the internal end of the auditory canal, forming the boundary to the middle ear; vibrates when hit by sound waves

8_____ submembranous structure in auditory and vestibular hair cells that determines their polarity

9_____ oval opening in the bone separating the middle ear from the inner ear; the stapes fits into it and thus transmits energy waves into the fluid of the inner ear

10_____ cilia that cover a surface of hair cells in the receptor areas of the ear

11_____ fluid found within the scala media, or cochlear duct

12_____ fluid found in the scala vestibuli and scala tympani of the cochlea

13_____ membrane of the cochlea that separates the scala media from the scala tympani and serves as a base for the organ of Corti

14_____ membrane of the cochlea that separates the scala media from the scala vestibuli

15_____ one of three tiny bones in each middle ear connected, as a chain, to the tympanum and the oval window of the inner ear; the malleus, incus, and stapes

16 _____ one of three half-circle canals (in three different planes) connected to the vestibule of the inner ear with receptor areas for one type of equilibrium (rotation direction/speed)

17 _____ portion of the inner ear at the base of the cochlea, containing the utricle and saccule, with receptors for one type of equilibrium (linear acceleration and position relative to gravity)

18 _____ portion of tissue within the cochlea that contains sensory hair cells for the reception of sound

19 _____ portion of the outer ear that constitutes a flexible flap of skin and cartilage

20 _____ single knoblike cilium on each hair cell in the vestibular receptor area surrounded by smaller stereocilia similar to those in the organ of Corti

21 _____ sensory receptor cell for sound found in the organ of Corti

22 _____ "lower" of three fluid chambers forming the cochlea, it begins at the apex of the cochlear tube and proceeds to the round window

23 _____ middle of three fluid chambers forming the cochlea, it is also called the cochlear duct

24 _____ the auditory tube; a partially collapsed canal leading from the middle ear to the pharynx that allows equalization with external air pressure

25 _____ "upper" of three fluid chambers forming the cochlea, it begins at the oval window and proceeds to the apex of the cochlear tube

26 _____ tube that leads inward through the outer ear and ends at the eardrum

Terms related to structures/substances of the eye

anterior cavity
aqueous humor (AYK-wee-us)
choroid layer (KOR-oyd)
ciliary body (SIL-ee-air-ee)
complex cell
cornea (KORN-ee-ah)
fovea (FOH-vee-ah)
ganglion cells
macrocolumn (MAK-roh-kahl-um)
off pathway

on pathway
optic disk
photopigment (foh-toh-PIG-ment)
photoreceptor (foh-toh-ree-SEP-tor)
posterior cavity
retina (RET-in-ah)
rhodopsin (roh-DAHP-sin)
simple cell
vitreous humor (VIT-ree-us)

1 _____ a column of sensory cortex dedicated to the analysis of a particular portion of the visual field; an organization unit composed of microcolumns

2 _____ a thick, transparent fluid that fills the posterior cavity of the eyeball

3 _____ a modified epithelial cell specialized for detection of light energy; rods and cones

4 _____ a small region of the retina containing a dense array of cones and no rods

5 _____ watery fluid that fills the anterior cavity of the eyeball; it is formed at the ciliary body and is reabsorbed at the canal of Schlemm

6 _____ ring of muscles in the choroid to which the edges of the lens attach via zonular fibers and which changes the shape of the lens

132

7_____ anterior portion of the eye's interior divided into anterior and posterior chambers, filled with watery aqueous humor

8_____ general name given to a molecule that absorbs light energy and then changes conformation; composed of a chromophore called retinal coupled with any of four proteins called opsins

9_____ in the visual cortex, a cell sensitive only to lines and edges

10_____ in the visual cortex, a cell sensitive to movements of lines and edges

11_____ in the retina, the neurons whose axons form the optic nerve

12_____ one of two pathways in the retina; in this pathway, light causes a decrease in afferent fiber activity (hyperpolarization)

13_____ one of two pathways in the retina; in this pathway, light causes an increase in afferent fiber activity (depolarization)

14_____ pigmented middle coat of the eyeball, vascular in the rear and forming the lens and iris in the front

15_____ portion of the inner eyeball behind the lens filled with vitreous humor and lined with retinal tissue

16_____ "blind spot" of the retina; a location at which the nerve fibers leave the eyeball via the optic nerve

17_____ first photopigment to be studied in detail; retinal is 11-cis retinal in the dark and all-trans retinal when bleached by light

18_____ inner coat of the eyeball, it is composed of nervous tissue (including photoreceptors and interneurons) originally derived from brain tissue

19_____ transparent anterior continuation of the posterior opaque sclera, the outer coat of the eyeball

Other Key Terms

hyperopia (hy-per-OH-pee-ah)
myopia (my-OH-pee-ah)
otitis media (oh-TY-tis MEE-dee-ah)
presbyopia (prez-bee-OH-pee-ah)

1_____ disorder common in older adults resulting in restriction of accommodation ability because of loss of lens elasticity

2_____ disorder exhibited by a flattened eyeball; farsightedness

3_____ disorder exhibited by an elongated eyeball; nearsightedness

4_____ inflammation of the middle ear

The Big Picture

Use the activities of this section to help you learn the broader concepts of this chapter.

Learning Exercises

1. Sound travels as waves of alternating compression and rarefaction of the medium through which they travel. Arrange these structures of the ear in the order in which sound waves travel through them during the process of hearing.

auditory canal
incus
malleus
organ of Corti
oval window
scala vestibuli
scala media
stapes
tympanic membrane

_____

_____

_____

_____

_____

_____

_____

_____

_____

2. Use these terms to fill in the blanks in the paragraph below. (Some terms are used more than once.)

Corti   perilymph
endolymph   resonance
high   stereocilia
low   tonotopism
media   tympani
oval   vestibular

Sound waves traveling up the cochlea from the _____ window cause the

_____ (fluid) of the scala _____ to vibrate at a certain

_____. This, in turn, causes the _____ membrane and

the _____ (fluid) in the scala _____ and the basilar

membrane to vibrate at the same frequency. If this frequency approximates the

134

_____ frequency of the organ of _____ , the resulting

displacement of the _____ results in a change in receptor potential that may cause

auditory information to reach the brain. Because each place along the organ of

_____ has a different _____ frequency,

_____ -pitched sounds are perceived by receptor cells toward the base of the

cochlea and _____ -pitched sounds are perceived nearer the apex of the cochlea.

This system of frequency interpretation makes possible a type of sensory processing called

_____ .

3.   Put each of these terms into its correct place in the table below. (The terms may be used in either
       column.)

filled with endolymph   relies on the flow of endolymph
has calcium carbonate crystals   sensitive to linear acceleration
has otolithic membranes   sensitive to gravity
has cristae   sensitive to rotational movement
has ampullae   sensitive to changes in direction

Semicircular canals	Utricle/saccule

4.   For each term in the list below, identify which structures are involved in formation of an image by writing "I" in the blank, and which are involved in generation/transmission of a sensory impulse by writing "S" in the blank.

amacrine cell ___   horizontal cell ___
bipolar cell ___   iris ___
ciliary body ___   lens ___
cornea ___   optic nerve ___
ganglion cell ___   pupil ___

5.   Use these terms to fill in the blanks in the paragraph below. (Each term may be used more than once.)

contrast   lateral inhibition
corresponding   macrocolumn
feature extraction   microcolumn(s)
ganglion   motion

    In the retina, _____ filters the image to increase

_____ . Retinal _____ cells, whose axons project to the

thalamus, are tuned to respond to spots on contrasting backgrounds. The central processing of visual

images involves _____ at increasing levels of analysis. Each orientation

_____ of the visual cortex contains cells that respond to lines of a single

orientation, with additional conditions of _____ and length that depend on cell

type. A complete analysis of the part of the image that falls on any two _____

points of the retina is carried out by a _____ containing orientation

_____ that analyze the input from each retina for all possible orientations.

6.   Use these terms to identify the visual structures indicated in Figure 10-1.

amacrine cell   optic nerve
bipolar cell   retina
cone   rod
ganglion cell   superior colliculus
horizontal cell   thalamus
optic radiations   visual cortex

Figure 10-1

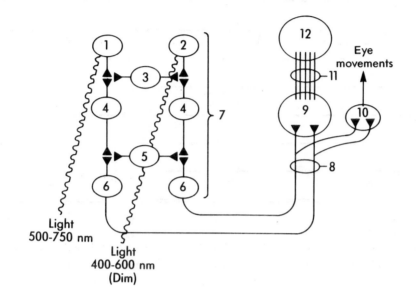

1 _____   7 _____

2 _____   8 _____

3 _____   9 _____

4 _____   10 _____

5 _____   11 _____

6 _____   12 _____

7. Put these characteristics of sensory modalities into the correct column in the table below (none applies to both).

cortical and limbic coprocessing
epithelial receptors
few submodalities

many submodalities
neuron receptors
specific cortical processing

Taste	Smell

Quick Recall
Review some of the major concepts of this chapter by doing these "quick recall" activities.

1. Name three main regions of the ear.

2. List two areas where equilibrium/motion receptors are located.

3. Name two ways in which sounds can be localized in space.

4. Name two structures that help focus images.

5. List the three major coats (layers) of the eyeball.

6. List four types of retinal interneurons.

7. Name the two kinds of photoreceptors and the types of vision they mediate.

8. Name the two forms of retinal.

9.   Name the two chemical senses.

Practice Test
Use this practice test to review the topics of this chapter and to prepare for your test on this material.

1.   The correct order of auditory ossicles is
      a.   incus, malleus, stapes
      b.   incus, stapes, malleus
      c.   malleus, incus, stapes
      d.   malleus, stapes, incus
      e.   stapes, malleus, incus

2.   Which of these structures serves to reduce the amplitude of sound waves?
      a.   chain of auditory ossicles
      b.   pinna
      c.   tensor tympani
      d.   organ of Corti
      e.   none of the above

3.   The apex of the cochlea features a canal that connects the perilymph chambers called the
      a.   helicotrema
      b.   organ of Corti
      c.   scala vestibuli
      d.   scala media
      e.   eustachian tube

4.   Tonotopism is possible because of
      a.   the resonance frequency of auditory tissues
      b.   varying compliance along the basilar membrane
      c.   varying tensions in the stapedius muscle
      d.   a and b are correct
      e.   a, b, and c are correct

5.   The otolithic membrane
      a.   contains calcium carbonate crystals
      b.   is involved in detecting rotation
      c.   is found in the ampulla
      d.   can cause nystagmus
      e.   a and b are correct

6.   Direction of a turning movement is best detected by
      a.   utricle
      b.   saccule
      c.   semicircular canals
      d.   otoliths
      e.   a, b, and d are correct

7. The lens of the eye
    a. decreases in flexibility with age
    b. is inflexible
    c. can be altered by ciliary muscles
    d. is opaque
    e. a and c are correct

8. Accommodation
    a. is synonymous with acuity
    b. is accomplished by the cornea
    c. is accomplished by the lens
    d. involves changing the radius of the eye
    e. a and d are correct

9. Which refracts light passing through the eye most?
    a. vitreous humor
    b. cornea
    c. lens
    d. aqueous humor
    e. cataracts

10. Complex neurons of the cortex respond primarily to
    a. movement only
    b. lines and edges
    c. movements, lines, and edges
    d. bright light
    e. low light

11. Macrocolumns are composed of
    a. cortical cells
    b. microcolumns
    c. ganglion cells
    d. horizontal cells
    e. a and b are correct

12. When rhodopsin is hit by light
    a. all-trans retinal is formed
    b. 11-cis retinal is formed
    c. all-trans opsin is formed
    d. the chromophore disintegrates
    e. it produces bleach

13. Bipolar cells
    a. connect receptors to ganglion cells
    b. may be hyperpolarized by the receptor
    c. may be depolarized by the receptor
    d. constitute either on or off pathways
    e. all of the above

14. The receptive field of ganglion cells are specialized to
    a. enhance response to uniformity of input
    b. enhance response to contrast of input
    c. suppress response to contrast of input
    d. suppress all information
    e. a and c are correct

15. Amacrine cells
    a. enhance perception of spatial input
    b. enhance perception of temporal input
    c. connect bipolar/ganglion cell synapses
    d. couple receptors
    e. b and c are correct

Answers

Here are answers (or references) to some of the questions presented above.

Word Parts: (your examples may be different) 1-basilar membrane, 2-chromophore, 3-otitis, 4-kinocilium, 5-otolith, 6-otolith, 7-photoreceptor, 8-semicircular canal, 9-resonance, 10-tectorial membrane, 11-tympanic membrane

Key Terms: Descriptive: 1. intensity difference 2. phase difference 3. olfactory 4. binaural 5. dark-adapted 6. pitch 7. pure tone 8. intensity 9. decibel 10. Hertz 11. resonant frequency
Processes: 1. spatial analysis 2. place coding 3. temporal analysis 4. bleaching 5. accommodation 6. impedance matching system 7. photopic vision 8. scotopic vision 9. visual acuity 10. rotational nystagmus **Structure/Ear:** 1. otolithic membrane 2. cupula 3. cochlea 4. otolith 5. tectorial membrane 6. ampulla 7. tympanic membrane 8. basal body 9. oval window 10. stereocilia 11. endolymph 12. perilymph 13. basilar membrane 14. vestibular membrane 15. auditory ossicle 16. semicircular canal 17. vestibule 18. organ of Corti 19. pinna 20. kinocilium 21. hair cell 22. scala tympani 23. scala media 24. eustachian tube 25. scala vestibuli 26. auditory canal **Structure/eye:** 1. macrocolumn 2. vitreous humor 3. photoreceptor 4. fovea 5. aqueous humor 6. ciliary body 7. anterior cavity 8. photopigment 9. simple cell 10. complex cell 11. ganglion cells 12. off pathway 13. on pathway 14. choroid layer 15. posterior cavity 16. optic disk 17. rhodopsin 18. retina 19. cornea **Other:** 1. presbyopia 2. hyperopia 3. myopia 4. otitis media

Learning Exercises: 1. auditory canal, tympanic membrane, malleus, incus, stapes, oval window, scala vestibuli, scala media, organ of Corti 2. oval, perilymph, tympani, vestibular, endolymph, media, resonance, Corti, stereocilia, Corti, resonance, high, low, tonotopism 3. SEMICIRCULAR CANALS: filled with endolymph, has cristae, has a ampullae, relies on the flow of endolymph, sensitive to changes in direction, sensitive to rotational movement; UTRICLE/SACCULE: filled with endolymph, has otolithic membranes, has calcium carbonate crystals, sensitive to gravity, sensitive to linear acceleration 4. I: ciliary body, cornea, iris, lens, pupil; S: amacrine cell, bipolar cell, ganglion cell, horizontal cell, optic nerve 5. lateral inhibition, contrast, ganglion, feature extraction, microcolumn, motion, corresponding, macrocolumn, microcolumns 6. 1-cone, 2-rod, 3-horizontal cell, 4-bipolar cell, 5-amacrine cell, 6-ganglion cell, 7-retina, 8-optic nerve, 9-thalamus, 10-superior colliculus, 11-optic radiations, 12-visual cortex 7. SMELL: many submodalities, neuron receptors, cortical and limbic coprocessing; TASTE: few submodalities, epithelial receptors, specific cortical processing

Quick Recall: (You should be able to answer these questions easily without correction or confirmation by this point in your studies. If you cannot, review your notes, the text chapter, and the previous study activities to find the answers.)

Practice Test: 1-c, 2-c, 3-a, 4-d, 5-a, 6-c, 7-e, 8-c, 9-b, 10-c, 11-e, 12-a, 13-e, 14-b, 15-e

Chapter 11
Skeletal, Cardiac, and Smooth Muscle

Focus
Review this section *first*. It will help you focus on the overall message of this chapter.

Chapter Outline
Read through the outline slowly. This activity will help your mind organize the topics of this chapter.

The structure of skeletal muscle
> Connective tissue boundaries of muscle cells
> The structure of sarcomeres
> Sliding filament model of muscle contraction

Muscle contraction at the molecular level
> Structure of the thin filaments
> Myosin subunit structure of thick filaments
> The power stroke of muscle contraction
> Muscle contractility

Excitation-contraction coupling
> The T-tubules of striated muscle
> The sarcoplasmic reticulum
> Calcium and excitation-contraction coupling
> Summation of contractions in single muscle fibers

The mechanics of muscle contraction
> Properties of isometric contractions
> Relation between maximum force and muscle length
> Skeletal muscle and skeletal levers coadaptation
> The latent period in afterloaded contractions

Muscle energetics and metabolism
> Muscle energy consumption and activity
> Skeletal muscle fiber types and energy metabolism
> The Cori cycle
> Effects of training on specific fiber types
> Muscle fatigue

Physiology of cardiac muscle
> Structure of cardiac muscle
> The heart as an electrical unit
> Lack of summation in cardiac muscle
> Excitation/contraction coupling in cardiac muscle
> Determinants of cardiac muscle force

Modulation of contractility in cardiac muscle by external inputs

The physiology of smooth muscle
    Classes of smooth muscle
    Length-tension relationships in smooth muscle
    Excitation-contraction coupling in smooth muscle
    Control of smooth muscle contractility
    Similarities and differences between the muscle types

Learning Objectives

These are the learning goals for this part of the course. After reading the text, attending class, and studying this chapter, you should be able to:

♦   identify the components of the contractile machinery of muscle

♦   understand the origin of force generation in muscle

♦   describe the structure of the sarcomere

♦   state the sliding filament model of muscle contraction

♦   describe the sequence of events mediating excitation-contraction coupling in muscle

♦   distinguish between isotonic and isometric contractions

♦   state the functional differences between cardiac and skeletal muscle

♦   understand the initiation and control of contraction in smooth muscle

♦   appreciate the different roles of calmodulin and caldesmon in smooth muscle contraction

♦   distinguish between multiunit and unitary smooth muscle

Language of Physiology

Physiology uses its own set of terms, many of which may be unfamiliar to you. This section will help you improve your mastery of key physiological terms.

Word Parts

Here are some combining forms often seen in physiological terms. Give an example of a term that contains each word part listed.

Word Part	Meaning	Example
-lemma	rind; peel	1_____
-metric	measurement	2_____
rigor-	stiffness	3_____
sarco-	flesh; muscle	4_____
tri-	three; triple	5_____

Key Terms

Read each of the terms in each grouping below aloud, using the pronunciation guide if necessary. This will help you to remember them better than if you read them silently. Then, write out the correct term next to each of the descriptions given.

Descriptive Terms

afterloaded (muscle)
antagonistic (muscle)
contractility (kahn-trak-TIL-it-ee)
elasticity (ee-las-TIS-it-ee)
fast-twitch (muscle)

multiunit (smooth muscle)
preloaded (muscle)
slow-twitch (muscle)
synergistic (muscle) (sin-erj-IST-ik)
unitary (smooth muscle)

1_____ term that describes smooth muscle fibers that have few gap junctions, so that only small groups of cells can act as units

2_____ term that describes a muscle that is already supporting a load, before it is stimulated to lift the load

3_____ term that describes smooth muscle fibers that are electrically and mechanically coupled to one another

4_____ term that describes a structure's tendency to return its original length after having stretched — for a muscle, it is exhibited as the passive tension curve

5_____ term that describes a muscle that does not begin to bear a load until after it has already begun to shorten

6_____ term that describes the extent to which a structure is able to generate force and shorten rapidly

7_____ describes a muscle that aids another muscle by pulling in more or less the same direction

8 _____ describes a muscle having a form of myosin with low ATPase activity, causing slow force development and shortening

9 _____ describes a muscle having a form of myosin with high ATPase activity, causing rapid force development and shortening

10 _____ describes a muscle whose movement opposes that of another muscle

Terms related to processes

atrophy (AT-roh-fee)
basic electrical rhythm [BER]
Cori cycle (KOHR-ee)
excitation
excitation-contraction coupling
fatigue
glycogen loading (GLY-koh-jen)
hypertrophy (hy-PER-troh-fee)
isometric contraction (ice-oh-MET-rik)

isotonic contraction (ice-oh-TAHN-ik)
latent period (LAY-tent)
myosin phosphorylation
   (fahs-for-il-AY-shun)
oxygen debt
piloerection (py-loh-ee-REK-shun)
sequestering (se-KWEST-er-ing)
tetanus (TET-a-nus)
twitch contraction

1 _____ skeletal muscle contraction in which the tension in a muscle organ increases, but the length remains the same

2 _____ process resulting in enlargement of a muscle organ by means of an increase in individual cell sizes; may result from heavy use of a muscle

3 _____ skeletal muscle contraction in which the length of the organ decreases, but the tension remains about the same

4 _____ dietary regimen in which a period of consumption of few carbohydrates is followed by consumption of many carbohydrates just before an athletic event

5 _____ process catalyzed by myosin light chain kinase (MLCK) in which a light chain of myosin gains phosphate, exposing a binding site for actin

6 _____ delay between excitation of a muscle and the beginning of observable shortening of that muscle

7 _____ process in which lactic acid forms during anaerobic respiration, incurring a physiological "debt" to later aerobically metabolize the lactic acid (in the liver)

8 _____ use-dependent decrease in the ability of muscle to generate force — may be of the "rapid" type seen after maximal exercise, or the "slow" type seen after prolonged submaximal exercise

9 _____ process of confining of a substance, as in the case of the sarcoplasmic reticulum's confinement of Ca^{++} ions within itself by means of ion pumping

10 _____ process resulting in a decrease in the size of a muscle organ — often the result of disuse

11 _____ process of coupling a signal (action potential) to the work process (contraction of the muscle) — occurs at the triad

12 _____ contraction of multiunit smooth muscles associated with hair follicles, causing the hairs to "stand" and producing "goose bumps"

13 _____ periodic waves of depolarization in visceral smooth muscle (serving as a pacemaker for GI motility)

14 _____ sustained contraction in a skeletal muscle, resulting from high-frequency stimulation

15 _____ contraction that results from a single action potential

16 _____ process by which lactic acid is converted to glucose and returned to the muscle

17 _____ passage of an action potential across the sarcolemma

Terms related to structures/substances

actin (AK-tin)
caldesmon (KAL-des-mon)
calsequestrin (kal-se-KWEST-rin)
collagen (KAHL-ah-jen)
creatine phosphate [CP]
  (KREE-ah-tin FAHS-fayt)
crossbridge
dense body
endomysium (en-doh-MY-zee-um)
epimysium (ep-ih-MY-zee-um)
fascicle (FAS-ih-kil)
insertion
intercalated disc (in-TER-kal-ayt-ed)
latchbridge
muscle triad (TRY-ad)
myofibril (my-oh-FYB-ril)
myoglobin (MY-oh-gloh-bin)

myosin light chain
myosin (MY-oh-sin)
myosin isozymes (ICE-oh-zym)
myosin heavy chain
origin
perimysium (pair-ih-MY-zee-um)
rigor complex
sarcolemma (sar-koh-LEM-ah)
sarcomere (SAR-koh-meer)
sarcoplasmic reticulum
  (sar-koh-PLAZ-mik ret-IK-yoo-lum)
tendon (TEN-don)
terminal cisternae (sis-TERN-ay)
thick filament
thin filament
transverse tubule

1 _____ small bundle of parallel muscle fibers within a skeletal muscle organ

2 _____ junction between the ends of cardiac muscle cells formed by a mesh of strong connecting fibers

3 _____ sheet of connective tissue, continuous with the tendon, that forms a covering of the entire skeletal muscle organ

4 _____ sheet of connective tissue that surrounds each individual muscle fiber, in a sheathlike fashion, within skeletal muscle organs

5 _____ sheet of connective tissue that surrounds bundles (fascicles) of muscle fibers within skeletal muscle organs

6 _____ contractile protein forming the thick filament of the myofibril; binds to actin

7 _____ type of crossbridge formed in smooth muscle that allows the tension to be maintained with little energy, but the action cycle is temporarily halted

8 _____ contractile protein forming much of the thin filament of the myofibril; binds to myosin

9 _____ protein within SR that reversibly binds to Ca^{++}, taking it out of solution temporarily, reducing the SR's Ca^{++} concentration

10 _____ protein capable of inhibiting crossbridge formation, and thus muscle contraction, by binding to the actin-tropomyosin complex

11 _____ protein found in many connective tissues, including those of tendons and ligaments; tends to form tough, flexible bundles or sheets

12 _____ high-energy molecule formed by joining creatine to a phosphate group — used by the muscle cell as an energy reserve

13 _____ protrusion ("head") of the myosin molecule, that reaches away from the thick filament and toward the thin filament, where it binds to actin

14 _____ organizational subunit of the myofibril, extending from one myofibril Z line to the next

15 _____ intracellular network of interconnected tubules (similar to ER in other cells) that tends to sequester Ca^{++} ions within itself

16 _____ organ composed of dense connective tissue, mostly collagen fibers, that forms a straplike band connecting a skeletal muscle organ to a skeletal bone organ

17 _____ invagination of the sarcolemma, forming a tubular inward extension of membrane deep into the muscle cell (lying very near the junctions between sarcomeres)

18 _____ oxygen-carrying protein within red muscle fibers

19 _____ any of several alternate forms of myosin, each with different ATPase activities

20 _____ describes one of two muscle attachments (to bone or another muscle), this one on the anchor point that does not move (or moves little) when the muscle shortens

21 _____ describes one of two muscle attachments (to bone or another muscle), this one on the anchor point that moves (or moves more) when the muscle shortens

22 _____ high-molecular-weight component of myosin containing the actin binding sites and ATPase activity

23 _____ in smooth muscle, the functional equivalent to skeletal muscle's Z lines, forming an attachment site for myosin molecules

24 _____ long aggregation of parallel myofilaments (organized into subunits called sarcomeres)

25 _____ lower-molecular-weight component of myosin located in the crossbridges that regulates myosin ATPase activity

26 _____ one of two myofilaments that compose the myofibril; this filament is composed largely of myosin molecules

27 _____ one of two myofilaments that compose the myofibril; this filament is composed of actin, with troponin and tropomyosin

28 _____ structure composed of a transverse tubule and two adjacent cisternae of the SR (one on each side), allowing changes in transverse tubule potential to affect the SR

29 _____ low-energy actin-myosin complex formed at the end of a power stroke that prevents the filaments from sliding past one another (producing temporary stiffness); it is usually broken quickly if ATP is available

30 _____ cell membrane of a skeletal muscle fiber

31 _____ lateral sacs of the sarcoplasmic reticulum found alongside the transverse tubules, forming the triad

Other Key Terms

leverage factor
sliding filament model

1 _____ model of muscle physiology proposed in 1955 that supposes that the thick and thin filaments slide past (overlap) one another with force to produce a contraction

2 _____ factor by which a muscle's force must exceed the load to produce movement

The Big Picture

Use the activities of this section to help you learn the broader concepts of this chapter.

Learning Exercises

1.   Use these terms to label the parts of a skeletal muscle cell (section) indicated in Figure 11-1.

capillary	nucleus	transverse tubule
mitochondrion	sarcolemma	Z line
muscle triad	sarcoplasmic reticulum	
myofibrils	terminal cisterna	

Figure 11-1

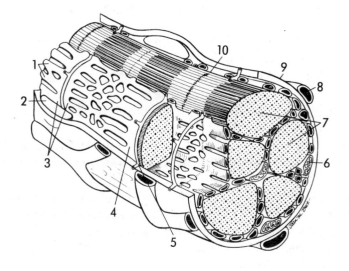

1 _____

2 _____

3 _____

4 _____

5 _____

6 _____

7 _____

8 _____

9 _____

10 _____

2. Use these terms to identify the parts of the contractile machinery of the skeletal muscle cell indicated in Figure 11-2.

A-band   thick
F-actin   thin
H-zone   tropomyosin
I-band   troponin
myosin head   Z-line
sarcomere

Figure 11-2

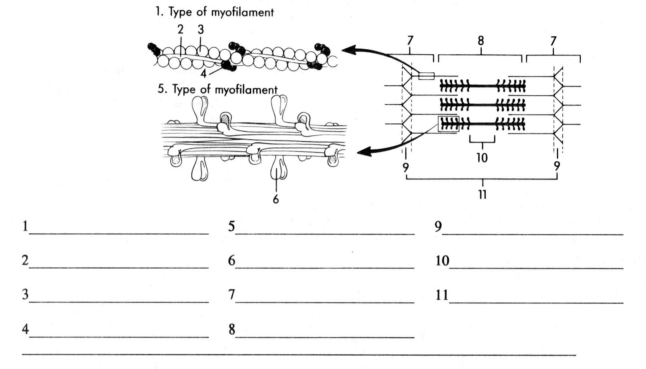

1. Type of myofilament
5. Type of myofilament

1 _____   5 _____   9 _____

2 _____   6 _____   10 _____

3 _____   7 _____   11 _____

4 _____   8 _____

---

3. Arrange these events of skeletal muscle fiber excitation, contraction, and relaxation in the order in which they occur.

A binding site (for myosin) is exposed on actin
Acetylcholine binds with receptors in the sarcolemma
Acetylcholine is released into the (neuromuscular) synaptic cleft
Action potential reaches the presynaptic (motor) axon terminal
An action potential travels across the sarcolemma (excitation)
Ca^{++} ions are released from the SR's terminal cisternae
Ca^{++} ions bind to troponin molecules in the thin filaments
Depolarization moves from transverse tubules to SR cisternae
Spread of depolarization into the transverse tubule system
The power stroke of muscle contraction (crossbridge cycling)
Uptake of Ca^{++} back into the SR, inactivating binding sites on actin

1 _____

2 _____

3 _____

4 _____

5 _____

6 _____

7 _____

8 _____

9 _____

10 _____

11 _____

4.   Fill in the blanks in this table comparing types of skeletal muscle fibers.

Characteristic	Type I	Type IIA	Type IIB
Contraction velocity	slow		
myosin ATPase		fast	
twitch duration	long		
Ca^{++} sequestration			rapid
capillaries	abundant		
glycolytic capacity	low		high
oxidative capacity		high	
myoglobin content			low
glycogen content	low		
fiber diameter		intermediate	
motor unit size			large
recruitment order			late

5. Compare and contrast skeletal, cardiac, and smooth muscle structure and function by completing missing sections of the table below.

Feature	Skeletal	Cardiac	Smooth
Organization			unitary or multiunit
Ca^{++} receptor	troponin C	troponin C	
Ca^{++} source	SR		
Force regulation			contractility modulation

6. The paragraphs that follow describe the physiology of contraction in smooth muscle cells. Use these terms to fill in the blanks appropriately. (Some terms are used more than once.)

action   excitation-contraction   myosin light chain
Ca^{++} latchbridge   kinase
caldesmon   myosin   thin
calmodulin

First, an _____ potential spreads across the membrane, causing

_____ channels to allow entry of extracellular _____

ions. These ions combine with at least two target proteins: the light chain of

_____ and a protein called _____.

_____ coupling in smooth muscle occurs in this sequence of events: The Ca^{++}-

_____ complex activates the enzyme _____. Then, that

enzyme phosphorylates one of the light chains of the _____ heads, causing a

binding site for actin to be exposed. The myosin crossbridges can now be activated by myosin binding to

actin, generating force.

A second level of control of contractility involves the _____ filament and

a molecule called _____. If insufficient Ca^{++} causes the crossbridge cycling to

cease but still maintains the contracted state, a special kind of crossbridge, the

152

_____ is formed. _____ is believed to form a link between actin and _____ heads that keeps the latchbridges from cycling. The ability to form _____s makes tension maintenance in smooth muscles very economical.

Quick Recall
Review some of the major concepts of this chapter by doing these "quick recall" activities.

1.   Name four connective tissue components of the skeletal muscle organ.

2.   List two types of myofilaments and their components.

3.   Name three phases of the twitch (single) contraction.

4.   Distinguish two types of skeletal muscle contraction.

5.   Name three different types of muscle tissue and compare them.

6.   Name four "storage" molecules within muscle cells.

Practice Test
Use this practice test to review the topics of this chapter and to prepare for your test on this material.

1.   The I-band of normal length, relaxed skeletal muscle fibers
      a.   lacks the protein myosin
      b.   lacks the protein actin
      c.   contains crossbridges
      d.   contains troponin
      e.   a and d are correct

2.   A sarcomere
      a.   is separated by Z-lines
      b.   is the repeating unit of striated muscle
      c.   shortens when a muscle shortens
      d.   contains thick and thin filaments
      e.   all of the above

3. Components of the thick filaments of a skeletal muscle fiber include
   a. actin
   b. tropomyosin
   c. calcium
   d. myosin
   e. a, b, and c

4. Troponin has binding sites for
   a. actin
   b. tropomyosin
   c. calcium
   d. myosin
   e. a, b, and c

5. Calcium released from the terminal cisternae binds to
   a. the sarcoplasmic reticulum
   b. troponin
   c. calcium
   d. myosin

6. The force of contraction in a skeletal muscle depends on
   a. filament overlap
   b. intracellular Ca^{++} concentration
   c. muscle length
   d. the species of myosin
   e. all of the above

7. During an isometric contraction
   a. ATP is hydrolyzed
   b. sarcomeres shorten
   c. crossbridges periodically generate force
   d. both a and c are correct
   e. a, b, and c are correct

8. The velocity of shortening in an isotonic contraction is
   a. less if the afterload is greater
   b. less if the preload is greater
   c. independent of the preload
   d. constant
   e. both a and b are correct

9. The total tension in a skeletal muscle can be increased by
   a. facilitation
   b. recruitment
   c. changes in initial length
   d. both a and b
   e. a, b, and c are all possible

10. In a given skeletal muscle
    a. the number of fibers in a motor unit is constant
    b. there is only one motor unit
    c. motor units are recruited in the order of increasing size
    d. individual motor units discharge at the same time
    e. none of the above

11. In cardiac muscle
   a. there are no sarcomeres
   b. there is no transverse tubule system
   c. cells are electrically coupled
   d. troponin is absent
   e. none of the above

12. Increasing the extracellular calcium concentration
   a. increases the force of contraction of cardiac muscle
   b. increases the force of contraction of skeletal muscle
   c. has no effect on the force of contraction of skeletal or cardiac muscle
   d. decreases the force of contraction of cardiac muscle

13. Smooth muscle contraction
   a. involves actin and myosin
   b. is regulated by calmodulin
   c. does not involve troponin
   d. is not activated by Ca^{++}
   e. a, b, and c are correct

14. Multiunit smooth muscle
   a. consists of electrically uncoupled cells like skeletal muscle
   b. has a clear pattern of striations
   c. has a well-developed tubular system
   d. consists of electrically coupled cells like cardiac muscle
   e. contains no myosin

15. Fast and slow skeletal muscle fibers differ in
   a. myosin content
   b. susceptibility
   c. pattern of striations
   d. actin content
   e. both a and b

Answers
Here are answers (or references) to some of the questions presented above.

Word Parts: (your examples may be different) 1-sarcolemma, 2-isometric, 3-rigor complex, 4-sarcomere, 5-triad

Key Terms: Descriptive: 1. multiunit (smooth muscle) 2. preloaded (muscle) 3. unitary (smooth muscle) 4. elasticity 5. afterloaded (muscle) 6. contractility 7. synergistic (muscle) 8. slow-twitch (muscle) 9. fast-twitch (muscle) 10. antagonistic (muscle)
Processes: 1. isometric contraction 2. hypertrophy 3. isotonic contraction 4. glycogen loading 5. myosin phosphorylation 6. latent period 7. oxygen debt 8. fatigue 9. sequestering 10. atrophy 11. excitation-contraction coupling 12. piloerection 13. basic electrical rhythm [BER] 14. tetanus 15. twitch contraction 16. Cori cycle 17. excitation
Structures/Substances: 1. fascicle 2. intercalated disc 3. epimysium 4. endomysium 5. perimysium 6. myosin 7. latchbridge 8. actin 9. calsequesterin 10. caldesmon 11. collagen 12. creatine phosphate [CP] 13. crossbridge 14. sarcomere 15. sarcoplasmic reticulum 16. tendon 17. transverse tubule 18. myoglobin 19. myosin isozymes 20. origin 21. insertion 22. myosin heavy chain 23. dense body 24. myofibril 25. myosin light chain 26. thick filament 27. thin filament 28. muscle triad 29. rigor complex 30. sarcolemma 31. terminal cisternae
Other: 1. sliding filament model 2. leverage factor

Learning Exercises: 1. 1-sarcoplasmic reticulum, 2-nucleus, 3-muscle triad, 4-terminal cisterna, 5-transverse tubule, 6- mitochondrion, 7-myofibrils, 8-capillary, 9-sarcolemma, 10-Z line 2. 1-thin, 2-tropomyosin, 3-F-actin, 4-troponin, 5-thick, 6-myosin head, 7-I-band, 8-A-band, 9-Z-line, 10-H-zone, 11-sarcomere 3. 1-Action potential reaches the presynaptic (motor) axon terminal, 2-Acetylcholine is released into the (neuromuscular) synaptic cleft, 3-Acetylcholine binds with receptors in the sarcolemma, 4-An action potential travels across the sarcolemma (excitation), 5-Spread of depolarization into the transverse tubule system, 6-Depolarization moves from transverse tubules to SR cisternae, 7-Ca^{++} ions are released from the SR's terminal cisternae, 8-Ca^{++} ions bind to troponin molecules in the thin filaments, 9-A binding site (for myosin) is exposed on actin, 10-The power stroke of muscle contraction (crossbridge cycling), 11-Uptake of Ca^{++} back into the SR, inactivating binding sites on actin 4. (answers are in Table 11-2 of the text) 5. (answers are in Table 11-5 of the text) 6. action, Ca^{++}, Ca^{++}, myosin, calmodulin, excitation-contraction, calmodulin, myosin light chain kinase, myosin, caldesmon, latchbridge, caldesmon, myosin, latchbridge

Quick Recall: (You should be able to answer these questions easily without correction or confirmation by this point in your studies. If you cannot, review your notes, the text chapter, and the previous study activities to find the answers.)

Practice Test: 1-e, 2-e, 3-d, 4-e, 5-b, 6-e, 7-d, 8-a, 9-e, 10-c, 11-c, 12-a, 13-e, 14-a, 15-e

Chapter 12
Somatic and Autonomic Motor Systems

Focus
Review this section *first*. It will help you focus on the overall message of this chapter.

Chapter Outline
Read through the outline slowly. This activity will help your mind organize the topics of this chapter.

Motor pathways of the peripheral nervous system
       Motor units
       Control of contractile force
       Innervation of skeletal muscle
       Pathways to the visceral effectors
       Dual autonomic innervation of visceral effectors
       Acetylcholine and norepinephrine as transmitters in the motor pathways
Somatic motor control at the spinal level
       The size principle of motor unit recruitment
       Spinal reflexes and postural stability
       Structure of the muscle spindle
       Muscle spindles as length and length change detectors
       Control of the stretch reflex by gamma motor neurons
       Coactivation of alpha and gamma motor neurons
       Golgi tendon organs — monitors of muscle tension
       The withdrawal reflex and crossed extension
Motor control centers of the brain
       Brainstem motor areas
       Decerebrate rigidity
       Role of the basal ganglia in stereotyped movements
       The cerebellum and coordination of rapid movements
       Regions of the motor cortex
       Motor programs in the CNS
       Readiness potentials
Connections between the brain and spinal motor neurons
       Comparison of the medial and lateral motor systems
       Descending motor pathways from the brain
The autonomic nervous system
       Brainstem autonomic control centers
       Spinal autonomic reflexes
       The role of dual autonomic inputs
       Membrane receptors for acetylcholine

Membrane receptors for norepinephrine
Autonomic receptor antagonists
Distribution of autonomic receptor types
Transmitter synthesis in adrenergic and cholinergic synapses

Learning Objectives

These are the learning goals for this part of the course. After reading the text, attending class, and studying this chapter, you should be able to:

♦ compare innervation of skeletal muscle fibers by somatic motor neurons with autonomic innervation of visceral smooth muscle and glands

♦ state the anatomical differences between the pathways followed by parasympathetic and sympathetic efferents to their effectors

♦ understand the role of dual innervation in the autonomic nervous system

♦ describe the different neurotransmitters used in the autonomic nervous system

♦ outline the spinal circuitry and functional role of the stretch reflex, withdrawal reflex, and the Golgi tendon reflex

♦ appreciate the role of subcortical structures in the initiation and control of movements

♦ distinguish between the lateral and proximal motor control systems

♦ understand the pharmacological differences between postsynaptic receptors in the autonomic nervous system

Language of Physiology

Physiology uses its own set of terms, many of which may be unfamiliar to you. This section will help you improve your mastery of key physiological terms.

Word Parts

Here are some combining forms often seen in physiological terms. Give an example of a term that contains each word part listed.

Word Part	Meaning	Example
dys-	bad; disordered; difficult	1 _____
myo-	muscle	2 _____
noc(i)-	to harm; hurt	3 _____
para-	by the side of; near	4 _____
ram-	branch	5 _____

Key Terms
Read each of the terms in each grouping below aloud, using the pronunciation guide if necessary. This will help you to remember them better than if you read them silently. Then, write out the correct term next to each of the descriptions given.

Descriptive Terms
adrenergic (ad-reen-ERJ-ik)
cholinergic (kohl-in-ERJ-ik)
muscarinic (mus-kar-IN-ic)
nicotinic (nik-oh-TIN-ik)

1_____ descriptive term used to associate a structure or process with the transmitters epinephrine and norepinephrine

2_____ descriptive term used to associate a structure or process with acetycholine

3_____ descriptive term referring to a structure or process associated with nicotine; for example, a type of cholinergic receptor in postganglionic ANS neurons

4_____ descriptive term referring to a structure or process associated with muscarine; for example, a type of cholinergic receptor in parasympathetic effector cells

Terms Related to Processes
alpha coactivation
  (koh-akt-ih-VAY-shun)
crossed extension
decerebration (dee-sair-eb-RAY-shun)
decomposition
denervation (dee-nerv-AY-shun)

dual innervation (in-er-VAY-shun)
motor program
myotatic reflex (my-oh-TAT-ik)
nociception (noh-sih-SEP-shun)
reciprocal inhibition
recruitment

1_____ situation in which an effector receives input from both sympathetic and parasympathetic fibers

2_____ stretch reflex

3_____ set of commands assembled in the brain before a movement begins, then appropriately timed and sequenced before being sent to motor units

4_____ process in which the activation of one muscle group inhibits the activation of the antagonistic (opposing) muscle group

5_____ cutting of the CNS below the cerebrum (for research purposes)

6_____ process in which muscular movements are fragmented into their component parts because of injury to the basal ganglia

7_____ reflex in which a noxious (painful) stimulus to one limb leads to oppositely directed movements on the two sides of the body

8_____ simultaneous activation of extrafusal muscle fibers (via alpha motor neurons) and intrafusal muscle fibers (via gamma motor neurons)

9_____ activation of additional motor units within a muscle organ; this process enables muscular contractions of varying force

10_____ cutting of the nerve pathway to or from a particular organ or structure

11_____ perception of pain or painful stimuli

159

Terms related to structure/substances

alpha [α] motor neuron
basal ganglia (BAY-sal)
cardiovascular centers
chromaffin cell (KROHM-ah-fin)
corticospinal tract
  (kor-tih-koh-SPY-nal)
epinephrine (ep-ih-NEF-rin)
extrafusal fiber (eks-trah-FYOO-sal)
extrapyramidal tract
  (eks-trah-peer-ah-MID-al)
gamma [γ] motor neuron
Golgi tendon organ (GOHL-jee)
gray ramus (RAM-us)
intrafusal fiber (in-trah-FYOO-sal)
motor unit
muscle spindle
myotome (MY-oh-tohm)

norepinephrine (nor-ep-ih-NEF-rin)
parasympathetic branch [of ANS]
paravertebral sympathetic ganglion
  (pair-ah-VERT-e-bral)
plexus (PLEKS-us)
postganglionic neuron
  (post-gang-lee-AHN-ik)
preganglionic neuron
  (pree-gang-lee-AHN-ik)
propriospinal interneuron
  (proh-pree-oh-SPY-nal)
sciatic nerve (sy-AT-ik)
sympathetic branch [of ANS]
vestibular nucleus (vest-IB-yoo-ler)
white ramus (RAM-us)

1 _____ transmitter substance secreted by most sympathetic postganglionic fibers (a small amount by chromaffin cells)

2 _____ segment of the body's muscles innervated by a single spinal nerve

3 _____ ganglion of the sympathetic division of the ANS found as part of a chain of ganglia alongside the vertebral column

4 _____ specialized receptor within muscles that provides information concerning muscle length and rate of change

5 _____ gray (nonmyelinated) nerve branch carrying sympathetic postganglionic fibers from the ganglion to join the spinal nerve

6 _____ collection of neurons in the brainstem (reticular formation) receiving input from vestibular (ear) hair cells, thus mediating antigravity reflexes

7 _____ network of axons formed by the intermingling of fibers from more than one spinal nerve (e.g., cervical, brachial, lumbar, sacral)

8 _____ white (myelinated) branch of the spinal nerve containing sympathetic preganglionic fibers proceeding toward the ganglion

9 _____ group of reflex centers in the pons that regulate blood pressure, including the dorsal vagal nuclei and the Edinger-Westphal nuclei

10 _____ motor neuron that innervates an extrafusal muscle fiber

11 _____ transmitter substance similar to norepinephrine but with a methyl group, secreted by chromaffin cells

12 _____ descending motor tract running directly from the cortex to spinal motor neurons; the pyramidal tract

13 _____ motor neuron which innervates an intrafusal muscle fiber

14 _____ any of several descending motor tracts outside the pyramidal (corticospinal) tract, including the rubrispinal tract

15 _____ division of the autonomic nervous system (ANS) whose preganglionic fibers start in cranial nerve nuclei and sacral segments of the spinal cord

16 _____ division of the autonomic nervous system (ANS) whose preganglionic fibers start in the intermediolateral gray horn of the thoracic and lumbar segments of the spinal cord

17 _____ group of ganglia in the telencephalon, including the caudate nucleus, putamen, and globus pallidus

18_____ in the autonomic nervous system, a neuron whose cell body is in the CNS but whose axon projects to a synapse within an autonomic ganglion in the PNS

19_____ in the autonomic nervous system, a neuron whose cell body is in an autonomic ganglion and whose axon projects to synapse with an effector

20_____ modified neuron in the adrenal medulla that does not have axons, but secretes sympathetic hormones directly into the blood

21_____ muscle fiber outside the muscle spindle; the "typical" muscle fiber; innervated by alpha motor neurons

22_____ muscle fiber within the muscle spindle having sensory nerve attachments and controlled by gamma motor neurons; one of two types — nuclear bag fiber and nuclear chain fiber

23_____ receptor within tendons (which connect muscles to bones) that detects changes in the tension produced by the attached muscles

24_____ spinal interneuron whose fibers extend through several segments, enabling it to coordinate several groups of muscles

25_____ set of muscle fibers (cells) innervated by all branches of the axon of a single motor neuron

26_____ largest nerve of the body, it emerges from the sacral plexus and innervates the posterior thigh, leg, and foot muscles

Other Key Terms

dyskinesia (dis-kin-EEZ-ee-ah)
evoked potential
motor homunculus (hoh-MUN-kyoo-lus)

muscle tone
readiness potential

1_____ form of evoked potential in the human association cortex just before a motor task, suggesting planning of motor activity by nonmotor cortex areas

2_____ any of a family of movement disorders, usually involving spontaneous, repeated, inappropriate movements of entire muscle groups

3_____ cortical map in the cerebral cortex (primary and premotor areas) that reflects topographic organization of motor control

4_____ general term for a change in the electrical potential in a sensory or motor area that corresponds to a sensation or movement

5_____ steady, low-level contractions in a skeletal muscle

The Big Picture

Use the activities of this section to help you learn the broader concepts of this chapter.

Learning Exercises

1. This table summarizes characteristics of the somatic and autonomic nervous systems. Fill in the blank portions.

Characteristic	Somatic	Autonomic
Effectors	_____	Cardiac, smooth muscle
Effect of motor nerves	Excitation	_____
Innervation of effector	_____	Typically dual
Number of neurons in path of effector	One	_____
Peripheral ganglia	_____	Yes
Transmitter	Acetylcholine	_____
Receptor types	Nicotinic	Cholinergic nicotinic _____ Adrenergic beta _____

2. Label the parts indicated in Figure 12-1 using these terms.

acetylcholine
cranial nerves/sacral segments
norepinephrine/epinephrine
parasympathetic postganglionic fiber
parasympathetic effector
parasympathetic ganglion

parasympathetic postganglionic fiber
sympathetic effector
sympathetic postganglionic fiber
sympathetic preganglionic fiber
sympathetic ganglion
thoracic/lumbar segments

Figure 12-1

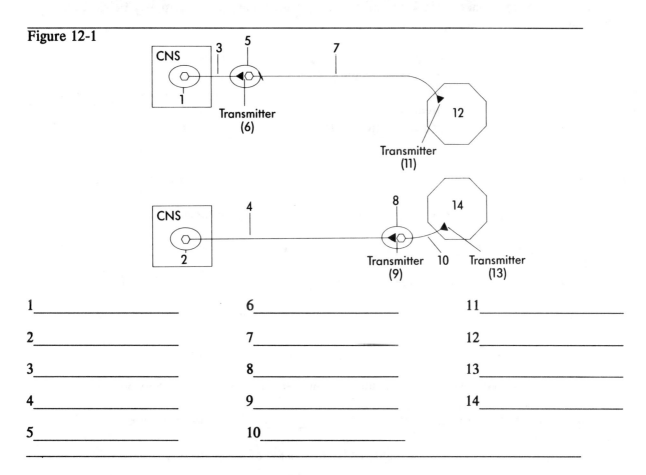

1 _____   6 _____   11 _____

2 _____   7 _____   12 _____

3 _____   8 _____   13 _____

4 _____   9 _____   14 _____

5 _____   10 _____

3. For each statement or term below, indicate those that apply to stretch reflexes by putting S in the blank, withdrawal reflexes by putting W in the blank, and Golgi tendon reflexes by putting G in the blank.

___ a nociceptive stimulus causes movement of a limb away from the stimulus

___ inhibits motor neurons in stretched muscle, while activating antagonists

___ involves distinctions between intrafusal and extrafusal fiber contraction

___ maintains muscle length, opposing passive increases in length

___ may also involve a crossed extension reflex

___ may provide overload protection to muscles with too much tension

___ may involve alpha-gamma coactivation

___ myotatic reflex

___ the knee-jerk reflex is an example

___ uses muscle spindle receptors

4. Use these terms to fill in the blanks of the following paragraphs. (Each term may be used more than once.)

basal ganglia	inhibitory	reticular
brainstem	motor homunculus	righting
cerebellum	motor programs	supplementary motor
coordinating	premotor cortex	area
decomposition	primary motor cortex	vestibular
execution		

The reticular formation of the _____ includes sources of descending

pathways. Of particular importance is the _____ nucleus, which coordinates

antigravity reflexes, such as the _____ reflex.

Subcortical forebrain nuclei that form the _____ receive input from the cortex

and send output to the cortex and _____ formation. These nuclei are thought to

be organizing centers for _____, sets of motor commands assembled in the brain

before being timed, sequenced, and sent out. Damage to these nuclei often results in inappropriate

movements because of the inappropriate _____ of motor programs.

The _____ is a highly ordered division of the brain, which probably explains

its ability to coordinate motor signals so well. All of the output of this division is

_____, which allows it to prevent decerebrate rigidity in intact animals. Damage

to this area of the brain usually results in the _____ of movements, showing that

it is a _____ center, not an organizing center like the basal ganglia.

The cortex has several motor control regions: the _____,

_____, and _____. The topographic organization of

some of these areas results in a cortical motor map or _____ in the cortex.

Experiments with decorticate primates suggests that the cortical motor regions are not required to initiate

_____.

5.   Put these characteristics of motor pathways into the correct category in the table below.

mainly gross movements/posture
involved mainly in fine movements
involves extrapyramidal tracts
involves the pyramidal tract
involves the corticospinal pathway
serves primarily proximal muscles

serves primarily distal muscles
tends to be rapid acting
tends to be slower acting
involves monosynaptic pathways
involves polysynaptic pathways

Lateral motor control system	Proximal motor control system

6.   Using your notes and textbook as resources, determine likely locations for each of these
        pharmacologically distinct receptor types found in the ANS.

Cholinergic receptors	
Nicotinic:	
Muscarinic:	

Adrenergic receptors	
Alpha$_1$:	
Alpha$_2$:	
Beta$_1$:	
Beta$_2$:	

Quick Recall

Review some of the major concepts of this chapter by doing these "quick recall" activities.

1.   List and describe three types of somatic motor reflexes.

2.   Name two transmitters used in the ANS.

3.   Name three centers in the brain involved in organizing and coordinating somatic muscle movements.

4.   Compare the medial and lateral motor control systems.

5.   List two types of cholinergic receptors.

6.   List two types of adrenergic receptors.

7.   Describe the two major branches of the ANS.

Practice Test

Use this practice test to review the topics of this chapter and to prepare for your test on this material.

1.   In the sympathetic branch of the ANS
     a.   all receptors are adrenergic
     b.   all receptors are cholinergic
     c.   pathways consists of two neurons
     d.   ganglia are always near the effector
     e.   a and c are correct

2.   Acetylcholine is the normal transmitter
     a.   in sympathetic ganglia
     b.   in parasympathetic ganglia
     c.   at parasympathetic effectors
     d.   at sympathetic effectors
     e.   a, b, and c are correct

3.   Muscle spindle receptors
     a.   are called Golgi organs
     b.   contain modified muscle fibers
     c.   are involved in withdrawal reflexes
     d.   contain extrafusal fibers
     e.   b and d are correct

4. Recruitment of motor units
    a. occurs in order of increasing size
    b. never occurs in skeletal muscle
    c. allows gradations in muscle tension
    d. is controlled by motor reflexes
    e. a, c, and d are correct

5. The Golgi tendon reflex tends to
    a. facilitate nerves to antagonistic muscles
    b. facilitate nerves to the muscle of origin
    c. facilitate nerves to synergistic muscles
    d. b and c are correct
    e. all are correct

6. Impulses to postganglionic cells can be blocked by
    a. acetylcholine
    b. epinephrine
    c. curare
    d. norepinephrine
    e. atropine

7. The motor system includes all but
    a. premotor cortex
    b. Broca's area
    c. basal ganglia
    d. cerebellum
    e. vestibular nucleus

8. The pyramidal tract is associated with
    a. fine muscular movements
    b. gross muscular movements
    c. posture
    d. b and c are correct
    e. a, b, and c are correct

9. Antigravity reflexes are mediated by the
    a. basal ganglia
    b. premotor cortex
    c. Golgi apparatus
    d. vestibular nucleus
    e. a and c are correct

10. Activation of the sympathetic branch may cause
    a. increased heart rate
    b. increased peristalsis in the gastrointestinal (GI) tract
    c. decreased sweating
    d. decreased blood glucose level
    e. increased intestinal motility

11. Alpha- or beta-blocking drugs affect
    a. parasympathetic effectors
    b. sympathetic effectors
    c. sympathetic ganglia
    d. parasympathetic ganglia
    e. none of the above

12. The basal ganglia
   a. are in the telencephalon
   b. are part of the lateral motor system
   c. organize motor programs
   d. a and c are correct
   e. a, b, and c are correct

13. The corticospinal tract
   a. can directly activate motor neurons
   b. forms pyramids in the medulla
   c. directs distal muscle groups
   d. a and c are correct
   e. a, b, and c are correct

14. Nociceptor stimulation results in
   a. withdrawal reflex
   b. Golgi tendon reflex
   c. stretch reflex
   d. inhibition of nerves to flexors
   e. a and d are correct

Answers

Here are answers (or references) to some of the questions presented above.

Word Parts: (your examples may be different) 1-dyskinesia, 2-myotome, 3-nociceptive, 4-paravertebral, 5-white ramus

Key Terms: Descriptive: 1.adrenergic 2.cholinergic 3.nicotinic 4.muscarinic
Processes: 1.dual innervation 2.myotatic reflex 3.motor program 4.reciprocal inhibition 5.decerebration 6.decomposition 7.crossed extension 8.alpha coactivation 9.recruitment 10.denervation 11.nociception
Structures/Substances 1.norepinephrine 2.myotome 3.paravertebral sympathetic ganglion 4.muscle spindle 5.gray ramus 6.vestibular nucleus 7.prevertebral ganglion 8.plexus 9.white ramus 10.cardiovascular centers 11.alpha motor neuron 12.epinephrine 13.corticospinal tract 14.gamma motor neuron 15.extrapyramidal tract 16.parasympathetic branch [of ANS] 17.sympathetic branch [of ANS] 18.basal ganglia 19.preganglionic neuron 20.postganglionic neuron 21.chromaffin cell 22.extrafusal fiber 23.intrafusal fiber 24.Golgi tendon organ 25.propriospinal interneuron 26.motor unit 27.sciatic nerve
Other: 1.readiness potential 2.dyskinesia 3.motor homunculus 4.evoked potential 5.muscle tone

Learning Exercises: 1. (check your answers with Table 11-1 in the text) 2. 1-thoracic/lumbar segments, 2-cranial nerves/sacral segments, 3-sympathetic preganglionic fiber, 4-parasympathetic postganglionic fiber, 5-sympathetic ganglion, 6-acetylcholine, 7-sympathetic postganglionic fiber, 8-parasympathetic ganglion, 9-acetylcholine, 10-parasympathetic postganglionic fiber, 11-norepinephrine/epinephrine, 12-sympathetic effector, 13-acetylcholine, 14-parasympathetic effector 3. W, G, S, S, W, G, S, S, S, S 4. brainstem, vestibular, righting, basal ganglia, reticular, motor programs, execution, cerebellum, inhibitory, decomposition, coordinating, premotor cortex, primary motor cortex, supplementary motor area, motor homunculus, motor programs 5. LATERAL: involved mainly in fine movements, involves the pyramidal tract, involves the corticospinal pathway, serves primarily distal muscles, tend to be rapid-acting, tends to involve monosynaptic pathways PROXIMAL: involved in mainly gross movements/posture, involves extrapyramidal tracts, serves primarily proximal muscles, tends to involve polysynaptic pathways, tends to be slower-acting 6. (answers to this section are in Tables 11-5 and 11-6 in the text)

Quick Recall: (You should be able to answer these questions easily without correction or confirmation by this point in your studies. If you cannot, review your notes, the text chapter, and the previous study activities to find the answers.)

Practice Test: 1-c, 2-e, 3-b, 4-e, 5-a, 6-c, 7-b, 8-a, 9-d, 10-a, 11-b, 12-e, 13-e, 14-d

Chapter 13
The Heart

Focus
Review this section *first*. It will help you focus on the overall message of this chapter.

Chapter Outline
Read through the outline slowly. This activity will help your mind organize the topics of this chapter.

An overview of the circulation
The structure and function of the heart
      Cardiac chambers and tissues
      The cardiac cycle
      Diastole
      Systole
The electrical activity of the heart
      The heart's pacemaker
      The action potentials of nonpacemaker cells
      Excitation/contraction coupling in cardiac muscle
      Spread of excitation in the heart
      Abnormalities of cardiac rhythm
      The electrocardiogram
A summary of events of the heart cycle
Pressures in the pulmonary and systemic loops
Intrinsic and extrinsic regulation of cardiac performance
      Intrinsic regulation of stroke volume—the Frank-Starling Law of the Heart
      Extrinsic regulation of the heart by the autonomic nervous system
Overview of interacting factors that affect cardiac performance

Learning Objectives
These are the learning goals for this part of the course. After reading the text, attending class, and studying this chapter, you should be able to:

♦   describe the components of the circulatory system: the heart, arteries, capillaries, and veins

♦   understand the role of valves in the heart

♦   distinguish the three types of cardiac muscle cells: pacemakers, conducting fibers, and contracting fibers (which generate the force of systole)

♦   describe the ionic basis of the action potentials of cardiac cells and the automatic generation of action potentials by cardiac pacemakers

♦   identify the five phases of the cardiac cycle: early diastole, atrial contraction, isovolumetric ventricular contraction, ejection, and isovolumetric ventricular relaxation

♦ understand how the Frank-Starling law of the heart can be derived from the length-tension relationship of cardiac muscle fibers

♦ understand how pacemaker discharge rate is affected by sympathetic and parasympathetic input

♦ identify the major factors that determine cardiac output

Language of Physiology
Physiology uses its own set of terms, many of which may be unfamiliar to you. This section will help you improve your mastery of key physiological terms.

Word Parts
Here are some combining forms often seen in physiological terms. Give an example of a term that contains each word part listed.

Word Part	Meaning	Example
brady-	slow	1_____
diastol-	relax; stand apart	2_____
ectop-	displaced	3_____
-lunar	moon; moonlike	4_____
sclero-	hard	5_____
systol-	contract; stand together	6_____
tachy-	fast	7_____

Key Terms
Read each of the terms in each grouping below aloud, using the pronunciation guide if necessary. This will help you to remember them better than if you read them silently. Then, write out the correct term next to each of the descriptions given.

Descriptive Terms
pulmonary (PUL-mah-nayr-ee)
systemic (sis-TEM-ik)

1_____   descriptive term conveying association with the lungs; in cardiovascular biology, referring to vessels carrying blood to and from the lungs

2_____   descriptive term used in cardiovascular biology to describe vessels or pathways associated with all body systems except the lungs

Terms related to measurement

cardiac function curve
cardiac output [CO]
Einthoven's triangle (IYNT-hoh-venz)
electrocardiogram
  (el-ek-troh-KARD-ee-oh-gram)

heart rate [HR]
mean arterial pressure
pulse pressure
standard limb leads (leedz)
stroke volume [SV]

1 _____ graphic representation (plot) of the relationship between cardiac output and venous pressure

2 _____ record of the electrical activity of the heart; it is abbreviated ECG, but to more easily distinguish it from EEG in verbal usage, the German abbreviation, EKG, can be used

3 _____ time-weighted average of the arterial pressure over the heart cycle (approximately equal to the sum of diastolic pressure and one third of the pulse pressure)

4 _____ pattern of electrode placement in ECG studies originally devised by Einthoven, involving three two-electrode measurements of potential difference: leads I, II, and III

5 _____ volume of blood pumped by a single ventricle per minute, determined by multiplying stroke volume by heart rate and expressed in L/min

6 _____ electrical axes of the three standard limb leads of the ECG, forming a "triangle" of electrical measurement

7 _____ rate of the heart's pumping cycles, expressed in beats (cycles) per minute [beats/min]

8 _____ difference in pressure between the systolic pressure and diastolic pressure in the arteries

9 _____ amount of blood expelled from the ventricle in one heart cycle, measured as the difference between end-diastolic volume and end-systolic volume and expressed as L/beat

Terms related to processes

atrioventricular (AV) delay
atrioventricular (AV) block
Ca^{++}-induced Ca^{++} release
chronotrophic effect (krahn-oh-TROH-fik)
diastole (dy-AS-toh-lee)

fibrillation (fib-rih-LAY-shun)
parasympathetic tone
plateau phase (pla-TOW)
systole (SIS-toh-lee)

1 _____ positive feedback mechanism in cardiac fibers in which small amounts of extracellular Ca^{++} entering the cells triggers the release of greater amounts of Ca^{++} from the SR

2 _____ term describing the effects of certain drugs or transmitters in terms of their effects upon the heart rate; a positive effect implies that heart rate has increased, a negative effect implies a decrease in heart rate

3 _____ pause of the cardiac action potential between initial depolarization (upstroke) and repolarization

4 _____ failure of action potentials to pass through the atrioventricular node from the atria to the ventricles (abnormal)

5 _____ steady input of parasympathetic signals to the normal resting adult heart, resulting in a heart rate of about 70 beats/min (rather than the ±100

beats/min likely without it)

6 _____ time required for action potentials to pass through the atrioventricular node from the atria to the ventricles

7 _____ period during which the ventricles are relaxed and both the atria and ventricles are filling with blood

8 _____ period during which first the atria then the ventricles contract

9 _____ uncoordinated pumping of myocardium resulting in ineffective pumping and leading to death within minutes unless treated (perhaps by means of defibrillation)

Terms related to structures/substances

aorta (ay-ORT-ah)
artery (ART-er-ee)
atrioventricular [AV] valve
   (ayt-ree-oh-ven-TRIK-yoo-ler)
atrioventricular [AV] node
atrium (AYT-ree-um)
capillary (KAP-ih-layr-ee)
chordae tendineae (KORD-ay TEN-din-ay)
conducting cardiac fibers
contractile cardiac fibers
ectopic pacemaker (ek-TAHP-ik)
endocardium (en-doh-KARD-ee-um)
epicardium (ep-ih-KARD-ee-um)
interventricular septum
   (in-ter-ven-TRIK-yoo-ler)

intraatrial septum (in-trah-AYT-ree-al)
myocardium (my-oh-KARD-ee-um)
pacemaker cardiac fibers
papillary muscles (PAP-ih-layr-ee)
pericardial fluid (payr-ih-KARD-ee-al)
pericardium (payr-ih-KARD-ee-um)
semilunar [SL] valve (sem-ee-LOON-er)
sinoatrial [SA] node
   (sine-oh-AYT-ree-al)
slow Na^+-Ca^{++} channels
thrombus (THROM-bus)
vein (vayn)
vena cava (VAYN-ah KAH-vah)
ventricle (VEN-trih-kil)

1 _____ large blood vessel carrying blood away from the heart and toward body tissues (systemic or pulmonary)

2 _____ conglomeration of pacemaker fibers located in the inferior portion of the interatrial septum

3 _____ sac with fibrous and serous components that surrounds the heart

4 _____ conglomeration of pacemaker fibers located near the junction of the superior vena cava and the right atrium

5 _____ clot of blood within a vessel, that may cause partial or complete blockage of blood flow

6 _____ large blood vessel carrying blood from body tissues (capillary circulation) toward and into the receiving heart chambers (atria)

7 _____ "out of place" pacemaking node that discharges action potentials from places (and at times) inappropriate for normal heart function

8 _____ ion channel in cardiac muscle that allows both Na^+ and Ca^{++} to pass through it, and whose activation rate is slower than the "fast" Na^+ channel of nerve and skeletal muscle fibers

9 _____ fingerlike projections of muscle from the interior ventricular wall that, by means of cords, prevent the edges of the AV valve cusp from everting when stressed

10 _____ heart valve that ensures one-way flow from the atrium into the ventricle;

on the left, also called the bicuspid or mitral valve — on the right, also called the tricuspid valve

11_____ inner layer of the heart wall, composed of endothelial tissue

12_____ one of two types of heart chamber, this one receiving blood and passing it to the other chamber type; there is one receiving chamber in the left [side of the] heart, one in the right heart

13_____ one of two (superior, inferior) large veins that empty systemic blood into the right atrium

14_____ one of two types of heart chamber, this one pushing blood out of the heart after having received it from the other chamber type; one pushing chamber in the left heart, one in the right heart

15_____ outer layer of the heart wall, synonymous with visceral layer of the serous pericardium

16_____ serous fluid found between the visceral and parietal layers of the pericardium, serving as a lubricant to prevent friction damage as the heart pumps

17_____ largest artery of the body; it exits the left ventricle

18_____ smallest of the blood vessels traveling through body tissues; form a network connecting arteries to veins

19_____ muscular portion of the heart wall

20_____ threads of connective tissue running from the tips of the AV valve cusps to fingerlike projections of muscle in the ventricles

21_____ type of cardiac fiber that is primarily suited to conducting action potentials, rather than to contracting or pacemaking; includes Purkinje fibers

22_____ type of cardiac fiber that is primarily suited to contraction, rather than to conduction or pacemaking

23_____ type of cardiac fiber that is primarily suited to initiating action potentials, rather than to conducting or contracting

24_____ valve in the heart that ensures one-way travel out of the ventricles, or in the vein, ensuring one-way travel toward the atria — in the heart, the left SL valve is called the aortic valve, the right one is called the pulmonary valve

25_____ wall of tissue separating the left ventricle from the right ventricle

26_____ wall of tissue separating the left atrium from the right atrium

Other Key Terms

arrhythmia (ah-RITH-mee-ah)
atherosclerosis (ath-er-oh-skleh-ROH-sis)
bradycardia (brad-ee-KARD-ee-ah)
congestive heart failure (kahn-JEST-iv)
Frank-Starling law of the heart
myocardial infarct
   (my-oh-KARD-ee-al IN-farkt)

premature ventricular contraction
  [PVC]
reentry (ree-ENT-ree)
tachycardia (tak-ee-KARD-ee-ah)

1 _____ general term describing any condition manifesting itself as a disorder of the heart's normal rhythm

2 _____ condition in which the central venous pressure and thus end-diastolic volume are high, progressively weakening the myocardium

3 _____ principle of cardiac function that states that the length-tension relationship of cardiac muscle causes cardiac output to be a function of venous return

4 _____ "heart attack," or damage to a region of the heart resulting from blockage of blood flow to muscle tissue (by a thrombus or other blocking condition)

5 _____ arrhythmia involving a slow heart rate

6 _____ arrhythmia involving extra systoles, possibly resulting from activity of ectopic pacemakers

7 _____ arrhythmia involving a rapid heart rate

8 _____ condition in which electrical activity in the heart is altered so that different regions excite one another in a vicious cycle

9 _____ formation of fatty deposits on the interior surface of arteries that can eventually obstruct the flow of blood

The Big Picture

Use the activities of this section to help you learn the broader concepts of this chapter.

Learning Exercises

1.   Use these terms to label the parts of Figure 13-1, the heart, as indicated.

SA node
R atrium
AV node
bundle of His
tricuspid valve

bundle branches
Purkinje fibers
interventricular   septum
L ventricle

papillary muscle
bicuspid valve
L atrium

Figure 13-1

1_____

2_____

3_____

4_____

5_____

6_____

7_____

8_____

9_____

10_____

11_____

12_____

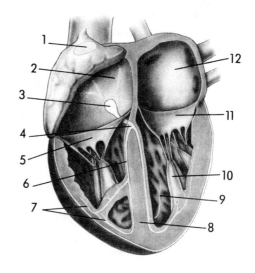

2. Figure 13-2 shows a frontal section of the heart. Use a pencil to trace the flow of blood through the heart (as you would do in a "maze" puzzle). You may want to use occasional arrows to indicate direction. Circle and label each valve as you pass through it.

Figure 13-2

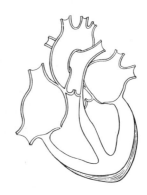

3. Fill in the blank portions of this table, which compares and contrasts sympathetic and parasympathetic heart effects.

	Sympathetic	Parasympathetic
Transmitter(s):		acetylcholine
Receptor type:	muscarinic	
Membrane effect (pacemaker cells):	faster closing of K^+ channels	
Membrane effect (contractile cells):	increased Ca^{++} entry increased Ca^{++} pumping	
Overall heart effect:	increased force of contraction	none

4. Using the brackets shown, label these portions of Figure 13-3:

P-Q interval
P wave
QRS complex
Q-T interval
T wave

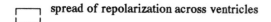
Figure 13-3

Using differently colored pencils, felt-tip pens, or highlighting markers, draw a box around (or shade over) those portions of this ECG graph that indicate the following:

☐ spread of depolarization across the atria

☐ spread of depolarization across the ventricles

☐ plateau phase of ventricles

☐ spread of repolarization across ventricles

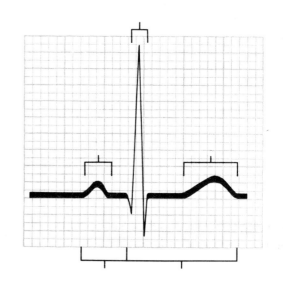

5.　Put these phases of the cardiac pumping cycle in the order in which they occur. Then write a brief description of the events that accompany each phase.

atrial contraction/late diastole　　　　　　　　isovolumetric ventricular contraction
ejection　　　　　　　　　　　　　　　　　　　passive filling
isovolumetric ventricular relaxation

_____:

_____:

_____:

_____:

_____:

6.　Label these portions of Figure 13-4, Part A, then answer the question regarding Part B.

AV valves open
AV valves close
SL valves open
SL valves close

1 _____

2 _____

3 _____

4 _____

What is the difference in volume between point X and point Y called?

_____

Figure 13-4

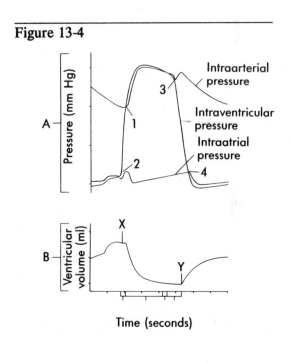

7.　Explain the Frank-Starling law of the heart (in terms of the length-tension relationship of cardiac fibers).

Quick Recall

Review some of the major concepts of this chapter by doing these "quick recall" activities.

1.   Name three different kinds of blood vessels.

2.   Name the four major valves of the heart.

3.   Name three different (functional) types of cardiac fiber.

4.   Name the major components of the heart's conduction system, in order.

5.   List the five phases of the cardiac pumping cycle, in order.

6.   List the major events of the ECG wave, in order.

7.   Give the equation relating factors that determine the stroke volume.

Practice Test

Use this practice test to review the topics of this chapter and to prepare for your test on this material.

1.   Cardiac contraction is normally regulated by
   a.   recruitment of motor units
   b.   facilitation of motor units
   c.   changes in initial fiber length
   d.   changes in contractility
   e.   both c and d are correct

2.   Velocity of ejection of blood is decreased by
   a.   increasing the end-diastolic volume
   b.   sympathetic stimulation
   c.   parasympathetic stimulation
   d.   increasing the aortic diastolic pressure
   e.   none of the above

3. Ventricular volume is lowest at the start of
   a. atrial contraction
   b. isovolumetric contraction
   c. reduced ejection
   d. isovolumetric relaxation
   e. reduced filling

4. In the normal excitation sequence of the heart, the structure activated just after the SA node is the
   a. apex
   b. AV node
   c. bundle of His
   d. Purkinje fibers
   e. ventricular muscle

5. The plateau phase of the heart cycle is caused primarily by
   a. slow influx of calcium
   b. slow influx of potassium
   c. slow influx of chloride
   d. a and b are correct
   e. none are correct

6. The AV valves are prevented from everting during ventricular contraction by
   a. chordae tendineae
   b. semilunar flaps
   c. papillary muscle
   d. trabeculae
   e. a and c are correct

7. The inner lining of the heart is called
   a. chordae tendineae
   b. mesothelium
   c. endocardium
   d. pericardium
   e. myocardium

8. In the ECG, the P-R interval reflects
   a. ventricular depolarization
   b. ventricular repolarization
   c. AV delay
   d. strength of atrial contraction
   e. heart rate

9. Cardiac output is
   a. determined in part by stroke volume
   b. determined in part by heart rate
   c. is expressed in L/beat
   d. a and b are correct
   e. a, b, and c are correct

10. The coronary circulation supplies the
    a. lungs
    b. systems other than the lungs
    c. myocardium
    d. brain
    e. b, c, and d are correct

11. The normal pacemaker of the heart is the
    a. SA node
    b. AV node
    c. ectopic pacemaker
    d. SL node
    e. bundle of His

12. Increased sympathetic innervation of the heart tends to
    a. increase heart rate
    b. decrease heart rate
    c. decrease calcium entry
    d. decrease closing of potassium channels
    e. a and d are correct

13. Ventricular activation is exhibited as the
    a. P-R interval
    b. P wave
    c. QRS wave
    d. T wave
    e. S-T interval

Answers

Here are answers (or references) to some of the questions presented above.

Word Parts: (your examples may be different) 1-bradycardia, 2-diastolic pressure, 3-ectopic pacemaker, 4-semilunar valve, 5-atherosclerosis, 6-systolic pressure, 7-tachycardia

Key Terms: Descriptive: 1. pulmonary 2. systemic **Terms related to Measurement:** 1. cardiac function curve 2. electrocardiogram 3. mean arterial pressure 4. standard limb leads 5. cardiac output [CO] 6. Einthoven's triangle 7. heart rate [HR] 8. pulse pressure 9. stroke volume [SV]
Processes: 1. Ca^{++}-mediated Ca^{++} release 2. chronotrophic effect 3. plateau phase 4. AV block 5. parasympathetic tone 6. AV delay 7. diastole 8. systole 9. fibrillation
Structures/Substances: 1. artery 2. atrioventricular [AV] node 3. pericardium 4. sinoatrial [SA] node 5. thrombus 6. vein 7. ectopic pacemaker 8. slow Na^+-Ca^{++} channels 9. papillary muscles 10. atrioventricular [AV] valve 11. endocardium 12. atrium 13. vena cava 14. ventricle 15. epicardium 16. pericardial fluid 17. aorta 18. capillary 19. myocardium 20. chordae tendineae 21. conducting cardiac fibers 22. contractile cardiac fibers 23. pacemaker cardiac fibers 24. semilunar [SL] valve 25. interventricular septum 26. intraatrial septum
Other: 1. arrhythmia 2. congestive heart failure 3. Frank-Starling law of the heart 4. myocardial infarct 5. bradycardia 6. premature ventricular contraction [PVC] 7. tachycardia 8. reentry 9. atherosclerosis

Learning Exercises: 1. 1-SA node, 2-R atrium, 3-AV node, 4-bundle of His, 5-tricuspid valve, 6-bundle branches, 6-Purkinje fibers, 7-interventricular septum, 8-L ventricle, 9-papillary muscle, 10-bicuspid valve, 11-L atrium 2. (refer to Figure 13-15 in the text) 3. (find answers in Table 13-4 of the text) 4. (for graph labels, see Figure 13-12 in the text) P wave-spread of depolarization across the atria, QRS complex-spread of depolarization across the ventricles, between S and T-plateau phase of ventricles, T wave-spread of repolarization across ventricle 5. passive filling, atrial contraction/late diastole, isovolumetric ventricular contraction, ejection, isovolumetric ventricular relaxation (events of each phase are summarized in Table 13-3 of the text). 6. 1-SL valves open, 2-AV valves close, 3-SL valves close, 4-AV valves open, x-y -> stroke volume 7. the length-tension relation of heart muscle is such that increased stretch by increased filling (increased end-diastolic volume) increases the force of systole and thus the stroke volume. The mechanism allows the heart to autoregulate its stroke volume to make cardiac output equal to venous return over a wide range of end-diastolic volumes.

Quick Recall: (You should be able to answer these questions easily without correction or confirmation by this point in your studies. If you cannot, review your notes, the text chapter, and the previous study activities to find the answers.)

Practice Test: 1-e, 2-c, 3-a, 4-b, 5-a, 6-a, 7-e, 8-c, 9-c, 10-d, 11-c, 12-a, 13-a, 14-c

Chapter 14
Blood and the Vascular System

Focus
Review this section *first*. It will help you focus on the overall message of this chapter.

Chapter Outline
Read through the outline slowly. This activity will help your mind organize the topics of this chapter.

Blood—a liquid tissue
      Blood composition
      Hemostasis
Structures of blood vessels
      Types of blood vessels
      The walls of arteries and veins
      The structure of capillaries
The mechanics of blood flow
      Definition of blood flow
      Relationship of blood flow to driving force and resistance
      Effects of vessel dimensions and branching on resistance and flow
      Importance of arterioles for control of blood flow distribution and peripheral resistance
Transfer of fluid and solutes between capillaries and tissues
Exchange of nutrients and wastes across capillary walls
Fluid exchange between capillaries and interstitial spaces
The lymphatic system

Learning Objectives
These are the learning goals for this part of the course. After reading the text, attending class, and studying this chapter, you should be able to:

◆   identify the components of the blood and define hematocrit

◆   describe the process of blood clotting (hemostasis), noting the differences between intrinsic and extrinsic pathways

◆   appreciate the role of the arteries in maintaining blood flow into the vasculature during diastole

◆   understand why veins are referred to as capacitance elements of the circulation

◆   distinguish between linear velocity of flow, average flow, and volume flow rate

- describe how vessel length, blood viscosity, and vessel radius affect vessel flow resistance

- understand the determinants of total peripheral resistance

- describe the effects of extrinsic autonomic control on vascular smooth muscle

- describe the factors that determine capillary fluid exchange

- understand the anatomy and circulation of the lymphatic system

Language of Physiology

Physiology uses its own set of terms, many of which may be unfamiliar to you. This section will help you improve your mastery of key physiological terms.

Word Parts

Here are some combining forms often seen in physiological terms. Give an example of a term that contains each word part listed.

Word Part	Meaning	Example
erythro-	red	1_____
-gen	creates; forms	2_____
hema-, hemo-	blood	3_____
leuko-	white	4_____
mega-	large; million(th)	5_____
poie-	make; produce	6_____
thrombo-	clot	7_____

Key Terms

Read each of the terms in each grouping below aloud, using the pronunciation guide if necessary. This will help you to remember them better than if you read them silently. Then, write out the correct term next to each of the descriptions given.

Terms related to measurement

capacitance (ka-PAS-it-ans)
continuity equation of flow
hematocrit (hee-MA-toh-krit)

perfusion pressure (per-FYOO-jen)
total peripheral resistance [TPR]

1_____   in the absence of sources or sinks, the volume flow of fluids or gases, expressed as the product of the linear velocity and cross-sectional area, remains constant

2_____   in the cardiovascular system, this term refers to the change in volume produced by a given change in pressure

3 _____   pressure actively generated by the heart

4 _____   the equivalent flow resistance of all systemic organs "felt" by the heart

5 _____   the percentage of the total blood volume that is red cells (normally 40 to 50% in males, 35 to 45% in females

Terms related to processes

edema (eh-DEE-mah)   hemostasis (hee-moh-STAY-sis)
erythropoiesis (ee-rith-roh-poy-EE-sis)   intrinsic pathway (in-TRIN-zik)
extrinsic pathway (eks-TRIN-zik)   laminar flow (LAM-in-ar)

1 _____   accumulation of fluid in the interstitial spaces, causing tissue swelling

2 _____   one of two pathways that lead to blood clot formation—this one is initiated by components normally found within the blood itself

3 _____   one of two pathways that lead to blood clot formation—this one is initiated by chemical factors released from damaged tissue

4 _____   red blood cell production (in the bone marrow)

5 _____   steady, unswirling flow

6 _____   the process of blood clot formation

Terms related to structures/substances

albumin (al-BYOO-min)   metarteriole (met-art-TEER-ee-ohl)
anticoagulant (an-tee-koh-AG-yoo-lent)   plasma (PLAZ-mah)
arachidonic acid (a-rak-ih-DON-ik)   plasmin (PLAZ-min)
arteriolar-venular shunt   precapillary sphincter
  (ar-teer-ee-OH-ler--VAYN-yoo-lar)   (pree-KAP-ih-layr-ee SFINK-ter)
arteriole (ar-TEER-ee-ohl)   prothrombin (proh-THROM-bin)
clot   thoracic duct (tho-RAS-ik)
embolism (EM-bol-izm)   thrombin (THROM-bin)
erythrocyte (ee-RITH-roh-site)   thrombocyte (THROM-boh-site)
fibrinogen (fy-BRIN-oh-jen)   thromboplastin (throm-boh-PLAS-tin)
Hageman factor (HAY-ge-man)   thrombus (THROM-bus)
immunoglobulin (im-yoo-noh-GLOB-yoo-lin)   tunica intima (TOON-ik-ah IN-tim-ah)
leukocyte (LOO-koh-site)   tunica externa (TOON-ik-ah eks-TERN-ah)
lymph node (limf)   tunica media (TOON-ik-ah MEED-ee-ah)
megakaryocyte (may-gah-KAR-ee-oh-site)   venule (VAYN-yool)

1 _____   cufflike circle of smooth muscle at the origin of each capillary that controls blood flow through the capillary

2 _____   large lymphatic duct that drains lymph from vessels from the entire body except the right shoulder/neck/head region (that are served by the right lymphatic duct)

3 _____   network of fibrin molecules that forms a patch (more lasting than a platelet plug) over a break in a blood vessel

4 _____   blood clot that forms at an inappropriate site within vessels, possibly blocking them

5 _____   term applied to a clotting factor (III) released by damaged cells that accelerates formation of a blood clot

6 _____   small vein (approximately 20 to 30 μm)

7 _____   small diameter (approximately 70 μm) artery branch, not quite as small as a capillary

8 _____   fatty acid released by platelets when they bind to a damaged surface; may be subsequently converted to thromboxane A_2, a prostaglandin that attracts additional platelets to the site

9 _____   vessel that (like many metarterioles) bypasses capillary circulation - by connecting arterioles to venules or arteries to veins

10 _____   alternate name for all red blood cells (RBCs)

11 _____   enzyme formed from plasminogen that dissolves blood clots when they are no longer needed

12 _____   arteriole branch (approximately 10 to 20 μm) whose walls are wrapped with smooth muscle only at intervals and which connects directly to venules (thereby shunting blood away from capillary circulation)

13 _____   any of several substances, such as prostacyclin or heparin, that act in some way to prevent or inhibit the clotting mechanism, thus helping to regulate this process

14 _____   any of a category of plasma proteins that serve as transport proteins (for lipids and steroid hormones) and play a role in body fluid balance

15 _____   any of many organs of the immune system/lymphatic system found at intervals along lymphatic vessels, that contain lymphocytes and thus act as immune "filters" of tissue fluids

16 _____   any of a category of plasma proteins that mediate specific immunity

17 _____   clotting factor XII; a plasma protein whose activation is the initial event in the formation of a blood clot

18 _____   general name for all white blood cells (WBCs)

19 _____   general name for the fluid portion of the blood

20 _____   inactive form of a plasma protein that (when activated by one of the clotting factors) catalyzes the conversion of fibrinogen to fibrin

21 _____   large cells within the bone marrow that fragment to form platelets

22 _____   name given to a clot or clot portion that breaks away from its site of attachment and moves into a smaller vessel, blocking it

23 _____   one of several plasma proteins involved in clotting, this one polymerizes to form fibrin

24 _____   platelet; type of small blood cell fragment involved in the clotting process

25 _____   active form of a plasma protein that catalyzes the conversion of fibrinogen to fibrin

26 _____   middle layer (of three) of arteries and veins, formed by a coat of circular smooth muscle

27_____   inner layer of arteries and muscles, consisting of a single layer of
endothelial cells

28_____   outer layer of arteries and veins, formed by a coat of longitudinal smooth
muscle

The Big Picture

Use the activities of this section to help you learn the broader concepts of this chapter.

Learning Exercises

1. Identify these three major steps of hemostasis.

clot dissolution
clot formation
platelet plug

1_____   platelets at a site of injury become "sticky" when exposed to a damaged
surface and congregate at the site, plugging the opening

2_____   fibrinogen is converted to fibrin by means of a cascade of chemical
reactions and forms a dense covering of the injury site

3_____   some factors released at the time of injury work slowly but eventually
trigger the dissolution of the fibrin covering of the injury site

2. Figure 14-1 is a simplified flowchart of the events of clot formation. Use these terms to identify
the substances and pathways represented in the chart.

extrinsic pathway
fibrin
Hageman factor
intrinsic pathway
prothrombin activator
prothrombin
thrombin

Figure 14-1

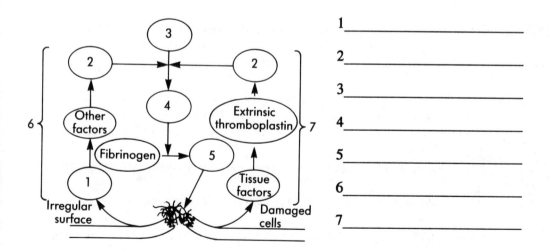

1_____

2_____

3_____

4_____

5_____

6_____

7_____

3.   Use these terms to fill in the following paragraphs.

average flow velocity	flow velocity
blood flow	pressure
capacitance	systole
compliance	volume flow rate

The ratio of volume to _____ in a vessel is determined by its compliance.

Arteries are low-_____ elements containing a small volume of blood under high

pressure. The arterial walls store energy during _____ and then recoil to

maintain _____ into the vasculature during diastole. Veins are the high-

compliance, _____ elements of the circulation.

Depending on context, "flow" indicates the volume of blood passing a point over time

(_____), the linear velocity of a single drop of blood

(_____), or the average velocity of all drops in a stream

(_____).

4.   For each of the situations described, indicate whether the result is likely to be an increase in
vessel flow resistance or a decrease in vessel flow resistance (assuming all factors not mentioned
remain stable). To further clarify the relationship of resistance to the factor described, state the
algebraic function that defines the relationship (use the right margin).

1 - An increase in vessel radius = _____ flow resistance

2 - A decrease in vessel length = _____ flow resistance

3 - A decrease in vessel radius = _____ flow resistance

4 - An increase in blood viscosity = _____ flow resistance

5 - A decrease in blood viscosity = _____ flow resistance

6 - Branching of the vessel = _____ flow resistance

5. Use these terms to fill in the following paragraphs. (Some terms may be used more than once.)

autonomic   sympathetic
constriction   systemic
dilation   total peripheral resistance
perfusion

The sum of the resistances of the arterioles in the various branches of the

_____ loop is the major determinant of the _____. TPR

is increased by arteriolar _____ and is decreased by arteriolar

_____.

Extrinsic control of vascular smooth muscle is generally mediated by the

_____ branch of the _____ nervous system, which mainly

causes _____ of vessels. Arterioles and precapillary sphincters are autoregulated

by local metabolic factors that match _____ of individual vascular beds to their

metabolism.

6. Identify these parts of Figure 14-2, which represents a systemic capillary.

arterial end   negative interstitial pressure
blood pressure   venous end
blood colloid osmotic pressure

1_____   Figure 14-2

2_____

3_____

4_____

5_____

Quick Recall
Review some of the major concepts of this chapter by doing these "quick recall" activities.

1. List the components of blood and describe their ratio.

2. List the major events of hemostasis.

3. List the major vessel types and compare them.

4. Name four factors that affect blood flow through vessels.

5. Name two mechanisms of control of blood flow through tissues.

6. List outwardly directed and inwardly directed forces affecting movement of fluids between blood plasma and interstitial fluid.

7. Describe the origin, pathway, and ultimate disposition of lymph.

8. Describe the lymph node and give its chief function.

Practice Test

Use this practice test to review the topics of this chapter and to prepare for your test on this material.

1. Blood contains
   a. plasma
   b. albumin
   c. erythrocytes
   d. interstitial fluid
   e. a, b, and c are correct

2. The hematocrit
   a. is the fraction of blood volume that is RBCs
   b. is normally 30% to 60%
   c. decreases in polycythemia
   d. a and b only
   e. a, b, and c

3. Plasminogen
   a. is activated by Hageman factor
   b. is inactivated by Hageman factor
   c. stimulates clot formation
   d. is the active form of plasmin
   e. a and c are correct

4. Immunoglobulin
   a. is a normal component of blood
   b. is present only during infections
   c. carries oxygen
   d. is a plasma protein
   e. a and d are correct

5. Arterioles
   a. are capacitance elements
   b. are resistance vessels
   c. are a type of capillary
   d. contain many semilunar valves
   e. a and d are correct

6. The thinnest layer of the venous wall
   a. varies from vein to vein
   b. is the tunica media
   c. is the endothelium
   d. is the tunica salada
   e. is missing in most veins

7. At the center of a large blood vessel
   a. blood does not flow
   b. linear blood velocity is near zero
   c. linear blood velocity is at its largest
   d. a and b may both be correct
   e. none are correct

8. The hydrostatic pressure at the ends of each of two rigid tubes is equal. Tube A is 81 times longer than tube B. Tube B has radius r. What is the radius of A, if flow in A = flow in B?
   a. 9 r
   b. 1/9 r
   c. 81 r
   d. 3 r
   e. 1/3 r

9. Six tubes with identical flow resistance R are connected in parallel. The total resistance of the combination is
   a. cannot be determined
   b. 1/6 R
   c. 6 R
   d. .6 R
   e. 1296 R

10. The major pressure drop in the systemic circulation occurs as blood flows
    a. through the lungs
    b. through the arterioles
    c. through the capillary wall
    d. through the venules
    e. through the capillaries

11. Increased compliance of arterial walls
    a. decreases pulse pressure
    b. increases mean arterial pressure
    c. decreases volume of arterial blood
    d. a and c are correct
    e. a, b, and c are correct

12. Capillaries are about _ (inside diameter).
    a. 70 μm
    b. 700 μm
    c. 10 μm
    d. 140 μm
    e. 1 μm

13. If plasma osmotic pressure is increased by intravenous administration of dextran
    a. edema may be seen in the extremities
    b. there will be a net capillary reabsorption of fluid
    c. the hematocrit would be decreased
    d. the mean arterial blood pressure would decrease
    e. both b and c are correct

Answers

Here are answers (or references) to some of the questions presented above.

Word Parts: (your examples may be different) 1-erythrocyte, 2-fibrinogen, 3-hematocrit, 4-leukocyte, 5-megakaryocyte, 6-erythropoiesis, 7-thrombocyte

Key Terms: Measurement: 1.continuity equation of flow 2.capacitance 3.perfusion pressure 4.total peripheral resistance [TPR] 5.hematocrit
Processes: 1.edema 2.intrinsic pathway 3.extrinsic pathway 4.erythropoiesis 5.laminar flow 6.hemostasis
Structures/Substances: 1.precapillary sphincter 2.thoracic duct 3.clot 4.thrombus 5.thromboplastin 6.venule 7.arteriole 8.arachidonic acid 9.arteriolar-venular shunt 10.erythrocyte 11.plasmin 12.metarteriole 13.anticoagulant 14.albumin 15.lymph node 16.immunoglobulin 17.Hageman factor 18.leukocyte 19.plasma 20.prothrombin 21.megakaryocyte 22.embolism 23.fibrinogen 24.thrombocyte 25.thrombin 26.tunica media 27.tunica intima 28.tunica externa

Learning Exercises: 1. 1-platelet plug, 2-clot formation, 3-clot dissolution 2. 1-Hageman factor, 2-prothrombin activator, 3-prothrombin, 4-thrombin, 5-fibrin, 6-intrinsic pathway, 7-extrinsic pathway (for more detail to these pathways, refer to Figure 14-6 in the Text) 3. pressure, compliance, systole, blood flow, capacitance, volume flow rate, flow velocity, average flow velocity, 4. 1-decreased ($R=x/r^4$ or $R=Lv/r^4$) 2-decreased ($R=xL$ or $R=Lv/r^4$) 3-increased ($R=x/r^4$ or $R=Lv/r^4$) 4-increased ($R=xv$ or $R=Lv/r^4$) 5-decreased (($R=xv$ or $R=Lv/r^4$) 6-decreased ($R_{total}=R'/N$)
5. systemic, total peripheral resistance, constriction, dilation, sympathetic, autonomic, constriction, perfusion 6. 1-arterial end, 2-blood colloid osmotic pressure, 3-blood pressure and negative interstitial pressure, 4-venous end

Quick Recall: (You should be able to answer these questions easily without correction or confirmation by this point in your studies. If you cannot, review your notes, the text chapter, and the previous study activities to find the answers.)

Practice Test: 1-e, 2-a, 3-a, 4-e, 5-b, 6-c, 7-c, 8-d, 9-c, 10-b, 11-a, 12-c, 13-b

Chapter 15
Regulation of the Cardiovascular System

Focus
Review this section *first*. It will help you focus on the overall message of this chapter.

Chapter Outline
Read through the outline slowly. This activity will help your mind organize the topics of this chapter.

Cardiovascular reflexes
    Components of the cardiovascular system
    Extrinsic control of vascular smooth muscle
    Intrinsic control of vascular smooth muscle
    Differences between vascular beds
    The baroreceptor reflex
    The role of blood volume regulation in blood pressure regulation
    Hypertension
Interaction of the heart and vessels
    Effect of cardiac output on central venous pressure
    Cardiovascular operating point
    Vascular determinants of cardiac output and mean arterial pressure
The cardiovascular system in exercise and disease
    Standing upright: the baroreceptor reflex and venous pumps
    Hemorrhage and hypovolemic shock
    Performance in sustained exercise: the cardiovascular limit
    Vascular changes in regulation of core body temperature

Learning Objectives
These are the learning goals for this part of the course. After reading the text, attending class, and studying this chapter, you should be able to:

♦   describe the autonomic innervation of blood vessels, distinguishing special features of blood vessels in skeletal muscle, the coronaries, and the external genitalia

♦   diagram the baroreceptor reflex

♦   describe how antidiuretic hormone, the atrial natriuretic hormone system and the renin-angiotensin-aldosterone system regulate mean arterial blood pressure

- appreciate the significance of the cardiovascular operating point in the regulation of central venous pressure, mean arterial pressure, and cardiac output

- understand how standing results in a drop in venous return and how mean arterial pressure is maintained by the baroreceptor reflex, venous valves, and the skeletal and respiratory pumps

- outline the changes that follow moderate hemorrhage

- describe the cardiovascular responses to exercise

- list factors that might be expected to lead to hypertension

Language of Physiology

Physiology uses its own set of terms, many of which may be unfamiliar to you. This section will help you improve your mastery of key physiological terms.

Word Parts

Here are some combining forms often seen in physiological terms. Give an example of a term that contains each word part listed.

Word Part	Meaning	Example
angio-	vessel	1_____
carot-	sleep; stupor	2_____
natri-	sodium	3_____
ortho-	straight	4_____
-rhage, -rhagia	breaking out	5_____
-tensin, -tension	pressure	6_____
varic-	enlarged vessel	7_____
vaso-	vessel	8_____
vol-	volume	9_____

Key Terms

Read each of the terms in each grouping below aloud, using the pronunciation guide if necessary. This will help you to remember them better than if you read them silently. Then, write out the correct term next to each of the descriptions given.

Terms Related to Processes

cardiac reserve
cardiac function curve
cardiovascular operating point
hemorrhage
hypertension
hypervolemia (hy-per-vol-EE-mee-ah)
hypotension
hypovolemia (hy-poh-vol-EE-mee-ah)

orthostatic hypotension
  (orth-oh-STAT-ik)
respiratory pump
skeletal muscle pump
vascular function curve
vasoconstriction (vaz-oh-kon-STRIK-shun)
vasodilation (vaz-oh-dy-LAY-shun)

1_____ decrease in the radius of a vessel

2_____ system formed by the combination of muscle contractions and the presence of unidirectional venous valves, propelling blood toward the heart as a sort of "pump"

3_____ increase in the radius of a vessel

4_____ condition resulting from a weak or absent baroreceptor reflex, in which standing is likely to cause fainting as a result of venous pooling and the subsequent drop in stroke volume

5_____ describes the actions of breathing in terms of their "pumping" of venous blood back to the heart (by means of the drop in intrapleural pressure during inspiration)

6_____ increased blood plasma volume

7_____ loss of blood from the circulatory system (through bleeding)

8_____ on a graph that plots both the vascular function curve and the cardiac function curve, the point where the two curves intersect

9_____ reduced arterial blood pressure, possibly causing underperfusion of critical organs

10_____ reduced blood plasma volume

11_____ graph of the relationship between cardiac output (venous return) and central venous pressure, thus describing the behavior of the peripheral vessels

12_____ amount that the cardiac output can increase above the normal resting level as a result of changes in venous return

13_____ chronic elevation of arterial blood pressure

14_____ graph of the relationship between cardiac output and venous pressure

Terms related to structures/substances

aldosterone (ahl-doh-STAYR-ohn)
angiotensin III (an-jee-oh-TEN-sin)
angiotensin II
angiotensin I
angiotensinogen
  (an-jee-oh-ten-SIN-oh-jen)
atrial natriuretic hormone [ANH]
  (nayt-ree-yoo-RET-ik)

carotid sinus (kah-ROT-id)
diuretic (dy-yoo-RET-ik)
renin
varicose vein
vasopressin (vaz-oh-PRES-in)

1 _____ a hormone released in response to increased atrial pressure (blood volume) that increases the rate of loss of plasma solutes and water in the urine

2 _____ a substance that tends to increase loss of fluid and solutes (via the urine)

3 _____ a vein that has become swollen because of an increase in its compliance

4 _____ a hormone released by endocrine cells of the kidney that catalyzes production of angiotensin and secretion of aldosterone

5 _____ a plasma protein that is converted to angiotensin I by the catalyzing action of renin

6 _____ a substance formed by angiotensin II when it is converted in the adrenal cortex; it stimulates aldosterone secretion

7 _____ a substance formed by angiotensinogen when acted upon by renin

8 _____ a substance formed by angiotensin I when acted upon by converting enzymes in the lung, liver, and other organs

9 _____ adrenal (steroid) hormone that decreases the rate of Na^+ loss in urine

10 _____ alternate name for antidiuretic hormone (ADH); it regulates water conservation by the kidneys, thirst sensation, and is a vasoconstrictor

11 _____ enlarged portion of the carotid artery (just superior to the heart) that contains the carotid baroreceptors

The Big Picture

Use the activities of this section to help you learn the broader concepts of this chapter.

Learning Exercises

1. Identify each of the substances listed below as a "dilator" or "constrictor," in terms of its effect(s) upon systemic blood vessels.

EXTRINSIC

Sympathetic neurotransmitters

1_____ α adrenergic

2_____ β adrenergic

3_____ cholinergic

Parasympathetic neurotransmitters

4_____ cholinergic

Hormones

5_____ vasopressin

6_____ angiotensin I, II

INTRINSIC

Metabolic

7_____ decreased O_2

8_____ decreased pH

9_____ increased K^+

Paracrine

10_____ prostaglandins

11_____ bradykinin

12_____ histamine

13_____ adenosine

2. Draw the major pathways of the baroreceptor reflex on Figure 15-1. Use solid lines to indicate nervous pathways and dotted lines to indicate endocrine pathways. Be sure to use arrows to indicate direction.

Figure 15-1

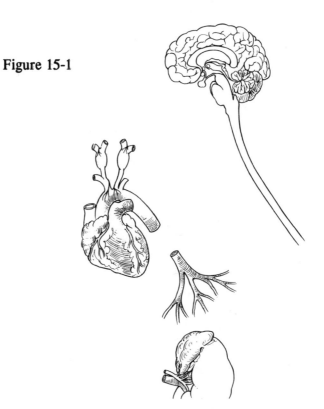

3. Use these terms to identify the substances indicated in Figure 15-2.

aldosterone   angiotensinogen
angiotensin I   antidiuretic hormone
angiotensin II   atrial natriuretic hormone

Figure 15-2

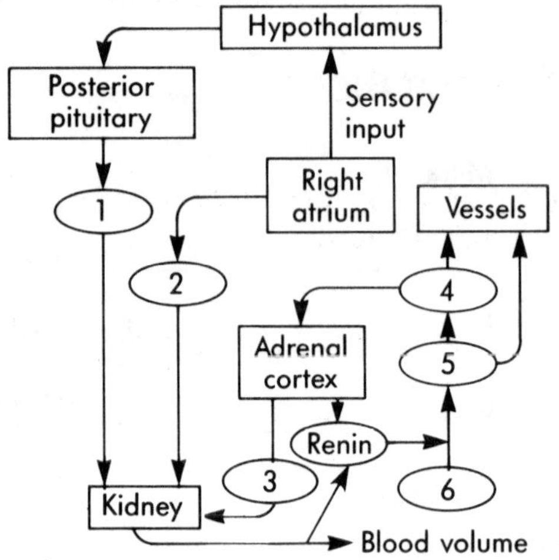

1 _____

2 _____

3 _____

4 _____

5 _____

6 _____

4. Use these terms to fill in the blanks in the paragraphs that follow. (Some terms may be used more than once.)

baroreceptor   muscular   respiratory
central venous   operating point   return
compliance   output   standing
compliant   pressure   total peripheral
hemorrhage   rate   resistance

The properties of the cardiovascular system are _____, blood volume,

venous _____, heart _____, and contractility. Given a

particular set of values for these properties, the cardiovascular _____ is the one

flow value for which the cardiac output equals the venous _____. A change in

one or more of the system's properties changes the outcome of the interaction between heart and

circulation and affects the system variables: _____ pressure, mean arterial

pressure and cardiac _____.

_____ results in pooling of the blood in _____

veins of the lower body, a drop in venous _____ and central venous pressure,

196

with a consequent drop of mean arterial _____ in the arteries superior to the

heart. Mean arterial pressure is maintained by the _____ reflex and with the

assistance of the _____ pump and _____ pump of the

veins. The responses to moderate _____ resemble those involved in standing,

except that lost fluid, plasma proteins, and blood cells must be replaced.

5. For each of the parameters listed, indicate whether it would be expected to "increase" or "decrease" from its resting level during submaximal exercise.

1_____ cardiac output   6_____ total peripheral resistance

2_____ arterial pressure   7_____ muscle blood flow

3_____ systolic pressure   8_____ flow to abdominal viscera

4_____ diastolic pressure   9_____ cutaneous blood flow

5_____ stroke volume

Quick Recall

Review some of the major concepts of this chapter by doing these "quick recall" activities.

1. List the autonomic innervations of the:

skeletal muscle vessels

coronary vessels

vessels of the external genitals

2. Name the locations of important baroreceptors.

3. List three major hormone systems that regulate mean arterial pressure.

4.   List the cardiovascular effects of standing upright.

5.   Outline the cardiovascular changes that follow moderate hemorrhage.

6.   List the cardiovascular responses to exercise.

7.   List factors that might be expected to lead to hypertension.

Practice Test
Use this practice test to review the topics of this chapter and to prepare for your test on this material.

1.   When blood volume is increased
        a.   the mean circulatory filling pressure increases
        b.   venous compliance increases
        c.   total peripheral resistance increases
        d.   the slope of the venous pressure curve changes
        e.   a and d are correct

2.   The slope of the venous pressure curve is
        a.   increased by increasing blood volume
        b.   independent of total peripheral resistance
        c.   increased by increases in venous compliance
        d.   a and c are correct
        e.   none are correct

3.   If the total peripheral resistance decreases
        a.   venous volume increases
        b.   cardiac output increases
        c.   mean filling pressure increases
        d.   venous pressure decreases
        e.   both b and c occur

4.   When myocardial contractility increases
        a.   cardiac output increases
        b.   blood pressure increases
        c.   cardiac reserve increases
        d.   venous pressure increases
        e.   all of the above

5.   During strenuous exercise
        a.   stroke volume increases
        b.   contractility increases
        c.   venous compliance increases
        d.   heart rate increases
        e.   all of the above

6. Venous valves
   a. reduce the hydrostatic pressure in the legs
   b. are found in areas subject to phasic muscular compression
   c. are absolutely required to maintain venous return
   d. become less effective with prolonged standing
   e. a, b, and d are correct

7. Baroreceptors
   a. discharge at a higher frequency when the mean arterial pressure is elevated
   b. discharge at a higher frequency when the arterial pressure is increasing
   c. are located in the carotid arteries
   d. decrease their firing rate following hemorrhage
   e. all of the above

8. Components of the baroreceptor reflex include
   a. a decrease in the total peripheral resistance
   b. an increase in venous compliance
   c. an increase in myocardial contractility
   d. an increase in heart rate
   e. both c and d

9. Aortic systolic pressure is decreased when
   a. myocardial contractility is decreased
   b. end-diastolic volume is increased
   c. total peripheral resistance is increased
   d. afferent nerves from aortic baroreceptors are stimulated
   e. a and d are correct

10. Which circulatory beds vasoconstrict when blood pressure decreases?
    a. cerebral
    b. cutaneous
    c. coronary
    d. renal
    e. both b and d

11. Serum renin increases when there is a fall in blood
    a. $[Ca^{++}]$
    b. pressure
    c. osmolarity
    d. pH
    e. ACTH

12. The volume receptor reflex involves
    a. decreased ADH secretion
    b. an increase in urine osmolarity
    c. an increase in sympathetic activity
    d. both b and c
    e. a, b, and c

13. Total peripheral resistance
    a. is less than renal resistance
    b. increases following acute blood loss
    c. is increased by parasympathetic activity
    d. is increased if the arterial blood pressure increases
    e. a and b are correct

14. The central venous pressure would be increased by
    a. increasing myocardial contractility
    b. administration of a liter of plasma
    c. decreasing venous compliance
    d. decreasing the total peripheral resistance
    e. b and d are correct

15. If the afferent arteriole to the kidney has a resistance that is higher than normal
    a. serum renin levels will be elevated
    b. mean arterial blood pressure will be decreased
    c. glomerular filtration rate will be increased
    d. plasma Na^+ will be elevated
    e. both a and d

Answers
Here are answers (or references) to some of the questions presented above.

Word Parts: (your examples may be different) 1-angiotensin, 2-carotid sinus, 3-natriuretic hormone, 4-orthostatic hypotension, 5-hemorrhage, 6-angiotensin, hypertension, 7-varicose vein, 8-vasodilation, 9-hypovolemia

Key Terms: Processes: 1. vasoconstriction 2. skeletal muscle pump 3. vasodilation 4. orthostatic hypotension 5. respiratory pump 6. hypervolemia 7. hemorrhage 8. cardiovascular operating point 9. hypotension 10. hypovolemia 11. vascular function curve 12. cardiac reserve 13. hypertension 14. cardiac function curve **Structures/Substances:** 1. atrial natriuretic hormone [ANH] 2. diuretic 3. varicose vein 4. renin 5. angiotensinogen 6. angiotensin III 7. angiotensin I 8. angiotensin II 9. aldosterone 10. vasopressin 11. carotid sinus

Learning Exercises: 1. 1-constrictor, 2-dilator, 3-dilator, 4-dilator, 5-constrictor, 6-constrictor, 7-dilator, 8-dilator, 9-dilator, 10-either, 11-dilator, 12-dilator, 13-dilator (see Tables 15-1 and 15-2 in the text for clarification) 2. (compare your figure to Figure 15-3 in the text) 3. 1-antidiuretic hormone, 2-atrial natriuretic hormone, 3-aldosterone, 4-angiotensin II, 5-angiotensin I, 6-angiotensinogen 4. total peripheral resistance, compliance, rate, operating point, return, central venous, output, standing, compliant, return, pressure, baroreceptor, respiratory, muscular, hemorrhage 5. 1-I, 2-I, 3-I, 4-D, 5-I, 6-D, 7-I, 8-D, 9-I

Quick Recall: (You should be able to answer these questions easily without correction or confirmation by this point in your studies. If you cannot, review your notes, the text chapter, and the previous study activities to find the answers.)

Practice Test: 1-e, 2-a, 3-e, 4-e, 5-e, 6-e, 7-e, 8-e, 9-a, 10-e, 11-b, 12-d, 13-e, 14-c, 15-e

Chapter 16
Respiratory Anatomy and the Mechanics of Breathing

Focus

Review this section *first*. It will help you focus on the overall message of this chapter.

Chapter Outline

Read through the outline slowly. This activity will help your mind organize the topics of this chapter.

Structure and function in the respiratory system
    The lungs and thorax
    The structures of the airway
    Sound production
    Protective functions of the airway
    Asbestosis and lung cancer: consequences of exposure to smoke and
    pollutants
    Acini and alveoli
Respiratory volumes and flow rates
    Lung volumes and capacities
    Alveolar ventilation and the anatomical dead space
The mechanics of breathing
    The lung–chest wall system
    Respiratory movements, pressure changes, and air flow
    The work of breathing
    The roles of pulmonary surfactant
    Pulmonary resistance and compliance in disease
Adaptations of the pulmonary circulation
    Pressure and flow in the pulmonary loop
    Capillary filtration and reabsorption in the lung
    Ventilation-perfusion matching

Learning Objectives

These are the learning goals for this part of the course. After reading the text, attending class, and studying this chapter, you should be able to:

◆ describe the components of the respiratory system, identifying the classes of airways, gas exchange elements, and the muscle responsible for ventilation

- ◆ describe the defense mechanisms of the lung

- ◆ understand how the terminal bronchioles are neurally and hormonally regulated

- ◆ appreciate the factors that affect gas exchange in the lung

- ◆ define the lung volumes and capacities and provide approximate normal values for them

- ◆ understand the factors that affect respiratory minute volume

- ◆ explain why intrapleural pressure is always less than alveolar pressure

- ◆ distinguish between the elastic and flow-resistive components of the work of breathing

- ◆ understand the roles of pulmonary surfactant

- ◆ summarize the basic characteristics of obstructive and restrictive lung disease

- ◆ compare pulmonary and systemic blood flow

- ◆ describe the conditions under which there may be an imbalance in the ventilation-perfusion ratio of regions of the lung, and show how this affects the O_2 and CO_2 content of alveolar gas

Language of Physiology

Physiology uses its own set of terms, many of which may be unfamiliar to you. This section will help you improve your mastery of key physiological terms.

Word Parts

Here are some combining forms often seen in physiological terms. Give an example of a term that contains each word part listed.

Word Part	Meaning	Example
alveol-	small hollow, cavity	1
bronch-	windpipe, air passage	2
dia-	across	3
-phragm	partition	4
pleur-	the side; rib	5
pneumo-	lung; breath	6
spiro-, -spire	breathe	7

Key Terms

Read each of the terms in each grouping below aloud, using the pronunciation guide if necessary. This will help you to remember them better than if you read them silently. Then, write out the correct term next to each of the descriptions given.

Terms related to measurement

alveolar minute volume (al-VEE-oh-lar)
anatomical dead space
expiratory reserve volume [ERV]
forced expiratory volume [FEV]
forced vital capacity [FVC]
functional residual capacity [FRC]
inspiratory capacity
inspiratory reserve volume [IRV]

residual volume [RV]
respiratory minute volume
respiratory rate
spirometry (spir-AHM-et-ree)
tidal volume [TV]
total lung capacity [TLC]
ventilation-perfusion ratio [V/Q]
vital capacity [VC]

1 _____   = VC + RV (approximately 5800 ml in a normal adult male)

2 _____   technique for measuring lung volume changes during inspiration and expiration

3 _____   total amount of air entering and leaving the respiratory system per minute (= TV x respiratory rate; typically 5000 ml/minute)

4 _____   rate of breathing cycles, expressed in breaths/minute

5 _____   volume of air remaining in the lungs after a maximal forced expiration (approximately 1200 ml)

6 _____   maximum amount of air that can be moved into and out of the lungs by muscular effort (= TV + IRV + ERV; approximately 3100 ml in females, 4600 ml in males)

7 _____   ratio of alveolar ventilation (V) to alveolar blood flow (Q); for the whole respiratory system, it equals alveolar minute volume divided by cardiac output (about 0.8)

8 _____   volume of air alternately inspired and expired in a single breath (approximately 500 ml)

9 _____   portion of the respiratory minute volume that ventilates the alveoli (and not the anatomical dead space)

10 _____ volume of air that can be expelled from the lung after the end of a passive expiration (approximately 1100 ml)

11 _____ region of the lung that cannot exchange gas

12 _____ volume of air that can be inspired after a normal inspiration (in the range of 3000 ml)

13 _____ volume of air forcefully expired (after forceful inspiration) during a specific period of time (a "dynamic" lung volume usually measured at 1-second intervals)

14 _____ total amount of air expelled during the FEV test, normally about equal to the vital capacity [VC]

15 _____ volume of air that can be inspired after normal expiration (= TV + IRV; typically about 3500 ml)

16 _____ volume of air that remains in the lung after a passive expiration (approximately 2300 ml)

Terms related to processes

mucociliary escalator
  (myoo-koh-SIL-ee-ayr-ee)
passive expiration

physiological dead space
physiological shunt
recruitment

1_____ case of V/Q mismatch in which a portion of the lung is inadequately ventilated (with air) but is well perfused (with blood), creating a situation in which blood is functionally "shunted" from areas in which gas exchange may occur

2_____ case of V/Q mismatch in which a portion of the lung is ventilated (with air) but is inadequately perfused (with blood), creating a "dead space" where no effective gas exchange can occur

3_____ process in the ciliated epithelial lining of the airway in which mucus is continually secreted and moved upward (toward the pharynx), carrying trapped particles with it

4_____ expiration involved in "quiet breathing," not driven by any muscle contractions but by the elastic recoil of the lungs and chest wall

5_____ in pulmonary physiology, the process of filling previously collapsed pulmonary blood vessels as cardiac output increases and the pulmonary pressure begins to rise

Terms related to structures/substances

acinus (AS-in-us)
allergen (AL-er-jen)
alveolar duct (al-VEE-oh-lar)
alveoli (al-VEE-oh-ly)
bronchus (BRON-kus)
conduction zone
diaphragm
diffusion zone
intercostal muscle
intrapleural space (in-trah-PLOO-ral)

larynx (LAYR-inks)
parenchyma cell (pah-REN-kih-mah)
pharynx (FAYR-inks)
pleura (PLOO-rah)
pulmonary surfactant
respiratory bronchiole (BRON-kee-ohl)
terminal bronchiole (BRON-kee-ohl)
thoracic cavity (thoh-RA-sik)
trachea (TRAY-kee-ah)
Type II alveolar cell (al-VEE-oh-lar)

1_____ phospholipid that, because of its amphipathic nature, reduces the surface tension of the fluid that lines the alveoli, thus reducing the force required to inflate the lung

2_____ sheet of skeletal muscle that forms the inferior boundary of the thoracic cavity and powers breathing

3_____ tiny (less than 0.5 mm) extension of a terminal bronchiole that has some alveoli in its walls

4_____ special type of epithelial cell in the lung that manufactures pulmonary surfactant

5_____ small, muscular extension of the respiratory bronchiole; it is the smallest airway leading to an alveolus

6_____ any of many skeletal muscles that connect one rib to the next

7_____ any of about 150,000 tiny, collapsible branches of the bronchi surrounded by multiunit smooth muscle cells; they connect the bronchi to the respiratory bronchioles

8 _____   any substance that triggers an inappropriate response of the immune system (allergic reaction)

9 _____   any of several air passages connecting the trachea to the alveoli in a treelike branched network; the largest are "primary," next largest "secondary," next "tertiary," and so on

10 _____   chest cavity; superior portion of the ventral body cavity, it houses the lungs and heart

11 _____   in the lung, a functional unit resembling a bunch of grapes arising from a terminal bronchiole and including all the attached respiratory bronchioles, alveolar ducts, and alveoli

12 _____   sheet of epithelial tissue that lines the interior of the thorax (parietal layer) and surrounds each lung (visceral layer)

13 _____   "windpipe"; a single air passage topped by the larynx and splitting into two bronchi inferiorly

14 _____   portion of the lung that conducts air (bulk flow) over long distances, consisting of the bronchial tree and bronchioles

15 _____   portion of the lung in which gases diffuse between the air in the respiratory passage and blood in the surrounding capillaries (this zone consists of the respiratory bronchioles, alveolar ducts and alveoli)

16 _____   space between the parietal pleura and the visceral pleura that is filled with lubricating intrapleural fluid

17 _____   throat; the portion of the upper respiratory tract just superior to the larynx

18 _____   "voice box"; the portion of the upper respiratory tract at the superior end of the trachea, containing the vocal folds

19 _____   tiny sac-like membranous structures in the lung across which gas exchange takes place

20 _____   type of cell in the lung that forms a mesh of elastic connective tissue that supports the alveoli

Other Key Terms

Boyle's Law
fibrosis (fy-BROH-sis)
Law of Laplace (la-PLAHS)
obstructive pulmonary disease

pneumothorax (noo-moh-THOR-aks)
respiratory distress syndrome
restrictive pulmonary disease

1 _____   category of pulmonary disease that includes conditions involving an increase in airway resistance

2 _____   scientific law that relates the pressure (P) inside a sphere to the tension (T) in its walls: $P = T/2r$

3 _____   category of pulmonary disease that includes conditions involving a decrease in lung compliance

4 _____   condition involving an increase in fibrous tissue, that in the lung reduces compliance

5 _____   also called hyaline membrane disease, a condition involving inadequate pulmonary surfactant, which causes low lung compliance (and thus respiratory distress)

6 _____   condition in which air enters the intrapleural space, causing the lung to collapse to its minimal volume

7_____ one of the so-called gas laws; it states that (at a constant temperature) the product of the pressure and volume of a gas is constant

The Big Picture
Use the activities of this section to help you learn the broader concepts of this chapter.

Learning Exercises

1. Label the portions of the airways shown in Figure 16-1 as indicated.

acinus	primary (main) bronchi	terminal bronchiole
alveolar duct	respiratory bronchiole	tertiary (segmental)
alveoli	secondary (lobar)	bronchus
larynx	bronchus	trachea

Figure 16-1

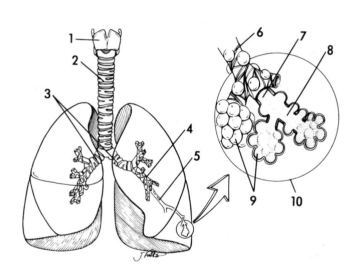

CONDUCTION ZONE

1_____

2_____

3_____

4_____

5_____

6_____

DIFFUSION ZONE

7_____

8_____

9_____

10_____

2. For each of the factors listed, indicate whether each would tend to "constrict" the bronchiolar airways or "dilate" the bronchiolar airways.

1_____parasympathetic input (acetylcholine)

2_____sympathetic input (epinephrine, norepinephrine)

3_____antihistamines

4_____irritants (smoke, dust, chemicals)

5_____prostaglandins D_2, $F_2\alpha$

6_____histamine

7_____adrenergic antagonists (theophylline)

8_____increased CO_2 in alveolar air

9_____leukotrines

3. Identify the lung volumes and capacities represented by the spirometry graph shown in Figure 16-2.

expiratory reserve volume   residual volume
functional residual capacity   tidal volume
inspiratory reserve volume   total lung capacity
inspiratory capacity   vital capacity

Figure 16-2

1_____

2_____

3_____

4_____

5_____

6_____

7_____

8_____

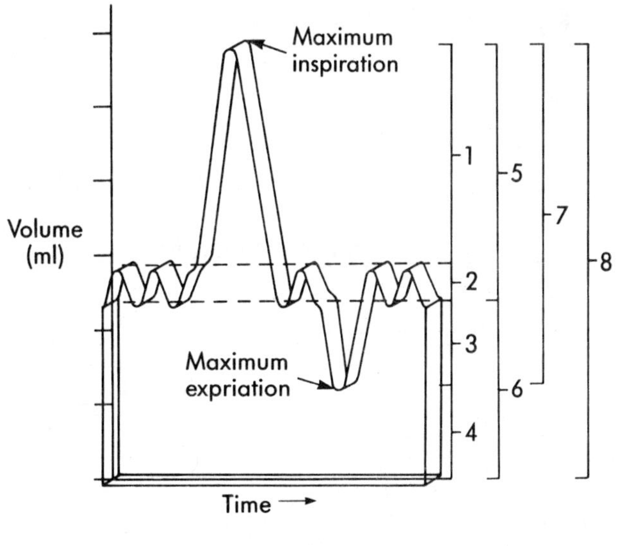

4.   Use the terms given to fill in the blanks in the paragraphs that follow.

muscles   ventilation   alveoli
pressure   elastic   reduced
Boyle's   flow-resistive   reduced
mechanically   tidal   large
alveolar   respiratory
recoil   surfactant

Respiratory _____ cause volume changes of the thorax, which result in

_____ changes in the thorax according to _____ Law.

The lungs and chest wall are _____ coupled by intrapleural fluid. The

intrapleural pressure is always less than _____ pressure because of inward elastic

_____ of the lung.

The total work in _____ is the sum of work done in changing the volume

of the lung –chest wall (_____ component) and the work done to move air

through the system (_____ component). Both components depend on

_____ volume and _____ rate, which are adjusted to

minimize the work of breathing.

Pulmonary _____ reduces the surface tension of the air-water interface in

the _____, with two major consequences for the lung. First, the work of

expanding the alveoli is _____. Second, the tendency of small alveoli to merge

into larger ones is _____, so that the _____ surface area

of the alveoli is maintained.

5. Compare pulmonary and systemic blood flow by filling in the blanks in the table below.

	Systematic	Pulmonary
Blood flow resistance	high	1
Arterial pressure required	2	low
Independent of cardiac output?	no	3
Pumping by which ventricle?	4	5

6. Because of unequal airflow to different parts of the lung, the respiratory system tries to maximize efficiency of gas exchange through a process called *ventilation-perfusion matching*. This process is summarized in the table below. Fill in the missing parts.

	V/Q ratio too high	V/Q ratio too low
Change in alveolar O_2	increased	
Change in alveolar CO_2		
Response of pulmonary arterioles	dilate	
Response of bronchioles		dilate

Quick Recall
Review some of the major concepts of this chapter by doing these "quick recall" activities.

1. Name the major anatomical components of the respiratory system.

2. List the major defense mechanisms of the lungs.

3. Name the control mechanisms of bronchiolar diameter.

4. List the major lung volumes (and their approximate normal values).

5. List the major lung capacities (and their approximate normal values).

6. List the factors that affect respiratory minute volume.

7. List some conditions that may cause an imbalance in the ventilation-perfusion ratio.

8.   Name two roles of pulmonary surfactant.

9.   Describe how sound is produced by the respiratory system.

Practice Test
Use this practice test to review the topics of this chapter and to prepare for your test on this material.

1. The conducting portion of the respiratory system
    a.   secretes mucus
    b.   removes debris
    c.   constitutes a dead space
    d.   warms and humidifies the air
    e.   all of the above

2. Gas exchange with the pulmonary blood occurs in the
    a.   bronchi
    b.   bronchioles (all)
    c.   alveoli
    d.   terminal bronchioles
    e.   both c and d are correct

3. Which of the following lung spaces cannot be measured with a spirometer?
    a.   vital capacity
    b.   residual volume
    c.   tidal volume
    d.   functional residual capacity
    e.   both b and d

4. The difference between the total lung capacity and the residual volume is the
    a.   vital capacity
    b.   inspiratory reserve volume
    c.   tidal volume
    d.   expiratory reserve volume
    e.   functional residual capacity

5. The intrapleural pressure
    a.   is always below atmospheric
    b.   is always less than the intra-alveolar pressure
    c.   decreases on inspiration
    d.   both b and c are correct
    e.   all are correct

Use these data for Nos. 6 and 7: a person has a residual volume of 1000 ml; total lung capacity of 6000 ml; functional residual capacity of 2000 ml; tidal volume of 500 ml

6. The vital capacity of this individual is
    a.   2000 ml
    b.   3000 ml
    c.   4000 ml
    d.   5000 ml
    e.   6000 ml

7. The expiratory reserve volume of this subject is
    a.   500 ml
    b.   1000 ml
    c.   1500 ml
    d.   2200 ml
    e.   none of the above

8. Pulmonary
    a.   mean blood pressure is greater than systemic mean blood pressure
    b.   vascular resistance is greater than systemic vascular resistance
    c.   vascular resistance is independent of cardiac output
    d.   blood vessels have little autonomic innervation

9. Pulmonary surfactant
    a.   lines the gas side of the alveolar-capillary membrane
    b.   has an area-dependent surface tension
    c.   reduces the force required to expand the lungs
    d.   eliminates the tendency for large alveoli to empty into smaller ones
    e.   all of the above are correct

10. Lung compliance is
    a.   increased by a decrease in surfactant
    b.   decreased in emphysema
    c.   larger at larger lung volumes
    d.   less in a fluid-filled lung
    e.   none of the above

11. During a resting tidal expiration in a normal person
    a.   alveolar pressure is subatmospheric
    b.   intrapleural pressure is subatmospheric
    c.   the expiratory muscles are active
    d.   the diaphragm is contracting
    e.   none of the above

12. In a standing individual
    a.   ventilation of the apex is less than ventilation of the base
    b.   perfusion of the base is less than perfusion of the apex
    c.   the apical alveoli are less compliant
    d.   there is a ventilation-perfusion gradient
    e.   all of the above are correct

13. Increasing airway resistance will
    a.   increase the elastic work of breathing
    b.   increase the flow resistive work of breathing
    c.   result in a greater alveolar pressure during expiration
    d.   favor airway collapse
    e.   b, c, and d are all correct

14. Forced expiration is
    a.   an active process requiring expenditure of muscular energy
    b.   a passive process involving relaxation of the inspiratory muscles
    c.   aided by the abdominal muscles
    d.   aided by the diaphragm
    e.   a, c, and d are correct

15. During severe exercise, work of breathing increases because
    a.   tidal volume increases
    b.   breathing frequency increases
    c.   expiration is, in part, active
    d.   airflow turbulence increases
    e.   all of the above

Answers

Word Parts: (your examples may be different) 1-alveoli, 2-bronchiole, 3-diaphragm, 4-diaphragm, 5-intrapleural space, 6-pneumothorax, 7-spirometry

Key Terms: Measurement: 1. total lung capacity [TLC] 2. spirometry 3. respiratory minute volume 4. respiratory rate 5. residual volume [RV] 6. vital capacity [VC] 7. ventilation-perfusion ratio [V/Q] 8. tidal volume [TV] 9. alveolar minute volume 10. expiratory reserve volume [ERV] 11. anatomical dead space 12. inspiratory reserve volume [IRV] 13. forced expiratory volume [FEV] 14. forced vital capacity [FVC] 15. inspiratory capacity 16. functional residual capacity [FRC]
Processes: 1. physiological shunt 2. physiological dead space 3. mucociliary escalator 4. passive expiration 5. recruitment
Structures/Substances 1. pulmonary surfactant 2. diaphragm 3. respiratory bronchiole 4. type II alveolar cell 5. alveolar duct 6. intercostal muscle 7. terminal bronchiole 8. allergen 9. bronchus 10. thoracic cavity 11. acinus 12. pleura 13. trachea 14. conduction zone 15. diffusion zone 16. intrapleural space 17. pharynx 18. larynx 19. alveoli 20. parenchyma cell
Other: 1. obstructive pulmonary disease 2. Law of Laplace 3. restrictive pulmonary disease 4. fibrosis 5. respiratory distress syndrome 6. pneumothorax 7. Boyle's law

Learning Exercises: 1. 1-larynx, 2-trachea, 3-primary bronchi, 4-secondary bronchus, 5-tertiary bronchus, 6-terminal bronchiole, 7-respiratory bronchiole, 8-alveolar duct, 9-alveoli, 10-acinus 2. 1-constrict, 2-dilate, 3-dilate, 4-constrict, 5-constrict, 6-constrict, 7-dilate, 8-dilate, 9-constrict 3. 1-inspiratory reserve volume, 2-tidal volume, 3-expiratory reserve volume, 4-residual volume, 5-inspiratory capacity, 6-functional residual capacity, 7-vital capacity, 8-total lung capacity 4. muscles, pressure, Boyle's, mechanically, alveolar, recoil, ventilation, elastic, flow-resistive, tidal, respiratory, surfactant, alveoli, reduced, reduced, large 5. 1-low, 2-high, 3-yes, 4-left, 5-right 6. (check your answers with Table 16-6 in the text)

Quick Recall: (You should be able to answer these questions easily without correction or confirmation by this point in your studies. If you cannot, review your notes, the text chapter, and the previous study activities to find the answers.)

Practice Test: 1-e, 2-c, 3-e, 4-a, 5-e, 6-d, 7-b, 8-c, 9-e, 10-d, 11-e, 12-e, 13-e, 14-e, 15-e

Chapter 17
Gas Exchange and Gas Transport in the Blood

Focus
Review this section *first*. It will help you focus on the overall message of this chapter.

Chapter Outline
Read through the outline slowly. This activity will help your mind organize the topics of this chapter.

Physics and chemistry of gases
  Molecular properties of liquids and gases
  The gas laws
  Water vapor
  Gases in solution
Gas exchange in alveoli
  The composition of alveolar gas
  The gas composition of pulmonary blood
Oxygen transport in the blood
  Hemoglobin and the problem of oxygen solubility
  Oxygen loading in the lungs
  Oxygen unloading in systemic capillaries
  Effects of CO_2, pH, temperature, and 2,3-DPG on O_2 unloading
  O_2 transfer from mother to fetus
  Myoglobin — an intracellular O_2 binding protein
Carbon dioxide transport and blood buffers
  The CO_2-H_2CO_3-HCO_3^- equilibrium
  Blood buffers and control of plasma pH
  CO_2 loading in systemic capillaries — the Haldane effect
  CO_2 unloading in the lungs

Learning Objectives
These are the learning goals for this part of the course. After reading the text, attending class, and studying this chapter, you should be able to:

♦ apply the gas laws to gas mixtures in the respiratory tract and gases dissolved in the blood and tissues

♦ understand the concept of partial pressure

♦ describe how O_2 is transported in the blood by hemoglobin

- appreciate why the sigmoid oxyhemoglobin dissociation curve maximizes O_2 loading in the lungs and unloading in the tissues

- describe the factors that shift the oxyhemoglobin dissociation curve to the right

- compare the oxyhemoglobin dissociation curve for adult hemoglobin to those for fetal hemoglobin and myoglobin

- describe how CO_2 in the blood is carried as HCO_3^-

- be able to apply the Henderson-Hasselbalch equation to bicarbonate transport in the blood

Language of Physiology

Physiology uses its own set of terms, many of which may be unfamiliar to you. This section will help you improve your mastery of key physiological terms.

Word Parts

Here are some combining forms often seen in physiological terms. Give an example of a term that contains each word part listed.

Word Part	Meaning	Example
a-, an-	without, not	1
glob-	ball	2
oxy-	oxygen	3

Key Terms

Read each of the terms in each grouping below aloud, using the pronunciation guide if necessary. This will help you to remember them better than if you read them silently. Then, write out the correct term next to each of the descriptions given.

Terms related to measurement

° Kelvin

oxyhemoglobin dissociation curve
  (aks-ee-hee-moh-GLOH-bin)

partial pressure

relative saturation

respiratory quotient [RQ]

solubility

vapor pressure

1_____ term that refers to the percent saturation of hemoglobin at a given partial pressure of O_2

2_____ amount (mass) of a solute that can be dissolved in a given amount of solvent

3_____ graphic representation of the relationship between the partial pressure of oxygen and the relative saturation of hemoglobin with O_2

4_____ ratio of CO_2 produced during metabolism to O_2 consumed

5 _____ pressure that one gas (in a mixture of gases) would exert if it were present alone in the same volume (as the mixture)

6 _____ pressure exerted by a solid or liquid that is at equilibrium with its own vapor (gaseous form) — for instance, 47 mm Hg for water at 37° C

7 _____ unit of temperature on the absolute temperature scale (Kelvin scale)

Terms related to structures/substances

2,3 diphosphoglycerate [2,3-DPG]
  (2-3-dy-fahs-foh-GLIH-ser-ayt)
carbaminohemoglobin
  (carb-ah-mee-no-hee-moh-GLOH-bin)
carbonic anhydrase
  (kar-BAHN-ik an-HYD-rayz)
deoxyhemoglobin
  (dee-aks-ee-hee-moh-GLOH-bin)

fetal hemoglobin
heme group (heem)
hemoglobin [Hb]
oxyhemoglobin
  (aks-ee-hee-moh-GLOH-bin)

1 _____ nonprotein portion of the hemoglobin molecule; the portion of hemoglobin to which up to four O_2 molecules bind

2 _____ oxygen binding protein found within the erythrocytes of normal adult human blood

3 _____ hemoglobin molecule whose heme group is fully saturated with (four) O_2 molecules

4 _____ form of hemoglobin found in developing fetuses, different from the Hb of normal adults

5 _____ form of hemoglobin that has lost one or more of its attached O_2 molecules

6 _____ metabolite of RBCs that increases at low PO_2 and is able to shift the oxyhemoglobin dissociation curve

7 _____ form of Hb to which CO_2 is bound

8 _____ enzyme in RBCs and other cells that increases the rate of carbonic acid (H_2CO_3) formation from CO_2 and H_2O

Other Key Terms

alveolar gas equation (al-VEE-oh-lar)
Bohr effect
Charles' law
chloride shift
gas equation
Dalton's law
Gay-Lussac's law (gay-LOO-sak's)
Haldane effect
Henderson-Hasselbalch equation
  (HEN-der-son HA-sel-balk)

Henry's law
ideal [gas]
iron deficiency anemia
pernicious anemia
sickle cell anemia
thalassemia (thal-ah-SEE-mee-ah)
universal gas constant

1 _____ gas law that states that (at equilibrium) the concentration of a dissolved gas depends on the partial pressure of the gas and its solubility

2 _____ term that refers to the effect of reduced O_2 in Hb on the dissociation curve of CO_2: deoxygenated Hb results in greater CO_2 loading

3 _____ derivative of Charles' law, this gas law states that volume changes proportionally to temperature, consequently changing pressure also

4 _____ genetic RBC disorder in which a substituted amino acid in the Hb β-chain causes Hb to aggregate into large polymers at a low PO_2 (distorting the RBC shape)

5 _____ deficiency of Hb in erythrocytes stemming from a dietary deficiency of iron (Fe)

6 _____ term that describes a gas or gas mixture that has a low density at physiological temperatures, thus having few interactions of gas molecules

7 _____ term that refers to the movement of Cl^- from plasma into the RBC in exchange for HCO_3^-, preventing buildup of HCO_3^- in the RBC (which would oppose dissociation of CO_2)

8 _____ gas law that applies the combined gas equation to mixtures of gases as well as pure gases (since a mole of pure gas has the same number of particles as a mole of a mix of gases), stating that the total pressure of a mixture is equal to the partial pressures of each of the component gases

9 _____ genetic RBC disorder in which defective Hb α-chains or β-chains cause lower amounts of Hb per cell and abnormal O_2 binding characteristics

10 _____ algebraic expression that allows calculation of the alveolar partial pressure of O_2 when the inspired partial pressure of O_2, alveolar partial pressure of CO_2, and alveolar ventilation are known

11 _____ algebraic expression summarizing Boyle's law, Charles' law, and Gay-Lussac's law ($PV = nRT$)

12 _____ impairment of red blood cell formation caused by a dietary deficiency of (or failure to absorb) vitamin B_{12}

13 _____ one of the gas laws, it states: at constant pressure, the volume of a gas is proportional to temperature

14 _____ constant R, used in the combined gas equation ($PV = nRT$)

15 _____ law of mass action applied to the reaction of CO_2 with H_2O to form bicarbonate and H^+. It describes the interrelationships between plasma pH, bicarbonate concentration, and the partial pressure of CO_2

16 _____ shift in the oxyhemoglobin dissociation curve produced by changes in pH, CO_2, or temperature

The Big Picture

Use the activities of this section to help you learn the broader concepts of this chapter.

Learning Exercises

1. There are four blood gas partial-pressure values missing in Figure 17-1 (marked 1,2,3,4). Put the correct values (in mm Hg) in the blanks provided.

Figure 17-1

1 _____

2 _____

3 _____

4 _____

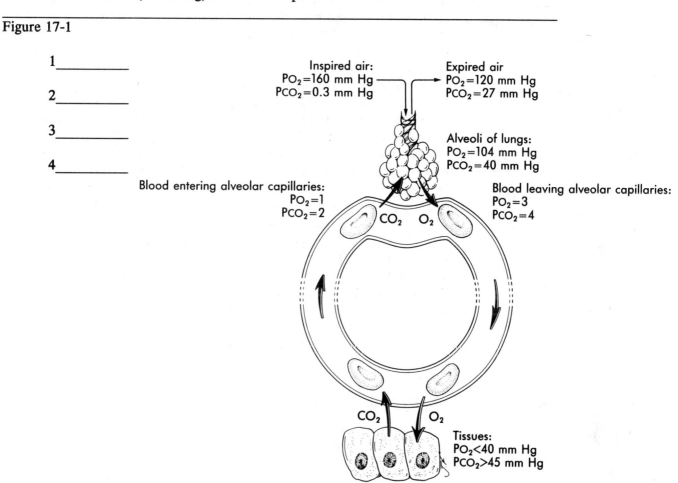

Inspired air:
PO_2=160 mm Hg
PCO_2=0.3 mm Hg

Expired air
PO_2=120 mm Hg
PCO_2=27 mm Hg

Alveoli of lungs:
PO_2=104 mm Hg
PCO_2=40 mm Hg

Blood entering alveolar capillaries:
PO_2=1
PCO_2=2

Blood leaving alveolar capillaries:
PO_2=3
PCO_2=4

CO_2 O_2

CO_2 O_2

Tissues:
PO_2<40 mm Hg
PCO_2>45 mm Hg

2. Fill in the values (vol%) for gas transport in the blood in the table below.

	Transport form	Systemic arteries	Systemic veins
O_2	in (physical) solution	_____	_____
	as HbO_2	_____	_____
	Total O_2 transported	19.8 vol%	14.5 vol%
CO_2	in (physical) solution	_____	_____
	as bicarbonate	_____	_____
	as carbaminoHb	_____	_____
	Total CO_2 transported	49.0 vol%	54.0 vol%

Figure 17-2. Use this graph representing the oxyhemoglobin dissociation curve as a reference for the next few learning activities.

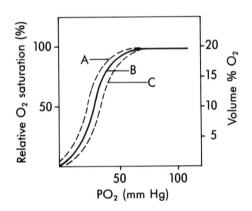

3. Use these terms to fill in the blanks in the paragraphs that follow.

2,3-DPG	increased	oxyhemoglobin
alveolar	left	dissociation
Bohr	myoglobin	right
decreased	oxygen	sigmoid
fetal	small	

Line B in the graph shown in Figure 17-2 represents the _____ curve

under systemic arterial conditions. The flat top portion of this _____

(S-shaped) curve allows Hb to load _____ to near 100% saturation even if

_____ PO_2 falls below normal. The steep portion of the curve allows a large

amount of oxygen to be delivered to the tissues with a relatively _____ drop in

PO_2.

Line C shows a _____ shift of the _____ curve.

This shift can be caused by _____ pH and _____ CO_2

(the _____ effect). The curve may also shift in this direction because of

increased RBC production of _____, and by _____

temperature. This type of shift decreases the affinity of hemoglobin for _____;

the greater the shift, the greater the _____ unloading.

Line A shows a _____ shift of the normal adult curve, which could

represent the O_2-dissociation characteristics of _____ in muscle cells, or

_____ hemoglobin. In either case, this type of shift infers a greater affinity of

Hb for _____. This allows oxygen to be drawn from the regular blood supply

for storage in the cell (in the case of _____) or allows it to be drawn from the

maternal blood easily (in the case of _____ Hb).

4. Use these terms to identify the numbered labels in Figure 17-3.

| carbonic anhydrase | HbO_2 | MbO_2 |
| CO_2 | HCO_3^- | |

Figure 17-3

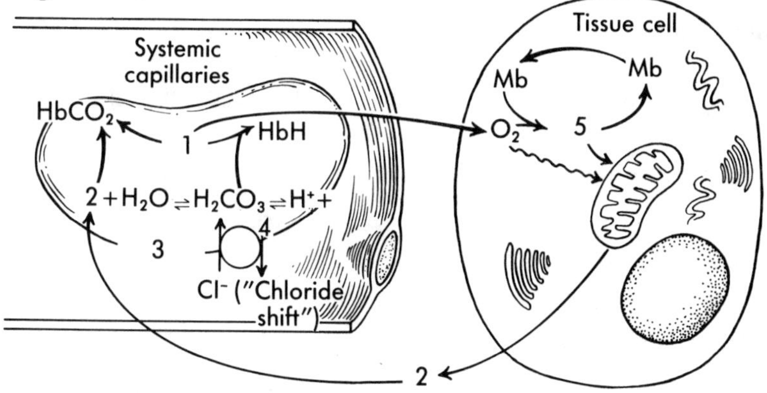

1 _____

2 _____

3 _____

4 _____

5 _____

5. Use the grid in Figure 17-4 below to draw a rough sketch of a typical graph of the CO_2-Hb dissociation curve in venous blood. Be sure to label the x-axis and y-axis correctly. When you have finished, answer the questions below.

a. Contrast the shape of this curve with the oxyhemoglobin dissociation curve.

b. Of what significance is this difference?

c. A shift of this curve to the left would be an expression of the _____ effect.

d. What factors would cause a left shift of the curve?

Quick Recall
Review some of the major concepts of this chapter by doing these "quick recall" activities.

1. Identify the relevance (applications) of each of these gas laws to the study of respiratory physiology:

Boyle's law

Charles' law

Dalton's law

Gay-Lussac's law

Henry's law

2.   Name the two principal forms in which oxygen is transported by the blood.

3.   Name the three principal forms in which carbon dioxide is transported by the blood.

4.   List the chemical events that cause blood pH to drop as CO_2 increases.

5.   List four buffering systems in the blood.

6.   Describe the shape of the O_2-Hb dissociation curve.

7.   List four factors that may cause a shift of the O_2-Hb dissociation curve to the right.

8.   Describe the shape of the CO_2-Hb dissociation curve.

Practice Test

Use this practice test to review the topics of this chapter and to prepare for your test on this material.

1.   A container of blood is placed in a large chamber containing oxygen at a partial pressure of 200 mm Hg and carbon dioxide at a partial pressure of 10 mm Hg. At equilibrium
        a.   the partial pressure of oxygen in the blood will be 200 mm Hg
        b.   the partial pressure of carbon dioxide in the blood will be 10 mm Hg
        c.   the amounts of dissolved oxygen and carbon dioxide will be similar
        d.   a and b are correct
        e.   a, b and c are correct

2.   The alveolar oxygen partial pressure in a person is 500 mm Hg. This would substantially
        a.   increase the rate of oxygen diffusion from the alveoli to the capillaries
        b.   increase the oxygen partial pressure in the pulmonary capillaries
        c.   increase the oxygen content of the blood
        d.   both a and b
        e.   a, b, and c

3. Diffusion limitation
   a. does not occur in a normal lung
   b. can result from alveolar fluid accumulation
   c. will affect oxygen more than carbon dioxide
   d. can decrease the arterial partial pressure of oxygen
   e. all of the above

4. Adult Hb
   a. can bind four molecules of oxygen
   b. can bind more oxygen at a given partial pressure than fetal Hb
   c. can bind more oxygen at a given partial pressure than myoglobin
   d. exhibits cooperativity in its binding of oxygen
   e. a and d are correct

5. Which of the following increase the oxygen affinity of Hb?
   a. an increase in oxygen partial pressure
   b. a decrease in pH
   c. an increase in 2,3-DPG concentration
   d. an increase in the partial pressure of carbon dioxide
   e. none of the above

6. Under normal conditions, hemoglobin is 50% saturated with oxygen at a partial pressure of
   a. 10 mm Hg
   b. 26 mm Hg
   c. 40 mm Hg
   d. 100 mm Hg
   e. 150 mm Hg

7. Which of the following will significantly increase the arterial oxygen content?
   a. increasing the inspired partial pressure of oxygen
   b. increasing the Hb concentration
   c. increasing the alveolar ventilation
   d. increasing the cardiac output
   e. a and b are correct

8. The O_2-Hb dissociation curve for blood leaving an exercising muscle is shifted relative to that for arterial blood because the venous blood from the muscle has a
   a. higher CO_2 partial pressure
   b. higher pH
   c. higher temperature
   d. a and c are correct
   e. a, b, and c are correct

9. In an anemic individual there will be a lower arterial
   a. blood oxygen content
   b. oxygen partial pressure
   c. hemoglobin saturation %
   d. both a and b
   e. a, b, and c

10. The arterial-venous O_2 difference for mixed venous blood
    a.   is normally 5 vols%
    b.   is increased when alveolar ventilation is increased
    c.   is increased during exercise
    d.   is independent of cardiac output
    e.   both a and c are correct

11. Most carbon dioxide is transported as
    a.   bicarbonate
    b.   carbonic acid
    c.   carbamino compounds
    d.   dissolved carbon dioxide
    e.   none of the above

12. The dissociation curve for carbon dioxide
    a.   is a rectangular hyperbola
    b.   is approximately linear
    c.   depends on hemoglobin oxygen saturation
    d.   a and c are correct
    e.   b and c are correct

The following data are to be used for the last three questions:
Arterial PO_2 = 40 mm Hg
Venous PO_2 = 26 mm Hg
Hb concentration = 15 mg/100 ml blood
P_{50} for Hb = 26 mm Hg

13. The arterial oxygen content is approximately
    a.   5 vols%
    b.   10 vols%
    c.   15 vols%
    d.   20 vols%
    e.   cannot be determined

14. The arterial-venous oxygen content difference is approximately
    a.   2.5 vols%
    b.   5 vols%
    c.   10 vols%
    d.   20 vols%
    e.   cannot be determined

15. The % saturation of hemoglobin in the venous blood is approximately
    a.   10%
    b.   20%
    c.   50%
    d.   75%
    e.   cannot be determined

Answers

Here are answers (or references) to some of the questions presented above.

Word Parts: (your examples may be different) 1-carbonic anhydrase, 2-hemoglobin, 3-oxyhemoglobin

Key Terms: Measurement: 1. relative saturation 2. solubility 3. oxyhemoglobin dissociation curve 4. respiratory quotient [RQ] 5. partial pressure 6. vapor pressure 7. ° Kelvin
Structures/Substances: 1. heme group 2. hemoglobin [Hb] 3. oxyhemoglobin 4. fetal hemoglobin 5. deoxyhemoglobin 6. 2,3 diphosphoglycerate [2,3-DPG] 7. carbaminohemoglobin 8. carbonic anhydrase
Other: 1. Henry's law 2. Haldane effect 3. Gay-Lussac's law 4. sickle cell anemia 5. iron deficiency anemia 6. ideal [gas] 7. chloride shift 8. Dalton's law 9. thalassemia 10. alveolar gas equation 11. gas equation 12. pernicious anemia 13. Charles' law 14. universal gas constant 15. Henderson-Hasselbalch equation 16. Bohr effect

Learning Exercises: 1. 1-40mm Hg, 2-45mm Hg, 3-104mm Hg, 4-40mm Hg 2. (compare your table to Table 17-2 in the text) 3. oxyhemoglobin dissociation, sigmoid, oxygen, alveolar, small, right, oxyhemoglobin dissociation, decreased, increased, Bohr, 2,3-DPG, increased, oxygen, oxygen, left,
myoglobin, fetal, oxygen, myoglobin, fetal 4. 1-HbO_2, 2-CO_2, 3-carbonic anhydrase, 4-HCO_3^-, 5-MbO_2 5. (your curve should be similar to that in Figure 17-12 in the text) a-this curve is linear, the other is sigmoid (nonlinear), b-CO_2 dissociation is directly proportional to PCO_2, whereas O_2 dissociation varies nonlinearly with PO_2, c-Haldane, d-O_2 dissociation from Hb, increasing the formation of reduced Hb and carbamino compounds (both of which increase the CO_2-carrying capacity)

Quick Recall: (You should be able to answer these questions easily without correction or confirmation by this point in your studies. If you cannot, review your notes, the text chapter, and the previous study activities to find the answers.)

Practice Test: 1-d, 2-e, 3-e, 4-e, 5-a, 6-b, 7-e, 8-d, 9-a, 10-e, 11-a, 12-e, 13-c, 14-b, 15-c

Chapter 18
Regulation of the Respiratory System

Focus
Review this section *first*. It will help you focus on the overall message of this chapter.

Chapter Outline
Read through the outline slowly. This activity will help your mind organize the topics of this chapter.

The rhythm of breathing
      The central motor program for the respiratory system
      How the CNS generates the basic rhythm of breathing
The chemical stimuli for breathing
      Arterial PCO_2 — the central chemoreceptors
      The choroid plexuses and the ventilatory setpoint
      Arterial PO_2 and pH — the carotid and aortic chemoreceptors
Integrated responses of the respiratory control system
      Interactions between peripheral and central chemoreceptors
      Breath-holding
      Acclimatization to altitude
      Acute acidosis
      Respiratory disease
      The ventilatory response to exercise

Learning Objectives
These are the learning goals for this part of the course. After reading the text, attending class, and studying this chapter, you should be able to:

◆ understand how respiratory motor movements are affected by centers in the medulla and pons

◆ list the factors affecting the intensity of respiratory drive, rate of breathing, and tidal volume

◆ explain how, by monitoring the pH of cerebrospinal fluid (CSF), the central chemoreceptors serve to regulate the arterial PCO_2

◆ appreciate how inputs from the peripheral chemoreceptors become important during hypoxia and acid-base imbalance

◆ describe the ventilatory responses to high-altitude exposure

- understand the role of the respiratory system in responding to acute metabolic acidosis and lung disease

- describe the factors that determine the ventilatory increase during exercise

Language of Physiology
Physiology uses its own set of terms, many of which may be unfamiliar to you. This section will help you improve your mastery of key physiological terms.

Word Parts
Here are some combining forms often seen in physiological terms. Give an example of a term that contains each word part listed.

Word Part	Meaning	Example
capn-	smoke	1
chemo-	chemical	2
chor-	skin	3
-ia, -sia	condition; process	4
-oid	like; in the shape of	5
plex-	twisted; woven	6

Key Terms
Read each of the terms in each grouping below aloud, using the pronunciation guide if necessary. This will help you to remember them better than if you read them silently. Then, write out the correct term next to each of the descriptions given.

Terms related to processes
Hering-Breuer reflex (HAYR-ing BROO-er)
respiratory drive

ventilatory response
(vent-ih-lah-TOR-ee)

1 _____ term that refers to the combined inputs to the brainstem centers that control respiration

2 _____ reflex involving stretch receptors in the lungs, in which sensory information is used to stop inspiration at the proper inflation point

3 _____ change in alveolar minute volume that results from any change in the inspired gas or the plasma chemistry

Terms related to structures/substances

aortic body
apneustic center (ap-NOOS-tik)
carotid body (kah-ROT-id)
central chemoreceptor
  (kee-moh-ree-SEP-tor)
choroid plexus (KOR-oyd)
conjugate base (KAHN-jug-at)

fixed acid
inspiratory center
irritant receptor
peripheral chemoreceptor
phrenic nerve
pneumotaxic center (noo-moh-TAKS-ik)

1_____ type of receptor in the respiratory epithelia responsible for the sensation of distress when noxious gases or particulates are inhaled

2_____ peripheral chemoreceptor in the arterial pathway, at the beginning of the aorta

3_____ respiratory reflex center in the medulla; the neurons in this area simulate phrenic nerves and intercostal nerves to external intercostal muscles and inhibit neurons in the expiratory area

4_____ respiratory reflex center in the pons; the neurons in this center, when stimulated, inhibit apneustic and inspiratory neurons

5_____ peripheral chemoreceptor in the arterial pathway, near the junction of the internal and external carotid arteries

6_____ respiratory reflex center in the pons, inferior to the pneumotaxic center; the neurons in this center chronically stimulate neurons in the inspiratory center

7_____ general term for a receptor outside the CNS that can detect changes in the chemistry of body fluids (e.g., changes in blood pH and PO_2)

8_____ general term for a receptor within the CNS that can detect changes in the chemistry of body fluids (e.g., changes in CSF pH)

9_____ one of several highly vascularized structures within the fluid chambers (ventricles) of the brain that filter blood to form cerebrospinal fluid

10_____ one of a pair of cervical spinal nerves that innervate the diaphragm

11_____ term referring to acid substances that, unlike CO_2, cannot be removed by means of the respiratory mechanism

12_____ base that is produced by the dissociation of an acid

Other Key Terms

acute mountain sickness
hypercapnia (hy-per-KAP-nee-ah)
hypocapnia (hy-poh-KAP-nee-ah)

hypoxia (hy-PAHKS-ee-ah)
metabolic acidosis (as-id-OHS-is)

1_____ condition of low blood pH, resulting from the presence of fixed acids (no matter what their origin)

2_____ condition of reduced plasma PCO_2

3_____ condition of increased PCO_2 in the arterial blood

4_____ general term for the condition of reduced arterial PO_2

5_____ hypoxia that results from rapid ascent from sea level, which reduces the atmospheric PO_2

The Big Picture

Use the activities of this section to help you learn the broader concepts of this chapter.

Learning Exercises

1. Fill in the blanks in this table of respiratory muscle movements, using either the term "contraction" or "relaxation."

Muscle (group)	Mode during inspiration	Mode during expiration
Diaphragm		
Internal intercostals		
External intercostals		
Abdominal muscles		

2. Use these terms to identify the numbered portions of the flow chart of respiratory control (Figure 18-1).

apneustic   motor   pneumotaxic
central   peripheral   spinal motor
Hering-Breuer

Figure 18-1

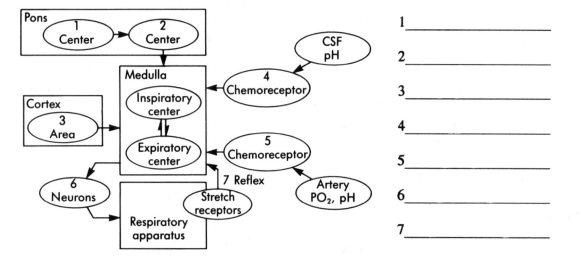

1 _____

2 _____

3 _____

4 _____

5 _____

6 _____

7 _____

3. Fill in the blanks below with "inhibits" or "excites."

pneumotaxic center   _____   apneustic center

inspiratory center   _____expiratory center

expiratory center   _____   internal intercostal muscles

inspiratory center   _____diaphragm

high blood PO_2 _____inspiratory center

low CSF pH   _____inspiratory center

feed-forward mechanism
(of exercise)   _____inspiratory center

4. Use these terms to fill in the blanks found in the paragraphs that follow. (Some terms are used more than once.)

blood-brain	H^+	plasma
central	HCO_3^-	proteins
choroid plexus	minute volume	ventilatory
CO_2		

CSF is formed by the vascular _____ of the brain ventricles. Because of

the nature of the _____ barrier, plasma _____ may enter

the CSF freely but not H^+ or _____ ions. However, once in the CSF, the

_____ reacts with H_2O to form carbonic acid, which dissociates into

_____ and HCO_3^- ions. These ions are then trapped in the CSF. Since CSF has

few _____, it is weakly buffered (and so is more pH sensitive than

_____ to PCO_2 changes). The reduced pH in CSF triggers

_____ chemoreceptors, which change the alveolar _____

by means of the _____ response.

Because the _____ barrier can regulate the influx of HCO_3^- into the CSF,

the CSF pH can be quickly restored to the _____ setpoint value. Subsequently,

the _____ chemoreceptors are "reset" (thus providing a type of adaptation to

chronic changes in blood pH).

5. A person with lung disease dies after receiving 100% oxygen. The steps leading to this tragedy are given below, but out of order. Put them into the correct sequence.

100% O_2 is administered
arterial PCO_2 is increased, and PO_2 is decreased
central receptors adapt to the elevated PCO_2
low blood pH and reduced PO_2 stimulate respiration
lung disease causes decreased alveolar ventilation
patient dies because respirations cease
peripheral receptors stop driving respiration because of increased PO_2
peripheral receptors alone respond to low PO_2, driving ventilation

1 _____

2 _____

3 _____

4 _____

5 _____

6 _____

7 _____

8 _____

6. Fill in the blank areas in this table with either "increased rate and volume" or "decreased rate and volume." As you fill in the table, think of what triggers the response and the result of the response on homeostasis.

Situation	Respiratory response
hypoxia	
acute metabolic acidosis	
sudden increase in altitude (from sea level)	
muscular exercise	

Quick Recall

Review some of the major concepts of this chapter by doing these "quick recall" activities.

1. List the three principal groups of respiratory muscles.

2. Name two mechanisms for producing rhythmicity of breathing.

3. Name four major respiratory control centers in the brainstem.

4. List factors affecting the intensity of respiratory drive, rate of breathing, and tidal volume.

5. Name the two primary types of chemoreceptors, distinguishing their locations.

6. List the respiratory responses to decreased PCO_2, increased PO_2.

7. List the respiratory responses to increased PCO_2, decreased PO_2.

Practice Test

Use this practice test to review the topics of this chapter and to prepare for your test on this material.

1. Respiration can be depressed by
   a. brainstem trauma
   b. overdoses of barbiturates
   c. breathing 5% CO_2
   d. a and b
   e. none of the above

2. Stretch receptors in the lung
   a. do not exist
   b. do not contribute to normal tidal breathing
   c. can play a role at high tidal volumes
   d. when activated, inhibit inspiration
   e. b, c, and d are correct

3. The peripheral chemoreceptors can be stimulated by
   a. large decreases in PO_2
   b. decreases in arterial pH
   c. increases in arterial CO_2
   d. both a and b
   e. a, b, and c

4.   Compared to the central chemoreceptors, the peripheral chemoreceptors are
      a.   less responsive to increases in arterial CO_2
      b.   more responsive to decreases in arterial pH
      c.   less responsive to decreases in arterial O_2
      d.   a and b
      e.   none of the above

5.   Arterial pH increases from 7.4 to 7.6. After a few minutes you would expect
      a.   increase in ventilation
      b.   decrease in CSF PCO_2
      c.   increase in plasma pH
      d.   a and b
      e.   none of the above

6.   The central chemoreceptors are
      a.   sensitive to oxygen
      b.   tonically active in a normal resting person
      c.   located behind the blood-brain barrier
      d.   b and c
      e.   a, b, and c are correct

7.   At sea level respiration is normally stimulated by
      a.   carbon dioxide
      b.   hydrogen ion
      c.   oxygen
      d.   peripheral chemoreceptors
      e.   none of the above

8.   A 40 mm Hg decrease in arterial PO_2 will
      a.   stimulate the peripheral chemoreceptors
      b.   stimulate the central chemoreceptors
      c.   stimulate the medullary respiratory control centers
      d.   a and c
      e.   none of the above

9.   On ascending to high altitude, a normal individual will exhibit
      a.   an increase in ventilation
      b.   an increase in arterial pH
      c.   a decrease in alveolar PCO_2
      d.   an increase in CSF pH
      e.   all of the above

10.   A fall in arterial PO_2 produces a larger ventilatory stimulation if
      a.   carbon dioxide levels are high
      b.   carbon dioxide levels are low
      c.   arterial pH is low
      d.   arterial pH is high
      e.   a and c

11. Ventilation increases during exercise mainly because
    a. the respiratory centers are stimulated by higher centers
    b. the peripheral chemoreceptors detect a fall in oxygen
    c. the central chemoreceptors detect an increase in carbon dioxide
    d. there is metabolic acidosis
    e. none of the above

12. The arterial PO_2 is 100 mm Hg; the arterial PCO_2 is 40 mm Hg; the arterial pH is 7.40. Ventilation is being driven
    a. mainly by the peripheral chemoreceptors
    b. mainly by the central chemoreceptors
    c. equally by the peripheral and central chemoreceptors
    d. by both, but the central drive is greater
    e. by both, but the peripheral drive is greater

13. The arterial PO_2 is 60 mm Hg; the arterial PCO_2 is 60 mm Hg; the arterial pH is 7.40. Ventilation is being driven
    a. mainly by the peripheral chemoreceptors
    b. mainly by the central chemoreceptors
    c. equally by the peripheral and central chemoreceptors
    d. by both, but the central drive is greater
    e. by both, but the peripheral drive is greater

14. The gradual increase in ventilation after ascent to a high altitude depends on
    a. production of more RBCs
    b. HCO_3^- transport at the blood-brain barrier
    c. peripheral chemoreceptor adaptation
    d. a, b, and c
    e. none of the above

15. The plasma pH drops in acidosis. Several minutes later, the CSF pH
    a. increases
    b. decreases
    c. remains unchanged

Answers

Here are answers (or references) to some of the questions presented above.

Word Parts: (your examples may be different) 1-hypercapnia, 2-chemoreceptor, 3-choroid plexus, 4-hypoxia, 5-choroid plexus, 6-choroid plexus

Key Terms: Processes: 1. respiratory drive 2. Hering-Breuer reflex 3. ventilatory response
Structures/Substances: 1. irritant receptor 2. aortic body 3. inspiratory center 4. pneumotaxic center 5. carotid body 6. apneustic center 7. peripheral
Other: 1. metabolic acidosis 2. hypocapnia 3. hypercapnia 4. hypoxia 5. acute mountain sickness chemoreceptor 8. central chemoreceptor 9. choroid plexus 10. phrenic nerve 11. fixed acid 12. conjugate base

Learning Exercises: 1. Diaphragm: contraction, relaxation; Internal intercostals: contraction, relaxation; External intercostals: relaxation, contraction; Abdominals: relaxation, contraction 2. 1-pneumotaxic, 2-apneustic, 3-motor, 4-

central, 5-peripheral, 6-spinal motor, 7-Hering-Breuer 3. inhibits, inhibits, excites, excites, inhibits, excites, excites 4. choroid plexus, blood-brain, CO_2, HCO_3^-, CO_2, H^+, proteins, plasma, central, minute volume, ventilatory, blood-brain, ventilatory, central 5. 1-lung disease causes decreased alveolar ventilation, 2-arterial PCO_2 is increased and PO_2 is decreased, 3-low blood pH (and reduced PO_2) stimulate respiration, 4-central receptors adapt to the elevated PCO_2, 5-peripheral receptors alone respond (to low PO_2), driving ventilation, 6-100% O_2 is administered, 7-peripheral receptors stop driving respiration (because of increased PO_2), 8-patient dies because respirations cease 6. (all cause an increase in rate and volume)

Quick Recall: (You should be able to answer these questions easily without correction or confirmation by this point in your studies. If you cannot, review your notes, the text chapter, and the previous study activities to find the answers.)

Practice Test: 1-d, 2-e, 3-e, 4-d, 5-e, 6-d, 7-a, 8-d, 9-e, 10-e, 11-a, 12-b, 13-d, 14-b, 15-a

Chapter 19
The Kidney

Focus
Review this section first. It will help you focus on the overall message of this chapter.

Chapter Outline
Read through the outline slowly. This activity will help your mind organize the topics of this chapter.

Structure of the excretory system
> Anatomy of the kidney, ureters, and bladder
> The urinary bladder: urine storage and urination
> Nephrons: the functional units of the kidney
> Renal blood vessels and the juxtaglomerular apparatus

Mechanisms of urine formation and modification
> Ultrafiltration and the composition of the glomerular filtrate

The glomerular filtration rate and its determinants
> Functions of the proximal tubule: reabsorption and secretion
> Functions of the distal tubule: formation of dilute urine
> The loops of Henle and the collecting duct: formation of concentrated urine
> Role of the vasa recta in urine concentration
> Endocrine control of urine concentration

Integrated function of the kidney
> Concept of renal clearance
> How Na^+ and K^+ are handled by the kidney
> The juxtaglomerular apparatus and tubuloglomerular feedback
> Renal contributions to acid-base regulation

Learning Objectives
These are the learning goals for this part of the course. After reading the text, attending class, and studying this chapter, you should be able to:

♦ describe the anatomy of the excretory system

♦ outline the reflex and voluntary pathways controlling urination

♦ understand the structure of the nephrons and distinguish between cortical and juxtamedullary nephrons

♦ describe the process of ultrafiltration across glomerular capillaries and describe the composition of the glomerular filtrate

♦ describe the mechanism for reabsorption of most of the filtered Na^+ and water in the proximal tubule and understand how this leads to the passive reabsorption of other small solutes

♦ understand the mechanisms of active reabsorption and secretion, defining the transport maximum

♦ appreciate how the loop of Henle acts to create an osmotic gradient in the kidney and understand the role of urea in urine concentration

♦ describe the transport processes occurring in the distal tubule and how these are affected by aldosterone

♦ understand how ADH affects the water permeability of the collecting duct

♦ appreciate the role of the vasa recta in preserving the medullary osmotic gradient

♦ define clearance and be able to solve problems involving clearance

♦ define tubuloglomerular feedback and trace the feedback loop

♦ explain how atrial natriuretic hormone modulates the rate of Na^+ loss in urine

Language of Physiology

Physiology uses its own set of terms, many of which may be unfamiliar to you. This section will help you improve your mastery of key physiological terms.

Word Parts

Here are some combining forms often seen in physiological terms. Give an example of a term that contains each word part listed.

Word Part	Meaning	Example
fenestr-	window; opening	1
glomer-	wound into a ball	2
juxta-	near; beside	3
pod-	foot	4
ren-	kidney	5
-uria	(refers to urine condition)	6

Key Terms

Read each of the terms in each grouping below aloud, using the pronunciation guide if necessary. This will help you to remember them better than if you read them silently. Then, write out the correct term next to each of the descriptions given.

Descriptive Terms

apical (surface) (AYP-ik-al)
basolateral (surface)
  (bay-zoh-LAT-er-al)

cortical (nephron)
juxtamedullary (nephron)
  (juks-tah-med-OOL-ar-ee)

1_____   descriptive term that refers to a nephron whose loop of Henle dips far into the renal medulla

2_____   descriptive term that refers to a nephron whose loop of Henle is largely within the renal cortex (only a tiny portion dips into the outer medulla)

3_____   descriptive term that refers to the surface of a tubule wall cell that faces away from the lining of the tubule

4_____   descriptive term that refers to the surface of a tubule wall cell that faces the inside of the tubule

Terms related to measurement

filtered load [L_x]
glomerular filtration rate [GFR]
  (gloh-MAR-yoo-lar)
renal blood flow [RBF]

renal clearance [C_x]
renal plasma flow [RPF]
transport maximum [T_m]

1_____   in the kidney, the maximum rate of tubular reabsorption of a given substance

2_____   in the kidney, the amount of a given substance that is filtered into the glomerulus (mg/min); = (P_x) (GFR), where P_x is the substance's plasma concentration

3_____   amount (liters) of plasma that are "completely" cleared of a given substance by the kidneys per minute; = (U_x) (V) / P_x, where U_x is urine concentration of substance x, V is rate of urine flow, and P_x is plasma concentration of x

4_____   amount of plasma that flows through the kidneys per unit time

5_____   volume of primary urine (filtrate) formed per unit time, normally expressed in liters/day

6_____   amount of (whole) blood that flows through the kidneys per unit time

Terms related to processes

classical hypothesis
countercurrent multiplication
countercurrent exchange
deamination (dee-am-in-AY-shun)
micturition (mik-shur-IH-shun)
pH trapping
reabsorption

renal handling
secretion
standing gradient hypothesis
transamination (tranz-am-in-AY-shun)
tubuloglomerular feedback
two-solute hypothesis

1_____ form of blood flow autoregulation in which the afferent and efferent renal arterioles dilate or constrict in response to changes in urine flow rate in the distal tubule

2_____ explanation for tubular reabsorption involving a process in which Na$^+$ transport across the basolateral surface (of tubule wall cells) creates an osmotic gradient for water (which then follows)

3_____ general term referring to the manner in which the kidney tubules deal with a particular substance (i.e., how it is "handled")

4_____ in the kidney tubule, the process of active transport of molecules from the peritubular blood, through the tubule wall, and into the urine

5_____ in the kidney, a process in which the blood vessels of the vasa recta act to conserve the high osmolarity in the medulla (by not removing too much of the excess solute)

6_____ in the kidney tubule, the process of active or passive movement of molecules from inside the tubule, across the tubule wall, and eventually into the peritubular blood

7_____ in the kidney, the process involving the loop of Henle that increases the osmolarity of the renal medulla (and thus allows production of hypertonic urine)

8_____ one of two major theories explaining countercurrent multiplication; this hypothesis holds that the NaCl gradient across the wall of the thin ascending limb of Henle and the urea gradient across the wall of the thick ascending limb both drive the increase in medullary osmolarity

9_____ one of two major theories explaining countercurrent multiplication; this hypothesis holds that salt ions are continually moved from the ascending limb of Henle into the descending limb, concentrating salt ions in the medullary fluid

10_____ transfer of amino groups (-NH$_2$) from one molecule to another

11_____ removal of amino groups (-NH$_2$) from a molecule

12_____ process of accumulating NH$_4^+$ in the tubular urine, resulting from the pH gradient across the tubule wall

13_____ urination; the process of voiding the urinary bladder upon relaxation of the skeletal muscle internal and external sphincters

238

Terms Related to Structures/Substances

basement membrane
Bowman's capsule
collecting duct (tubule)
distal tubule
fenestrated endothelium
glomerular filtrate (gloh-MAR-yoo-lar)
glomerulus (gloh-MAR-yoo-lus)
juxtaglomerular apparatus
  (juks-tah-gloh-MAR-yoo-lar)
loop of Henle (HEN-lee)
nephron (NEF-rahn)
peritubular capillary bed
  (par-ih-TOOB-yoo-ler)
podocyte (poh-doh-SITE)

proximal convoluted tubule
renal pelvis
renal pyramid
renal medulla
renal cortex
renal calyx (KAY-liks)
renal corpuscle
urea
ureter (YOO-ret-er)
urethra (yoo-REE-thrah)
urinary bladder
vasa recta

1 _____ wedge-shaped portion of the renal medulla, composed primarily of collecting ducts

2 _____ cuplike structure at the apex of each renal pyramid for the collection of urine from the collecting ducts

3 _____ twisted portion of the nephron between the Bowman's capsule and the loop of Henle

4 _____ large urine collection area in the kidney, it drains urine from the calyces and empties it into the ureter

5 _____ cell of the visceral wall of the Bowman's capsule, whose footlike extensions interlock and form slit pores (for filtration) between them

6 _____ large, extensible sac in the pelvic cavity that collects urine from each ureter and stores it until it is voided via the urethra

7 _____ tube that drains urine from the bladder to the outside of the body (it is longer in males, because it also serves to conduct semen through the penis)

8 _____ muscular tube that continually drains urine from the renal pelvis of the kidney inferiorly toward the urinary bladder

9 _____ nitrogenous compound that is a waste product of protein catabolism

10 _____ group of specialized epithelial cells of the distal tubule (macula densa) and the adjacent arteriolar wall (granular cells) that is responsible for glomerulotubular balance

11 _____ portion of the nephron after the loop of Henle that connects to the collecting duct; it has three portions: convoluted, connecting, and initial collecting regions

12 _____ portion of the nephron between the proximal and distal tubules, composed of a descending limb and an ascending limb

13 _____ balllike network of capillaries at the head of the nephron, it is fed by an afferent arteriole and drained by an efferent arteriole

14 _____ also called the basal lamina, it is a layer that connects the glomerular endothelium to the visceral wall of the Bowman's capsule (and may filter some plasma proteins)

15 _____ general term for the entire outer region of the kidney

16_____ general term for the entire inner region of the kidney

17_____ kidney tubule that drains urine from the distal tubule of the nephron

18_____ funnel-shaped beginning of the nephron, covering the glomerulus

19_____ portion of the peritubular capillary bed that surrounds the long loop of Henle in a juxtamedullary nephron

20_____ network of capillaries fed by the efferent arteriole and surrounding the outside of the nephron tubule

21_____ filtrate formed as fluid passes from the blood through the glomerular-capsular membrane and into the Bowman's capsule

22_____ renal tubule; a tiny functional unit within the kidney in which urine is formed

23_____ lining of glomerular capillaries that, because of its large pores, allows exit of fluids (but blocks the exit of blood cells)

24_____ structure formed by the glomerulus and Bowman's capsule together

Other Key Terms

Addison's disease

diabetes insipidus
 (dy-ah-BEET-ees in-SIP-id-us)

hemoglobinuria
 (hee-moh-gloh-bin-YOO-ree-ah)

proteinuria (proh-ten-YOO-ree-ah)

urinary retention

urinary incontinence (in-KAHN-tin-ens)

1_____ abnormal condition in which some factor prevents voiding of urine from the urinary bladder

2_____ abnormal condition in which large amounts of relatively dilute urine are produced (because of a lack of ADH regulation)

3_____ abnormal condition in which nerve damage or some other factor allows periodic (inappropriate) leakage of urine from the bladder

4_____ abnormal condition caused by inadequate secretion of adrenal cortical hormones, including aldosterone, that results in excessive sodium loss by the kidneys

5_____ general term for the condition of abnormally high protein content in the urine, as in kidney disease

6_____ condition of excessive hemoglobin content in the urine, as sometimes observed after severe exercise (urine may appear brownish)

The Big Picture
Use the activities of this section to help you learn the broader concepts of this chapter.

Learning Exercises

1. Use these terms to label Figure 19-1, a frontal section of the kidney.

calyx   renal pelvis   renal pyramid
renal medulla   renal cortex   ureter

Figure 19-1

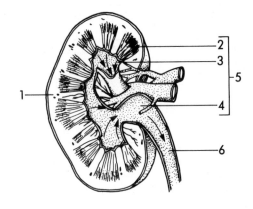

1 _____

2 _____

3 _____

4 _____

5 _____

6 _____

2. Use these terms to label Figure 19-2, which represents control of urination.

external sphincter   parasympathetic   stretch receptor
internal sphincter   pathway   ureter
                  spinal motor pathway   urethra

Figure 19-2

1 _____

2 _____

3 _____

4 _____

5 _____

6 _____

7 _____

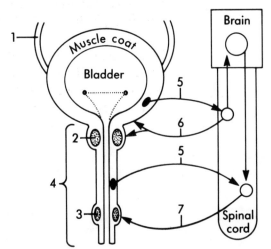

3. Use these terms to label the nephron in Figure 19-3.

afferent arteriole
Bowman's capsule
collecting duct
connecting portion
convoluted portion
descending limb (of Henle)
distal tubule
efferent arteriole

glomerulus
initial collecting portion
juxtaglomerular apparatus
proximal tubule
renal corpuscle
thick ascending limb (of Henle)
thin ascending limb (of Henle)

Figure 19-3

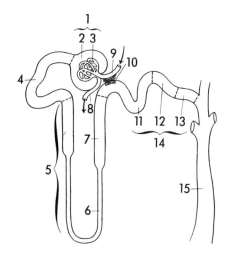

1 _____

2 _____

3 _____

4 _____

5 _____

6 _____

7 _____

8 _____

9 _____

10 _____

11 _____

12 _____

13 _____

14 _____

15 _____

4. Figure 19-4 represents the glomerular-capsular (filtration) membrane with blood plasma on the left and glomerular filtrate on the right. Show which particles normally filter through the membrane (in significant quantities) to become part of the glomerular filtrate by drawing an arrow from the particle, across the membrane, to the other side.

Figure 19-4   Plasma   Glomerular filtrate

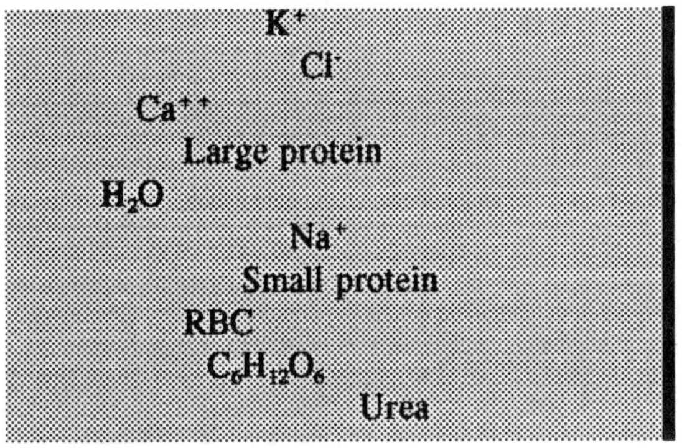

K^+

Cl^-

Ca^{++}

Large protein

H_2O

Na^+

Small protein

RBC

$C_6H_{12}O_6$

Urea

└─ Filtration membrane

Glomerulus   Bowman's capsule

5. Use these terms to fill in the blanks in the paragraphs that follow.

cotransport	osmosis	reabsorption
finite	osmotic	60
glomerular filtrate	passive	sodium
gradient	primary	transport maximum
interstitial	proximal	
more		

Of the 174 liters/day of _____ filtered into the Bowman's capsules, only

about _____ liters/day reaches the loops of Henle. The difference can be

accounted for by the process of _____ in the _____

tubule. This process is actually a combination of active and _____ transport

processes. First, many of the _____ ions are actively transported out of the

tubule and into the _____ fluid. This sets up an _____

gradient, which then causes water to follow passively, via _____. Once the

sodium and water are outside the tubule, other solutes are _____ concentrated

than they had been. This concentration _____ promotes the passive diffusion of

some of these other solutes, such as urea, out of the tubule also.

243

Some solutes, such as glucose, are reabsorbed via _____ that is coupled

to the sodium gradient. Any solute that relies directly or indirectly on active transport has an upper limit

(the _____) to the amount of solute that can be reabsorbed at any one time. This

is because there is a _____ number of transport sites.

6. Describe the changes in the relative water content of urine as it passes through the nephron by filling in the blank portions of the following table with "isotonic," "hypertonic," or "hypotonic" (describing the urine relative to normal plasma).

Nephron segment	Hormones not present Beginning	End	Hormones present Beginning	End
Proximal tubule				
Descending limb of Henle				
Thin ascending limb of Henle				
Thick ascending limb of Henle				
Distal (convoluted) tubule				
Distal (collecting) tubule				
Collecting duct				

7. Use these terms to fill in the blanks in the text regarding urine concentration. (Some terms are used more than once.)

active

actively

ADH

aldosterone

countercurrent

hypotonic

impermeable

isotonic

medulla

osmotic

thick ascending

urea

vasa recta

water

The loop of Henle concentrates solutes in the interstitial fluid of the kidney's

_____ via the _____ multiplier mechanism. This forms

an _____ gradient between the cortex and medulla. Current theory holds that

NaCl is _____ pumped from the _____ of the loop of

Henle and into the surrounding interstitial fluid. _____ cannot leave this portion of the tubule because the walls are impermeable to it. The medullary interstitial fluid (IF) is further concentrated with solute by the addition of _____, a nitrogenous metabolite that diffuses from the collecting duct. Because of the loss of NaCl to the IF, without a loss of water, urine leaving the loop of Henle is _____ to normal body fluids.

High medullary osmolarity is preserved by the _____ exchange mechanism of the _____ (the medullary portion of the peritubular capillary bed). Because the vessels dip down, then up, in a hairpin fashion, blood leaving the medulla is nearly _____ to the blood that enters. This means that little solute leaves the medulla, and thus the _____ gradient between it and the cortex is maintained.

Dilute urine formed in the loop of Henle is further diluted by the _____ reabsorption of Na^+, in exchange for K^+. The rate of Na^+ gain - K^+ loss is increased by the hormone _____. The dilute urine could then pass through the collecting ducts without a change in osmolarity, because these ducts are relatively _____ to water. However, in the presence of the hormone _____, the collecting ducts become water permeable. This allows _____ to leave osmotically (and enter the medullary IF), concentrating the urine.

Quick Recall
Review some of the major concepts of this chapter by doing these "quick recall" activities.

1. List the major organs of the urinary system.

2. List the events that lead to micturition once the bladder is full.

3. List the major portions of the nephron in anatomical order.

4. Write the formula for determining net filtration pressure.

5. Write the formula for determining filtered load of a solute.

6. Name two hormones that affect urine production.

Practice Test
Use this practice test to review the topics of this chapter and to prepare for your test on this material.

1. Which of the following never penetrates the medulla?
   a.   the distal tubule
   b.   the collecting duct
   c.   the glomerulus
   d.   the loop of Henle
   e.   a and c

2. Juxtamedullary nephrons
   a.   are more numerous than cortical nephrons
   b.   form the greatest tissue mass in the kidney
   c.   have loops of Henle that penetrate the inner medulla
   d.   b and c
   e.   a, b, and c

3. The internal urinary sphincter
   a.   is composed of smooth muscle
   b.   is composed of striated muscle
   c.   relaxes during urination
   d.   is under voluntary control
   e.   a and c

4. The glomerular filtration rate will increase when
   a.   there is occlusion of a ureter
   b.   the afferent arterioles constrict
   c.   plasma osmotic pressure decreases
   d.   the efferent arterioles are constricted
   e.   none of the above

5. If glomerular capillary hydrostatic pressure = 50 mm Hg
   plasma osmotic pressure = 15 mm Hg
   Bowman capsule hydrostatic pressure = 10 mm Hg
   tubular fluid osmotic pressure = 0 mm Hg
   then what is the net filtration pressure?
   a.   0 mm Hg
   b.   10 mm Hg
   c.   -10 mm Hg
   d.   25 mm Hg
   e.   125 mm Hg

6. Peritubular hydrostatic pressure is normally
   a.   below systemic capillary pressure
   b.   below glomerular hydrostatic pressure
   c.   at a level that favors net filtration
   d.   a and b
   e.   a, b, and c

7. To determine the clearance of a substance one must know
   a. the amount in the urine
   b. its plasma concentration
   c. the glomerular filtration rate
   d. a and b
   e. a, b, and c

8. The plasma inulin concentration is 0.25 mg/ml; urine flow is 1.0 ml/min; urine inulin concentration is 25 mg/ml. What is the GFR?
   a. 50 ml/min
   b. 75 ml/min
   c. 100 ml/min
   d. 125 ml/min
   e. 150 ml/min

9. If the filtered load of a substance X exceeds its transport maximum
   a. reabsorption of X will be complete
   b. no reabsorption of X will occur
   c. some X will appear in the urine
   d. all are correct

10. The urine osmolarity will decrease when
    a. active NaCl transport in the ascending limb of Henle is inhibited
    b. the osmotic pressure in the renal medulla is decreased
    c. circulating levels of ADH decrease
    d. a and b
    e. a, b, and c

For Nos. 11 and 12:
glomerular filtration rate = 150 ml/min
plasma [glucose] = 5 mg/ml
T_m for glucose = 300 mg/min

11. The filtered load of glucose is
    a. 150 mg/min
    b. 300 mg/min
    c. 750 mg/min
    d. 1500 mg/min
    e. none of the above

12. The amount of glucose reabsorbed by the kidney is
    a. 75 mg/min
    b. 150 mg/min
    c. 300 mg/min
    d. 750 mg/min
    e. none of the above

13. The tubular fluid is always hypotonic in the
    a. proximal tubule
    b. early distal tubule
    c. collecting duct
    d. loop of Henle
    e. b and c

14. About 65% of the filtered load of most substances is reabsorbed in the
    a. proximal tubule
    b. distal tubule
    c. collecting duct
    d. loop of Henle
    e. none of the above

Answers

Here are answers (or references) to some of the questions presented above.

Word Parts: (your examples may be different) 1-fenestrated endothelium, 2-glomerulus, 3-juxtaglomerular, 4-podocyte, 5-renal, 6-proteinuria

Key Terms: Descriptive: 1. juxtamedullary (nephron) 2. cortical (nephron) 3. basolateral (surface) 4. apical (surface)

Measurement: 1. transport maximum $[T_m]$ 2. filtered load $[L_x]$ 3. renal clearance $[C_x]$ 4. renal plasma flow [RPF] 5. glomerular filtration rate [GFR] 6. renal blood flow [RBF]

Processes: 1. tubuloglomerular feedback 2. standing gradient hypothesis 3. renal handling 4. secretion 5. countercurrent exchange 6. reabsorption 7. countercurrent multiplication 8. two-solute hypothesis 9. classical hypothesis 10. transamination 11. deamination 12. pH trapping 13. micturition

Structures/Substances: 1. renal pyramid 2. renal calyx 3. proximal convoluted tubule 4. renal pelvis 5. podocyte 6. urinary bladder 7. urethra 8. ureter 9. urea 10. juxtaglomerular apparatus 11. distal tubule 12. loop of Henle 13. glomerulus 14. basement membrane 15. renal cortex 16. renal medulla 17. collecting duct (tubule) 18. Bowman's capsule 19. vasa recta 20. peritubular capillary bed 21. glomerular filtrate 22. nephron 23. fenestrated endothelium 24. renal corpuscle

Other: 1. urinary retention 2. diabetes insipidus 3. urinary incontinence 4. Addison's disease 5. proteinuria 6. hemoglobinuria

Learning Exercises: 1. 1-renal cortex, 2-renal pyramid, 3-calyx, 4-renal pelvis, 5-renal medulla, 6-ureter 2. 1-ureter, 2-internal sphincter, 3-external sphincter, 4-urethra, 5-stretch receptor, 6-parasympathetic pathway, 7-spinal motor pathway 3. 1-renal corpuscle, 2-Bowman's capsule, 3-glomerulus, 4-proximal tubule, 5-descending limb (of Henle), 6-thin ascending limb (of Henle), 7-thick ascending limb (of Henle), 8-efferent arteriole, 9-afferent arteriole, 10-juxtaglomerular apparatus, 11-convoluted portion, 12-connecting portion, 13-initial collecting portion, 14-distal tubule, 15-collecting duct 4. (all but RBC and large protein may pass through the membrane) 5. glomerular filtrate, 60, reabsorption, proximal, passive, sodium, interstitial, osmotic, osmosis, more, gradient, cotransport, transport maximum, finite 6. (Compare your table with the far left columns of Table 19-2 in the text.) 7. medulla, countercurrent, osmotic, actively, thick ascending, water, urea, hypotonic, countercurrent, vasa recta, isotonic, osmotic, active, aldosterone, impermeable, ADH, water

Quick Recall: (You should be able to answer these questions easily without correction or confirmation by this point in your studies. If you cannot, review your notes, the text chapter, and the previous study activities to find the answers.)

Practice Test: 1-e, 2-d, 3-e, 4-d, 5-d, 6-d, 7-d, 8-c, 9-c, 10-e, 11-c, 12-c, 13-b, 14-a

Chapter 20
Control of Body Fluid, Electrolyte, and Acid-Base Balance

Focus
Review this section *first*. It will help you focus on the overall message of this chapter.

Chapter Outline
Read through the outline slowly. This activity will help your mind organize the topics of this chapter.

The fluid compartments of the body
> The intracellular and extracellular compartments
> Fluid and salt balance
> Challenges to salt and water homeostasis

Mechanisms of regulation of water and Na^+ balance
> Neural and endocrine effects on glomerular filtration rate
> Control of renal water reabsorption by the antidiuretic hormone
> Control of sodium reabsorption and vascular tone by the renin-angiotensin-aldosterone hormone system
> Control of Na^+ and water loss by the atrial natriuretic hormone system
> Thirst and salt appetite

Potassium homeostasis
> Location of K^+ in the body
> Regulation of K^+ excretion by aldosterone
> Interaction between Na^+ and K^+ regulation and acid-base balance

Calcium and phosphate homeostasis
> Transfer of Ca^{++} and phosphate between bone, intestine, and kidney
> Endocrine regulation of total body calcium and phosphate

Acid-base homeostasis
> The importance of pH regulation
> Buffer systems
> Respiratory and renal contributions to regulation of plasma pH
> Renal compensatory responses in respiratory disease
> Renal compensatory responses in metabolic acidosis and alkalosis

Learning Objectives

These are the learning goals for this part of the course. After reading the text, attending class, and studying this chapter, you should be able to:

♦ describe how total body water is distributed between the intracellular, interstitial, and vascular compartments

♦ understand why cell volume is determined by cytoplasmic protein and extracellular fluid by total body Na^+

♦ list the routes for daily water turnover

♦ understand the effects of atrial natriuretic hormone on glomerular filtration rate and Na^+ reabsorption

♦ describe how antidiuretic hormone secretion responds to changes in plasma osmolarity and atrial stretch

♦ describe the factors affecting aldosterone secretion by the adrenal cortex and explain how aldosterone increases the recovery of filtered Na^+ in the distal tubule

♦ understand the mechanisms for the reabsorption of filtered K^+ and how plasma K^+ directly stimulates K^+ secretion

♦ describe how plasma Ca^{++} and phosphate are regulated by calcitonin, parathyroid hormone, and 1,25-dihydroxycholecalciferol

♦ appreciate how the extracellular fluid is buffered by the bicarbonate buffer system and how the state of this buffer system is controlled by the combined actions of lungs and kidneys

♦ describe how H^+ secretion first recovers filtered HCO_3^- and then results in the formation of "new" HCO_3^- from CO_2, increasing plasma $[HCO_3^-]$ and pH

Language of Physiology

Physiology uses its own set of terms, many of which may be unfamiliar to you. This section will help you improve your mastery of key physiological terms.

Word Parts

Here are some combining forms often seen in physiological terms. Give an example of a term that contains each word part listed.

Word Part	Meaning	Example
-bar	pressure	1
-blast	sprout; make	2
-clast	break; destroy	3
kal-	potassium	4
mala-	bad	5
osteo-	bone	6

Key Terms

Read each of the terms in each grouping below aloud, using the pronunciation guide if necessary. This will help you to remember them better than if you read them silently. Then, write out the correct term next to each of the descriptions given.

Terms related to processes

bulk fluid loss

insensible water loss

natriuresis (nat-ree-yoo-EES-is)

renin-angiotensin-aldosterone [RAA] system

1_____ term that names the mechanism, or system, of fluid regulation involving renin, angiotensin, and aldosterone

2_____ increase in the urinary loss of Na^+ from the body

3_____ normal massive loss of water by means of urination and defecation

4_____ normal small (but continuous) loss of water by means of evaporation from the respiratory tract and skin

Terms related to structures/substances

1,25-dihydroxycholecalciferol
  (1 25 dy-hyd-roks-ih-kol-ek-al-SIF-er-ol)
calcitonin (kal-sih-TOH-nin)
cholecalciferol (kol-ek-al-SIF-er-ol)
extracellular compartment

intracellular compartment
osteoblast (AHS-tee-oh-blast)
osteoclast (AHS-tee-oh-klast)
parathormone [PTH] (par-ah-THOR-mohn)

1_____ type of bone tissue cell that functions to deposit new hard bone matrix (calcium phosphate mineral) by using plasma calcium and phosphate

2_____ type of bone tissue cell that functions to dissolve old hard bone matrix (calcium phosphate mineral), thereby releasing calcium and phosphate ions to the plasma

3_____ protein hormone of the thyroid gland that stimulates bone deposition and thus decreases plasma $[Ca^{++}]$

4_____ abbreviated 1,25 DOHCC, this vitamin D derivative stimulates calcium and phosphate absorption in the intestines, a process required for normal growth and development

5_____ also called parathyroid hormone, a protein hormone that promotes breakdown of hard bone, increases renal reabsorption of Ca^{++}, and increases renal clearance of phosphate — all of which raise plasma $[Ca^{++}]$

6_____ one of two main fluid compartments of the body in which fluid is normally found; includes fluid inside all body cells

7_____ one of two main fluid compartments of the body in which fluid is normally found; includes fluids outside the body cells and can be further subdivided into the interstitial and vascular compartments

8_____ collective name for vitamin D_3 (from animal sources) and vitamin D_2 (from plant sources), both of which serve as precursors of 1,25-DOHCC

Other Key Terms

anion gap
buffer capacity
CO_2 isobar
Davenport diagram
dehydration
Gamblegram
high-renin hypertension
hypercalcemia (hy-per-kal-SEE-mee-ah)
hyperkalemia (hy-per-kal-EE-mee-ah)
hypernatremia (hy-per-nat-REE-mee-ah)
hypervolemia (hy-per-voh-LEE-mee-ah)

hypokalemia (hy-poh-kal-EE-mee-ah)
hypophosphatemia
  (hy-poh-fahs-fay-TEE-mee-ah)
hypovolemia (hy-poh-voh-LEE-mee-ah)
ketoacidosis (kee-toh-as-id-OH-sis)
metabolic alkalosis
osteomalacia (ahs-tee-oh-ma-LAY-sha)
pH optimum
respiratory acidosis
respiratory alkalosis
rickets

1_____ measure of plasma anions other than Cl^- and HCO_3^-

2_____ condition of impaired bone growth in children, caused by the absence of sufficient 1,25-DOHCC

3_____ bar graph that represents the cation and anion composition of blood plasma

4_____ condition of impaired bone growth in adults, caused by the absence of sufficient 1,25-DOHCC

5 _____ titration curve on a Davenport diagram for PCO_2 at a particular value

6 _____ graphic representation of the Henderson-Hasselbalch equation

7 _____ general term referring to low plasma $[K^+]$

8 _____ general term for the abnormal depletion of the body's total volume

9 _____ general term describing the condition of abnormally increased blood plasma volume

10 _____ general term describing the condition of abnormally decreased blood plasma volume

11 _____ general term referring to elevated plasma $[Na^+]$

12 _____ general term referring to high plasma $[K^+]$

13 _____ hypertension (high blood pressure) that results from renal arteriolar atherosclerosis (which chronically stimulates production of renin)

14 _____ narrow range of acidity (pH) in which a particular enzyme functions optimally

15 _____ total amount of acid or base a particular buffer is able to neutralize (based on total amount of buffer present)

16 _____ condition of high blood pH caused by subnormal PCO_2

17 _____ condition of low blood pH caused by high plasma PCO_2

18 _____ condition of increased extracellular $[Ca^{++}]$

19 _____ condition of decreased extracellular phosphate concentration

20 _____ condition of low blood pH caused by the presence of acid ketone bodies (products of fat catabolism)

21 _____ condition of high blood pH caused by increased amounts of fixed bases in the plasma, as in excess ingestion of bases or metabolic dysfunction

The Big Picture

Use the activities of this section to help you learn the broader concepts of this chapter.

Learning Exercises

1. Use the grid below (Figure 20-1) to make a bar graph comparing the % of total body water each fluid compartment holds (under normal conditions).

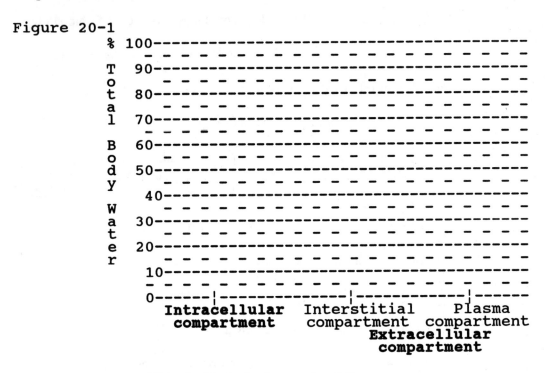

Figure 20-1

2. Use these terms to fill in the blanks in the text that follows.

compartments   extracellular   sodium
cytoplasmic protein   impermeant

The effective osmotic pressures of the intracellular and _____ fluids

are equal. The distribution of fluid between these two _____ is determined

by the _____ solute content of each. Thus cell volume is determined by its

major _____ solute, which is _____. Extracellular

volume is determined by its _____ solute, which is

_____.

3. Fill in the blanks in Figure 20-2 with the terms given.

atrial natriuretic   plasma   water
GFR   sodium

Figure 20-2

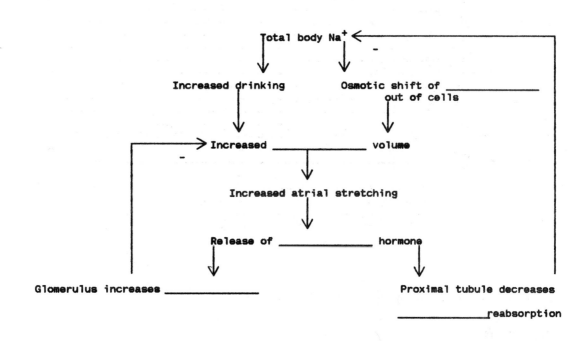

4. Use these terms to fill in the blanks in the text that follows.

antidiuretic   hyperosmotic   pituitary
atrial   increased   water

    The posterior _____ secretes the peptide

_____ hormone in response to _____ osmolarity of

plasma. Secretion of the hormone may be inhibited by increased _____

stretch. _____ hormone increases water reabsorption across the wall of the

collecting duct, stimulating _____ conservation and resulting in the

255

production of _____ urine. _____ hormone could be

said to be the hormone of _____ conservation.

5. Use these terms to label the parts of Figure 20-3.

renin   angiotensin II
angiotensinogen   aldosterone

Figure 20-3

1 _____

2 _____

3 _____

4 _____

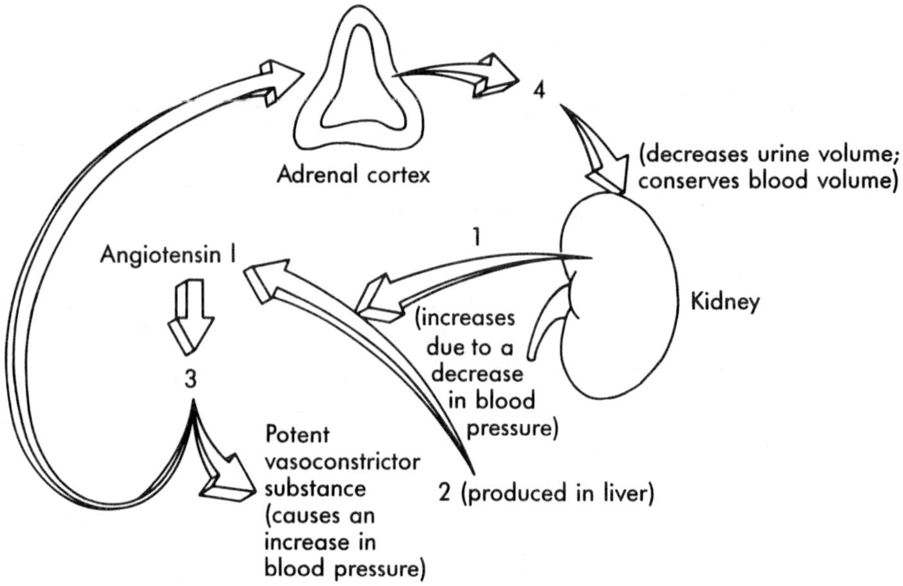

Adrenal cortex

Angiotensin I

3

Potent
vasoconstrictor
substance
(causes an
increase in
blood pressure)

1

(increases
due to a
decrease
in blood
pressure)

2 (produced in liver)

4

(decreases urine volume;
conserves blood volume)

Kidney

6. Use these terms to fill in the blanks in the text that follows.

aldosterone H^+ proximal
distal   handling

   All filtered K^+ is reabsorbed in the _____ tubule and loop of Henle. Thus

the _____ tubule's secretion of K^+ is the regulatory step in renal K^+

_____. Plasma K^+ directly stimulates _____ release, which in

turn stimulates _____ tubular K^+ secretion. If Na^+ reabsorption is constant, K^+

secretion and _____ secretion behave as if they were competitive; both are

stimulated by _____.

7. Fill in each blank below with either "increase" or "decrease."

Release of calcitonin tends to _____ plasma Ca^{++} level

Release of parathormone tends to _____ plasma Ca^{++} level

Increased 1,25-DOHCC tends to _____ plasma Ca^{++} level

Increased 1,25-DOHCC tends to _____ plasma $HPO_4^=$ level

In the kidney, PTH tends to _____ reabsorption of $HPO_4^=$

In the intestine, 1,25-DOHCC tends to _____ absorption of $HPO_4^=$

In bone, 1,25-DOHCC tends to _____ release of $HPO_4^=$

8. Fill in the table with "decreased," "normal," or "increased."

Condition	$[HCO_3^-]$	PCO_2	pH
Metabolic acidosis Before compensation			
After compensation	or normal	or normal	or normal
Metabolic alkalosis Before compensation			
After compensation	or normal	or normal	or normal
Respiratory acidosis Before compensation			
After compensation			less
Respiratory alkalosis Before compensation			
After compensation			or normal

9. Use these terms to fill in the blanks in the following paragraph. (Some terms are used more than once.)

acidosis HCO_3^-
alkalosis   lungs
base   pH
CO_2

Extracellular fluid pH is buffered by the _____ buffer system, whose

state is controlled by the combined action of the _____ and kidneys.

Respiratory compensation for metabolic acidosis/alkalosis involves increases or decreases in arterial

P_____, with corresponding effects on plasma

[_____] and _____. Renal compensation for

_____ involves an increase in tubular H^+ secretion. The H^+ secretion first

recovers all of the filtered _____, which results in the formation of "new"

HCO_3^- from _____, increasing plasma [HCO_3^-] and

_____. Renal compensation for _____ involves

decreased secretion of H^+, so that some _____ is not reabsorbed and

constitutes a net loss of _____ through the urine.

Quick Recall
Review some of the major concepts of this chapter by doing these "quick recall" activities.

1. List the three major fluid compartments of the body.

2. List the routes for daily water turnover.

3. Name three major hormones that regulate water and sodium balance.

4. List the steps of the RAA system.

5. Name the major intracellular cations and anions.

258

6. Name the major extracellular cations and anions.

7. Describe the effects of each of these on Ca^{++}-$HPO_4^=$ balances:

calcitonin

PTH

1,25-DOHCC

8. List the causes of each of these conditions and tell how the body deals with each disorder:

Metabolic acidosis

Metabolic alkalosis

Respiratory acidosis

Respiratory alkalosis

Practice Test
Use this practice test to review the topics of this chapter and to prepare for your test on this material.

1. In a normal individual
    a. the ratio of the intracellular fluid volume to the extracellular fluid volume is approximately 2:1
    b. the interstitial space is about 80% of the extracellular compartment
    c. intracellular osmolarity is approximately 300 mOsm/L
    d. both a and b are correct
    e. a, b, and c are correct

2. The relative sizes of the fluid compartments will be changed by
    a. intravenous administration of pure water
    b. intravenous administration of isotonic NaCl
    c. a and b
    d. none of the above

3. Intracellular osmolarity will be changed by
    a. intravenous administration of isotonic saline
    b. loss of isotonic urine
    c. prolonged vomiting
    d. profuse sweating
    e. both c and d

4. An individual gains 3 L of one-third isotonic saline (50 mM NaCl). From the point of view of body fluid balance, this is equivalent to gaining
    a. 1 L of isotonic saline
    b. 1 L of isotonic saline plus 2 L water
    c. 1 L of isotonic saline and losing 2 L of water
    d. 2 L of isotonic saline
    e. none of the above

5. Ingestion of hypertonic saline will
    a. dehydrate the cells by an amount equal to the amount ingested
    b. dehydrate the cells by an amount exceeding the amount ingested
    c. dehydrate the cells by an amount less than the amount ingested
    d. have no effect on intracellular water
    e. none of the above

6. An individual has a total body water content of 30 L. Plasma $[Na^+]$ = 150 mEq/L. Plasma osmolarity is 300 mOsm/L. This individual then drinks 3 L of pure water. The new value of plasma osmolarity is
    a. 300 mOsm/L
    b. 333 mOsm/L
    c. 272 mOsm/L
    d. 200 mOsm/L
    e. 400 mOsm/L

7. Sodium is
    a. actively reabsorbed in the proximal tubule
    b. actively reabsorbed in the distal tubule
    c. regulated by aldosterone in the distal tubule
    d. a and b
    e. a, b, and c

8. Aldosterone secretion
    a. increases when plasma Na^+ increases
    b. increases when plasma K^+ decreases
    c. is inhibited by renin
    d. inhibits the reabsorption of Na^+ from the distal tubule
    e. none of the above

9. Addition of strong acid can
    a. be buffered by Hb
    b. be buffered by carbonic acid/bicarbonate
    c. cause a decrease in plasma pH
    d. a and c
    e. a, b, and c

10. Renal reabsorption of bicarbonate
   a. is normally complete
   b. is inhibited by inhibitors of carbonic anhydrase
   c. involves the secretion of H^+
   d. depends on the filtered load of bicarbonate
   e. all of the above

11. The buffer systems of the body
   a. return the plasma pH toward normal
   b. include hemoglobin
   c. always result in depletion of bicarbonate
   d. a and b
   e. a, b, and c

12. Respiratory compensation for metabolic acid loads
   a. returns the plasma pH completely to normal
   b. involves an increase in ventilation
   c. involves a decrease in plasma bicarbonate
   d. b and c
   e. a, b, and c

13. The kidney can increase plasma bicarbonate levels by
   a. secreting excess H^+
   b. secreting bicarbonate ions
   c. reabsorbing Na^+
   d. a and b
   e. none of the above

14. Which of the following is correct?
   a. ammonia is produced within the renal tubule cells
   b. ammonia is lipid soluble and hence penetrates membranes readily
   c. ammonium ions do not cross membranes because of their charge
   d. all of the above

15. For individuals A, B, C, and D, which has metabolic acidosis?

	$[HCO_3^-]$	pH	PCO_2
A	40	7.58	43
B	21	7.65	20
C	36	7.20	95
D	10	7.25	30

Answers

Here are answers (or references) to some of the questions presented above.

Word Parts: (your examples may be different) 1-CO_2 isobar, 2-osteoblast, 3-osteoclast, 4-hyperkalemia, 5-osteomalacia, 6-osteoblast

Key Terms: Processes: 1. renin-angiotensin-aldosterone [RAA] system 2. natriuresis 3. bulk fluid loss 4. insensible water loss

Structures/Substances: 1. osteoblast 2. osteoclast 3. calcitonin 4. 1,25-dihydroxycholecalciferol 5. parathormone [PTH] 6. intracellular compartment 7. extracellular compartment 8. cholecalciferol

Other: 1. anion gap 2. rickets 3. Gamblegram 4. osteomalacia 5. CO_2 isobar 6. Davenport diagram 7. hypokalemia 8. dehydration 9. hypervolemia 10. hypovolemia 11. hypernatremia 12. hyperkalemia 13. high-renin hypertension 14. pH optimum 15. buffer capacity 16. respiratory alkalosis 17. respiratory acidosis 18. hypercalcemia 19. hypophosphatemia 20. ketoacidosis 21. metabolic alkalosis

Learning Exercises: 1. Intracellular-67%, Interstitial-25%, Plasma-8% (calculate from Figure 20-1 in text) 2. extracellular, compartments, impermeant, impermeant, cytoplasmic protein, impermeant, sodium 3. (compare to Figure 20-8 in text) 4. pituitary, antidiuretic, increased, atrial, antidiuretic, water, water, hyperosmotic, antidiuretic, water 5. 1-renin, 2-angiotensinogen, 3-angiotensin II, 4-aldosterone 6. proximal, distal, handling, aldosterone, distal, H^+, aldosterone 7. decrease, increase, increase, increase, decrease, increase, increase 8. (compare your table with Table 20-3 in the text) 9. HCO_3, lungs, CO_2, HCO_3^-, pH acidosis, HCO_3^-, CO_2, pH, alkalosis, HCO_3^-, base

Quick Recall: (You should be able to answer these questions easily without correction or confirmation by this point in your studies. If you cannot, review your notes, the text chapter, and the previous study activities to find the answers.)

Practice Test: 1-e, 2-b, 3-e, 4-b, 5-b, 6-b, 7-e, 8-e, 9-e, 10-e, 11-d, 12-d, 13-a, 14-d, 15-D

Chapter 21
Gastrointestinal Organization, Secretion, and Motility

Focus
Review this section *first*. It will help you focus on the overall message of this chapter.

Chapter Outline
Read through the outline slowly. This activity will help your mind organize the topics of this chapter.

Organization of the gastrointestinal system
       The anatomy of the mouth and esophagus
       The anatomy of the stomach
       Intestinal anatomy
       Histology of the gastrointestinal tract
       Surface area of the gastrointestinal tract
       The life cycle of cells of the mucosal epithelium
       Functions of the mucosa
       Gastrointestinal smooth muscle
       Patterns of motility in the GI tract
       Neural and hormonal control of motility
The role of the mouth and esophagus
       Function and control of salivary secretion
       Mechanism of salivary secretion
       Swallowing
Gastric secretion and motility
       Gastric secretion
       The cellular mechanism of acid secretion
       Control of gastric acid secretion by the enteric nervous system
       Gastric motility
Secretion and motility in the intestine
       Secretions of the intestine and pancreas
       Pancreatic enzymes
       The liver and bile
       Intestinal motility
       Defecation

Learning Objectives

These are the learning goals for this part of the course. After reading the text, attending class, and studying this chapter, you should be able to:

♦ describe the anatomy of the gastrointestinal tract and assign general physiological functions to each of its components

♦ identify the location and role of secretory and absorptive epithelial cells

♦ describe the blood supply to the gastrointestinal tract, identifying systemic blood vessels and lymph lacteals

♦ appreciate how muscular contractions mix and move chyme from one region of the gastrointestinal tract to another

♦ distinguish between segmentation and peristalsis

♦ understand the function of mucus in the gastrointestinal tract

♦ describe the composition of secretions in the stomach and small intestine and the nature of bile secreted by the liver

♦ understand the transport mechanisms responsible for acid and bicarbonate secretion

♦ describe the circulation and physiological role of bile salts

♦ understand how intestinal motility mixes the chyme with digestive secretions, promotes absorption of nutrients, and propels the chyme from one region of the intestine to another

Language of Physiology

Physiology uses its own set of terms, many of which may be unfamiliar to you. This section will help you improve your mastery of key physiological terms.

Word Parts

Here are some combining forms often seen in physiological terms. Give an example of a term that contains each word part listed.

Word Part	Meaning	Example
bili-	bile	1
entero-	intestine	2
-flux	flow	3
gastr-	stomach	4
sigm-	Greek Σ or Roman *S*	5
stal-	contract	6
zymo-	refers to "enzyme"	7

Key Terms

Read each of the terms in each grouping below aloud, using the pronunciation guide if necessary. This will help you to remember them better than if you read them silently. Then, write out the correct term next to each of the descriptions given.

Terms related to processes

alkaline tide
gastric reflux
mass movement
pancreatolysis (pan-kree-ah-TAHL-is-is)
peristalsis (payr-ih-STAL-sis)

segmentation
stress relaxation
stress activation
swallowing center

1 _____ reflex center in the brainstem that mediates the process of swallowing (pharyngeal and esophageal phases only, the oral phase is voluntary)

2 _____ series of local contractions in the GI wall that tend to mix the GI contents at a particular location (segment)

3 _____ in smooth muscle, a process in which increased tension (stretch) leads to contraction of the smooth muscle cells

4 _____ in the large intestine, a process in which segmentation ceases and a strong peristaltic wave sweeps along the colon, moving a mass of material into the rectum

5 _____ in smooth muscle, a process in which increased tension (stretch) leads to relaxation of the smooth muscle cells

6 _____ movement of acidic stomach contents into the lower esophagus (as a result of insufficient contraction of the cardiac sphincter), often causing the sensation of "heartburn" (acid burn)

7 _____ increase in plasma [HCO_3^-] resulting from the increase in H^+ secretion that accompanies a meal

8 _____ condition of the digestion of pancreatic cells by pancreatic enzymes (occurs only when the pancreatic duct is blocked)

9 _____ waves of contraction of the GI wall that travel for some distance along its length, tending to propel the GI contents further along the tract

Terms related to structures/substances

acini (as-EE-nee)
anus
bile
bolus
brush border
chyme (kym)
colon
crypts of Lieberkühn (LEE-ber-koon)
duct cells
duodenum (doo-oh-DEEN-um)
enteric nervous system (en-TAYR-ik)
enteroendocrine cell
 (en-ter-oh-EN-doh-krin)
esophageal hiatus
 (es-ahf-a-JEE-al hy-AYT-us)
esophagus (es-AHF-ah-gus)
G cell
gallbladder

gastrointestinal [GI] tract
 (gas-troh-in-TEST-in-al)
goblet cell
haustra (HOW-strah)
ileum (IL-ee-um)
jejunum (je-JOO-num)
lacteal (lak-TEEL)
mucosa (myoo-KOH-sah)
muscularis externa
myenteric plexus (my-en-TAYR-ik)
plicae circulares
 (PLY-kay sir-cyoo-LAR-eez)
rectum
serosa (se-ROH-sah)
stomach
submucosa (sub-myoo-KOH-sah)
submucosal plexus (sub-myoo-KOH-sal)
taeniae coli (TAYN-ee-ay KOH-lee)
villi

1 _____ 400 cm segment of the small intestine just distal to the jejunum and proximal to the large intestine

2 _____ 250 cm segment of the small intestine between the duodenum and the ileum

3 _____ semisolid material formed in the stomach by the mixing of partially digested food and gastric secretions

4 _____ muscular bladder near the underside of the liver, it stores and concentrates bile between meals (bile backs up into it from the common bile duct, which is closed by the sphincter of Oddi between meals)

5 _____ secretory epithelial cell of the digestive mucosa, it secretes glycoprotein mucine, which combines with water to form mucus

6 _____ layer of connective tissue, blood and lymphatic vessels, and exocrine glands between the muscularis externa and mucosa of the GI wall

7 _____ ball of (chewed) food that enters the pharynx during swallowing and then proceeds to the stomach

8 _____ mixture of substances synthesized by the liver (includes bile acids (or, conjugated acids, bile salts), lecithin, cholesterol, bilirubin, bile pigment, detoxified poisons, and $NaHCO_3$

9 _____ also called Meissner's plexus, it is a network of autonomic nerve fibers between the submucosa and muscularis externa of the GI wall

10 _____ also called Auerbach's plexus, it is a network of autonomic axons and ganglia in the muscularis of the GI tract wall, forming diffuse synaptic connections with the muscle fibers

11 _____ also called Kerkring's folds, they are circular ridges of the epithelium that forms the intestinal mucosa

12 _____ cells of the stomach and small intestine that act as chemoreceptors or mechanoreceptors and may also secrete endocrine or paracrine regulatory agents in response to stimulation (also called argentaffin cells)

13 _____ cells that line the ducts of exocrine glands and secrete an electrolyte solution

14 _____ enteroendocrine cells in the stomach that secrete the hormone gastrin

15 _____ general term for the digestive tract: esophagus, stomach, and intestines

16 _____ lymphatic capillary within each intestinal villus

17 _____ segment of the large intestine, formed by outpouchings of the wall, in which segmentation occurs

18 _____ external covering of the GI tract organs, formed by the visceral portion of the peritoneum (a serous membrane)

19 _____ muscular tube that connects the pharynx to the stomach, having an upper sphincter and lower (cardiac) sphincter

20 _____ luminal membranes of the stomach and intestinal mucosa, that are covered with many microvilli

21 _____ major portion of the large intestine, subdivided anatomically into ascending, transverse, descending, and sigmoid regions

22 _____ secretory cells of exocrine glands

23 _____ distal opening of the rectum (to the outside of the body), regulated by a pair of sphincters: internal (smooth muscle) and external (skeletal muscle)

24 _____ portion of the GI tract distal to the esophagus, it consists of a body and fundus (both specialized for temporary storage), antrum (specialized for mixing food and secretions) and the pylorus (which acts as a sphincter valve)

25 _____ last portion of the large intestine, it is a small storage area for feces, which empty out of this region via the anus

26 _____ two autonomic plexi of the GI wall (myenteric and submucosal), together acting to coordinate muscular and glandular function

27 _____ 20 cm initial segment of the small intestine just distal to the pylorus of the stomach

28 _____ muscular layer of the GI tract wall, formed by layers of smooth muscle fibers

29 _____ innermost layer of the GI wall, consisting of mucous epithelium, lamina propria, and the muscularis mucosa

30 _____ opening in the diaphragm through which the esophagus passes to reach the stomach

31 _____ three bands of smooth muscle in the wall of the large intestine, formed by the longitudinal muscle fibers of the muscularis externa

32_____ tiny (1 mm) fingerlike projections of the intestinal mucosa, which act to increase the absorptive surface area of the GI tract

33_____ tubelike openings at the bases of the intestinal villi lined with germinal cells that continually form new epithelial cells (which then migrate to cover the villi)

Terms related to digestive enzymes

α-amylase (AL-fah AM-il-ayz)   protease (PRO-tee-ayz)
enterokinase (en-ter-oh-KIN-ayz)   trypsin (TRIP-sin)
lipase (LY-payz)   zymogen (ZY-moh-jen)

1_____ general term for a class of enzymes that digest proteins and polypeptides

2_____ pancreatic protease formed by the activation of trypsinogen

3_____ membrane-bound enzyme of the intestinal epithelial cells that converts the inactive proteolytic enzyme trypsinogen to trypsin (which then converts other pancreatic zymogens)

4_____ general term for a class of enzymes that digest triglycerides (to form fatty acids and glycerol)

5_____ inactive precursor of a digestive enzyme (usually activated in the lumen of the GI tract) — the form in which many digestive enzymes are secreted

6_____ enzyme in saliva and pancreatic juice that catalyzes digestion of starches into monosaccharides and disaccharides

The Big Picture

Use the activities of this section to help you learn the broader concepts of this chapter.

Learning Exercises

1. Put these structures of the GI tract in the order in which food materials pass through them.

anus
ascending colon
cardiac sphincter
descending colon
duodenum

ileum
jejunum
mouth
pharynx
pylorus

rectum
sigmoid colon
stomach body
transverse colon
upper esophagus

1_____

2_____

3_____

4_____

5_____

6_____

7_____

8_____

9_____

10_____

11_____

12_____

13_____

14_____

15_____

2. Use these terms to identify the structures of the GI system in Figure 21-1.

colon
esophagus
gallbladder

liver
pharynx
rectum

salivary gland
small intestine
stomach

Figure 21-1

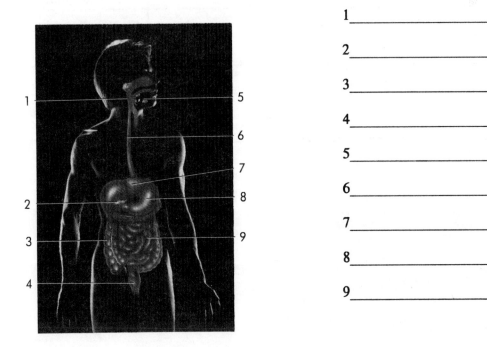

1_____

2_____

3_____

4_____

5_____

6_____

7_____

8_____

9_____

3. Fill in the blank areas in the table below, which summarizes the general functions of the primary GI organs.

Organ	Subdivision	General function(s)
_____		Gross mechanical breakdown; lubrication with saliva
_____		Swallowing, joins esophagus at a sphincter
_____		Movement of food from pharynx to stomach
_____	_____	Initial storage of food
	_____	Storage; secretion of gastric juice
	_____	Vigorous mixing of food with secretions to form chyme
_____	_____	Receives chyme from stomach and liver and pancreas secretions; important site for regulation/coordination of GI tract
	_____	Absorption of the majority of digestive end products
	_____	Fluid reabsorption; joins with large intestine
_____	_____	Fluid reabsorption
	_____	Fluid reabsorption
	_____	Fluid reabsorption
	_____	Storage of feces
	_____	Storage and elimination of feces

4. Identify the numbered structures in Figure 21-2, a cross-section of the intestinal wall.

artery   longitudinal muscle   serosa
circular muscle   lymphatic vessel   submucosa
crypts of Lieberkühn   mucosa   submucosal plexus
lacteals   muscularis externa   vein
lamina propria   myenteric plexus   villi

Figure 21-2

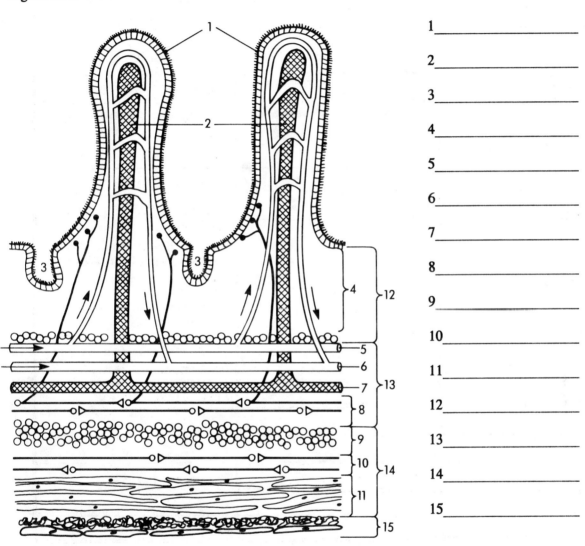

1 _____

2 _____

3 _____

4 _____

5 _____

6 _____

7 _____

8 _____

9 _____

10 _____

11 _____

12 _____

13 _____

14 _____

15 _____

5. Use these phrases to identify the characteristics of segmentation and peristalsis.

local
mainly for moving materials

mainly for mixing materials
occurs within haustra

occurs over long distances
pushes chyme out of stomach

Segmentation	Peristalsis

6. Fill in the blank portions of this table, which summarizes secretions into the GI lumen.

Gland/cell type	Secretion	Functional role
Salivary gland duct cell		
mucus cell		
serous cell		
Gastric gland parietal cell		
chief cell		
surface mucus		
mucus neck		
Pancreas acinar cell		
duct cell		
Liver		
Intestine most cells		
goblet cells		

272

7. Figure 21-3 represents the core of the mechanism for H$^+$ and HCO$_3^-$ secretion into the GI tract. Write in the molecular formulae that are missing.

Compartment A   Cell(s)   Compartment B

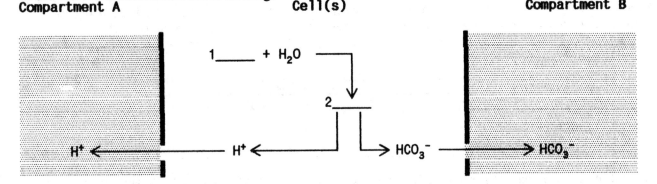

If this figure represents gastric secretion, Compartment ___ is the lumen and Compartment ___ is the blood.
If this figure represents intestinal secretion, Compartment ___ is the lumen and Compartment ___ is the blood.

8. Put a check mark by those situations that tend to stimulate mass movements and the defecation process.

1____presence of chyme in the duodenum

2____presence of food in the stomach

3____absence of food in the stomach

4____stretching of the rectum

5____sympathetic reflexes

6____parasympathetic reflexes

Quick Recall

Review some of the major concepts of this chapter by doing these "quick recall" activities.

1. Name the primary and accessory organs of the digestive system.

2. List the four principal layers of the GI wall.

3. Describe the movements of segmentation and peristalsis.

4. List the secretions found in the stomach lumen and their sources.

5. List the secretions found in the intestinal lumen and their sources.

6. List the structural adaptations of the GI tract that facilitate absorption.

7. Describe the cyclic path of bile salts.

Practice Test
Use this practice test to review the topics of this chapter and to prepare for your test on this material.

1.   The GI tract is regulated by
        a.   the myenteric plexus
        b.   the submucosal plexus
        c.   the parasympathetic branch of the ANS
        d.   GI hormones
        e.   all of the above

2.   The surface area for absorption in the GI tract is
        a.   limited to the duodenum and ileum
        b.   increased by microvilli
        c.   greater in the large intestine
        d.   approximately that expected for a smooth cylinder
        e.   b and c are correct

3.   Epithelial cells in the GI tract
        a.   have villi on their surface
        b.   are constantly being replaced
        c.   contain membrane-bound enzymes
        d.   b and c are correct
        e.   a, b, and c are correct

4.   The smooth muscle cells of the GI tract
        a.   are multi-unit
        b.   cannot generate action potentials
        c.   are activated by epinephrine
        d.   can develop force over a wide range of muscle lengths
        e.   do not contain myosin

5.   Activity of the smooth muscle cells of the GI tract is generally increased by
        a.   parasympathetic activity
        b.   stress activation
        c.   gastrin
        d.   all of the above

6.   Activity of the smooth muscle cells of the GI tract is generally decreased by
        a.   stress relaxation
        b.   cholecystokinin
        c.   secretin
        d.   increased slow wave activity
        e.   both a and c

7. In the process of swallowing
   a. there can be waves of secondary peristalsis
   b. the glottis is closed
   c. the lower esophageal sphincter opens
   d. b and c are correct
   e. a, b, and c

8. In the stomach
   a. motility is increased by sympathetic stimulation
   b. contractions are initiated by a pacemaker in the stomach body
   c. contractions decrease in velocity as the pylorus is approached
   d. a, b, and c

9. Bile assists primarily in the digestion of which nutrient?
   a. starches
   b. lipids
   c. proteins
   d. sugars
   e. a and d

10. Saliva contains an enzyme that digests
    a. lipids
    b. proteins
    c. starches
    d. vitamins
    e. none of the above

11. α-amylase is secreted by the
    a. stomach
    b. salivary glands
    c. pancreas
    d. liver
    e. b and c

12. Most digestion occurs in the
    a. duodenum
    b. stomach
    c. colon
    d. liver
    e. ileum

13. Slow waves in the small intestine
    a. have a lower frequency in the duodenum than in the ileum
    b. occur less frequently than in the stomach
    c. directly produce muscle contraction
    d. arise in the longitudinal muscle
    e. none of the above is correct

14. Segmentation in the small intestine is
    a. decreased by parasympathetic activity
    b. increased by sympathetic activity
    c. increased by local distension
    d. necessary to permit adequate time for reabsorption
    e. c and d

15.　The colon
　　　a.　　is characterized by prolonged segmentation
　　　b.　　is specialized for water reabsorption
　　　c.　　undergoes occasional mass movements
　　　d.　　a, b, and c

Answers

Here are answers (or references) to some of the questions presented above.

Word Parts (your examples may be different) 1-bilirubin, 2-enteroendocrine, 3-gastric reflux, 4-gastrin, 5-sigmoid colon, 6-peristalsis, 7-zymogen

Key Terms: Processes: 1. swallowing center 2. segmentation 3. stress activation 4. mass movement 5. stress relaxation 6. gastric reflux 7. alkaline tide 8. pancreatolysis 9. peristalsis

Structures/Substances: 1. ileum 2. jejunum 3. chyme 4. gallbladder 5. goblet cell 6. submucosa 7. bolus 8. bile 9. submucosal plexus 10. myenteric plexus 11. plicae circulares 12. enteroendocrine cell 13. duct cells 14. G cell 15. gastrointestinal [GI] tract 16. lacteal 17. haustra 18. serosa 19. esophagus 20. brush border 21. colon 22. acini 23. anus 24. stomach 25. rectum 26. enteric nervous system 27. duodenum 28. muscularis externa 29. mucosa 30. esophageal hiatus 31. taeniae coli 32. villi 33. crypts of Lieberkühn

Enzymes: 1. protease 2. trypsin 3. enterokinase 4. lipase 5. zymogen 6. α-amylase

Learning Exercises: 1. 1-mouth, 2-pharynx, 3-upper esophagus, 4-cardiac sphincter, 5-stomach body, 6-pylorus, 7-duodenum, 8-jejunum, 9-ileum, 10-ascending colon, 11-transverse colon, 12-descending colon, 13-sigmoid colon, 14-rectum, 15-anus 2. 1-pharynx, 2-gallbladder, 3-colon, 4-rectum, 5-salivary gland, 6-esophagus, 7-liver, 8-stomach, 9-small intestine 3. (Compare your table to Table 21-1 in the text.) 4. 1-villi, 2-lacteals, 3-crypts of Lieberkühn, 4-lamina propria, 5-artery, 6-vein, 7-lymphatic vessel, 8-submucosal plexus, 9-circular muscle, 10-myenteric plexus, 11-longitudinal muscle, 12-mucosa, 13-submucosa, 14-muscularis externa, 15-serosa 5. Peristalsis: mainly for moving materials, occurs over long distances, pushes material out of stomach; Segmentation: mainly for mixing materials, local, occurs within haustra 6. (Compare your table with Table 21-4 in the text.) 7. 1-CO_2, 2-HCO_3^- (gastric: A, B) (intestinal: B, A) 8. 1, 2, 4, 6

Quick Recall: (You should be able to answer these questions easily without correction or confirmation by this point in your studies. If you cannot, review your notes, the text chapter, and the previous study activities to find the answers.)

Practice Test: 1-e, 2-e, 3-e, 4-d, 5-d, 6-a, 7-e, 8-b, 9-b, 10-c, 11-e, 12-a, 13-a, 14-e, 15-d

Chapter 22
Absorption and Digestion

Focus
Review this section *first*. It will help you focus on the overall message of this chapter.

Chapter Outline
Read through the outline slowly. This activity will help your mind organize the topics of this chapter.

An overview of digestion and absorption
      Digestion, the task at hand
      Pathways for absorption from the gastrointestinal tract
      The liver and hepatic portal circulation
Carbohydrate digestion and absorption
      Dietary sources of carbohydrate
      Starch digestion by amylases and brush-border enzymes
      Monosaccharide absorption
Protein digestion and absorption
      Enzymes of protein digestion
      Mechanisms of amino acid absorption
Fat digestion and absorption
      Fat emulsification in the intestine
      Fat digestion by pancreatic lipases
      Micelle formation and fat absorption
      Chylomicron formation in intestinal epithelial cells
Absorption of iron and vitamins
      Iron absorption
      Vitamin absorption
Electrolyte and water absorption
      The scale of daily movement of material in the GI tract
      Mechanisms of solute and water transfer across the GI tract wall
      Mechanisms of diarrhea and constipation
Regulation of gastrointestinal function
      Gastrointestinal control systems
      Cephalic phase of digestion
      Gastric phase of digestion
      Control of gastric motility and stomach emptying
      Intestinal phase of digestion

Learning Objectives
These are the learning goals for this part of the course. After reading the text, attending class, and studying this chapter, you should be able to:

♦ understand how water, amino acids, and sugars are absorbed in the gastrointestinal tract

♦ appreciate the role of the transmembrane Na^+ gradient in carrier-mediated cotransport of most amino acids and sugars into the intestinal epithelial cells

♦ describe carbohydrate digestion in the mouth, stomach and small intestine, noting the role of brush-border enzymes in the small intestine

♦ trace the pathway of lipids from the intestinal lumen to the bloodstream

♦ describe how lipids are absorbed, resynthesized in the epithelial cells, and transported in the lymph

♦ describe the processes involved in iron absorption

♦ understand the mechanisms for absorption of water-soluble and fat-soluble vitamins, noting the specialized transport mechanisms for vitamins

♦ characterize the cephalic, gastric, and intestinal phases of digestion

♦ compare long-loop and short-loop reflexes in the control of digestion

♦ identify the major known gastrointestinal tract hormones--gastrin, motilin, gastric inhibitory peptide, secretin, and cholecystokinin--and describe how each regulates gastrointestinal tract function

Language of Physiology
Physiology uses its own set of terms, many of which may be unfamiliar to you. This section will help you improve your mastery of key physiological terms.

Word Parts
Here are some combining forms often seen in physiological terms. Give an example of a term that contains each word part listed.

Word Part	Meaning	Example
chyl-, chym-	juice; something poured	1
ferr-	iron	2
hepat-	liver	3
-in	signifies a protein	4
-ose	signifies a carbohydrate	5
sin-	cavity; recess	6

| -ule | (diminutive) | 7 |

Key Terms
Read each of the terms in each grouping below aloud, using the pronunciation guide if necessary. This will help you to remember them better than if you read them silently. Then, write out the correct term next to each of the descriptions given.

Terms related to processes

cephalic phase (se-FAL-ik)
conjugation (kahn-joo-GAY-shun)
enterogastric reflex
  (en-ter-oh-GAST-rik)
gastric phase

gastrocolic reflex (gas-troh-KOHL-ik)
gastroileal reflex (gas-troh-IL-ee-al)
intestinal phase
lipolysis (lip-AHL-is-is)
receptive relaxation

1 _____ parasympathetic reflex in which distension of the duodenal walls causes a reflex inhibition of gastric motility and an increase in pyloric tone

2 _____ reflex in which stomach activity causes relaxation of the ileocecal valve, emptying the small intestine's contents in anticipation of the stomach emptying its contents

3 _____ reflex in which stomach activity stimulates motility in the large intestine, causing the mass movements that often follow a meal

4 _____ in the liver, a process of adding a polar group (such as glucuronic acid, taurine, or glycine) to a non-water-soluble molecule so that it can later be cleared easily by the kidney

5 _____ process of the digestion of lipid molecules

6 _____ second of three major phases of digestion; it begins when food enters the stomach and triggers both local and long-loop parasympathetically-mediated reflexes

7 _____ relaxation of stomach's smooth muscle as food enters

8 _____ first phase of digestion, during which anticipation of eating food can trigger physiological preparations to begin its digestion

9 _____ third of three phases of digestion; it begins when food begins to enter the duodenum and triggers a series of regulatory reflexes

Terms related to structures/substances

acidophilus milk (as-id-oh-FIL-us)
amylopectin (am-il-oh-PEK-tin)
bile canaliculi (kan-al-IK-yoo-lee)
cellulose
cholecystokinin [CCK]
  (koh-le-sis-toh-KYN-in)
cholesterol ester
chylomicron (ky-loh-MY-krahn)
ferritin (FAYR-it-in)
gastric inhibitory peptide [GIP]

gastrin
hepatic vein (hep-AT-ik)
hepatic portal vein (hep-AT-ik)
hepatocyte (hep-AT-oh-syt)
intrinsic factor
lobule
mixed micelle (my-SEL)
motilin (moh-TIL-in)
secretagogue (se-KREE-tah-gawg)
secretin (se-KREE-tin)

1_____ GI hormone released by the stomach's G cells that acts to amplify the parasympathetic stimulation of the stomach's parietal cell secretion of acid and chief cell secretion of pepsinogen

2_____ substance released by intestinal K cells in response to the high osmotic pressure of food-filled chyme (rather than water); it also acts to slow stomach motility

3_____ GI hormone released from duodenal argentaffin cells when the pH exceeds 4.5, triggering increased stomach mixing (and pyloric tone)

4_____ GI hormone released by duodenal cells when the pH drops below 4.5 and/or when presented with hypertonic or high-fat chyme; it acts to stimulate bicarbonate secretion by the pancreas, inhibit stomach motility, and stimulate pepsinogen secretion

5_____ glycoprotein synthesized and released by stomach parietal cells; it binds to vitamin B_{12}, allowing its uptake into epithelial cells

6_____ type of mixed micelle formed within the intestinal epithelial cells that subsequently exits via exocytosis from the basolateral surface and moves into a lacteal

7_____ type of molecule formed by the joining of cholesterol to a single fatty acid chain; one of many types of dietary fat

8_____ polysaccharide of glucose that forms the walls of plant cells (the main structural component of plant tissue); it is indigestible by humans and is the major component of dietary fiber

9_____ duodenal hormone that causes the gall bladder to contract and inhibits gastric secretion in response to food entry into the duodenum

10_____ iron-binding protein within intestinal epithelial cells that stores iron absorbed from bile in the lumen of the GI tract

11_____ iron-carrying protein in the plasma that picks up iron released during processing of old RBCs

12_____ general term for liver cells

13_____ general term for a 50 to 100 nm structure composed of fatty acids, cholesterol, lysophosphatides, 2-monoglycerides, glycerol, lecithin, and bile salts in a spherical arrangement (with polar groups facing outward); a result of lipid digestion

14_____ large capillaries found between the hepatocyte sheets that form a liver lobule

15_____ milk that contains a culture of lactose-digesting bacteria

16_____ plant starch consisting of chains of glucose that, together with glycogen, contributes over 50% of total daily carbohydrate intake

17_____ substances such as free amino acids that stimulate gastric secretion by promoting release of gastrin and pepsin

18_____ small functional unit of the liver, composed of sheets of hepatocytes organized around a central vein

19_____ tiny ducts in the liver that collect the bile formed by hepatocytes and then converge to form the hepatic bile duct

20_____ vein that carries blood away from the liver and back toward the heart

21_____   vein that carries blood from GI wall capillaries to the liver

Terms related to digestive enzymes

chymotrypsin (ky-moh-TRIP-sin)   exopeptidase (eks-oh-PEP-tyd-ayz)
colipase (koh-LYP-ayz)   phospholipase (fahs-foh-LIP-ayz)
endopeptidase (en-doh-PEP-tyd-ayz)

1_____   pancreatic polypeptide that enhances lipase digestion of emulsified fats by increasing lipase adherence to lipid droplets, preventing lipase inhibition by bile salts, and optimizing the pH

2_____   endopeptidase secreted by the pancreas, along with trypsin

3_____   enzyme that digests phospholipids, yielding lysophosphatides and fatty acids

4_____   member of a class of peptide-bond-breaking enzymes that break bonds in the center of polypeptide chains (as opposed to the free ends)

5_____   member of a class of peptide-bond-breaking enzymes that break polypeptide chains at the free carboxy end (carboxypeptidase) or at the free amino end (aminopeptidase)

Other Key Terms

anorexia nervosa   hypervitaminosis
bulimia   (hy-per-vyt-ah-min-OH-is)
                       lactose intolerance

1_____   condition of self-inflicted starvation; its victims becoming severely malnourished, although they deny hunger

2_____   toxic condition caused by excess consumption of vitamins

3_____   condition in which the patient alternates between eating binges and fasting, accompanied by self-induced vomiting and abuse of laxatives and diuretics (to control weight)

4_____   condition in which the enzyme needed to degrade lactose is absent

The Big Picture

Use the activities of this section to help you learn the broader concepts of this chapter.

Learning Exercises

1. For each of the series of diagrams in the Figure 22-1 series on the following pages, sketch the manner in which the designated nutrient is absorbed. Use standard molecular formulae and/or chemical names, "+", and "------>" where appropriate. As an arrow crosses a cell membrane, show whether it is unfacilitated passive transport by using a plain arrow "------>" or carrier-mediated transport by using a circle and arrow "__O__>." Be sure to include molecules that are indirectly involved in transporting the nutrient (a Na⁺ gradient, for example).

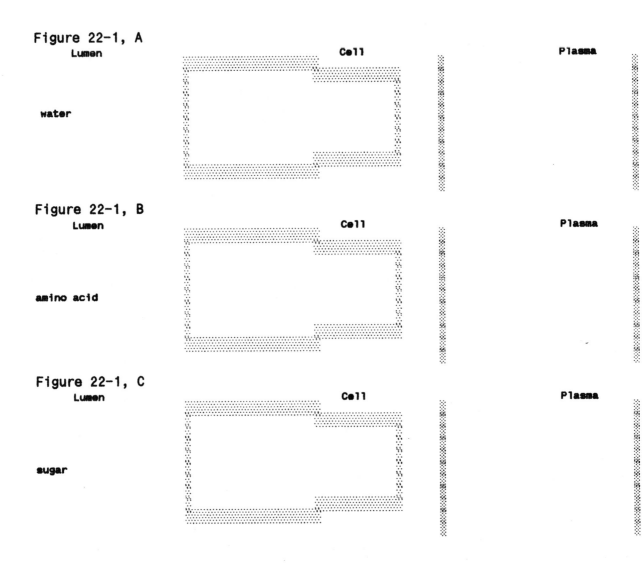

Figure 22-1, A
Lumen · · · Cell · · · Plasma

water

Figure 22-1, B
Lumen · · · Cell · · · Plasma

amino acid

Figure 22-1, C
Lumen · · · Cell · · · Plasma

sugar

Figure 22-1, D

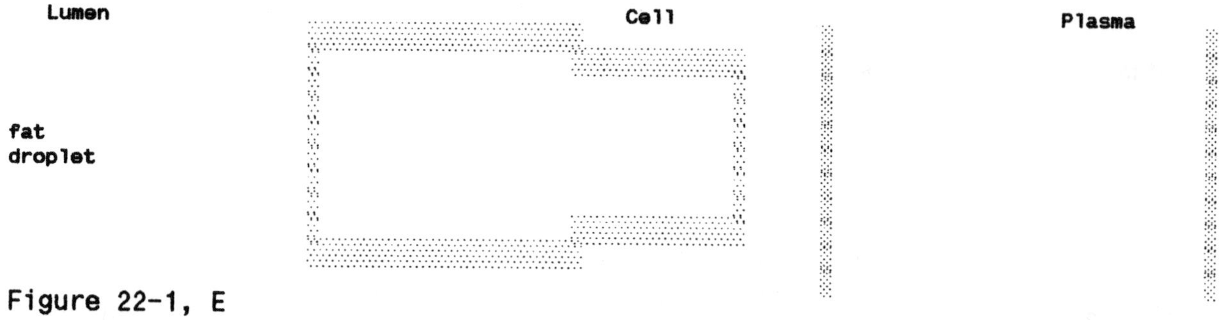

Lumen   Cell   Plasma

fat
droplet

Figure 22-1, E

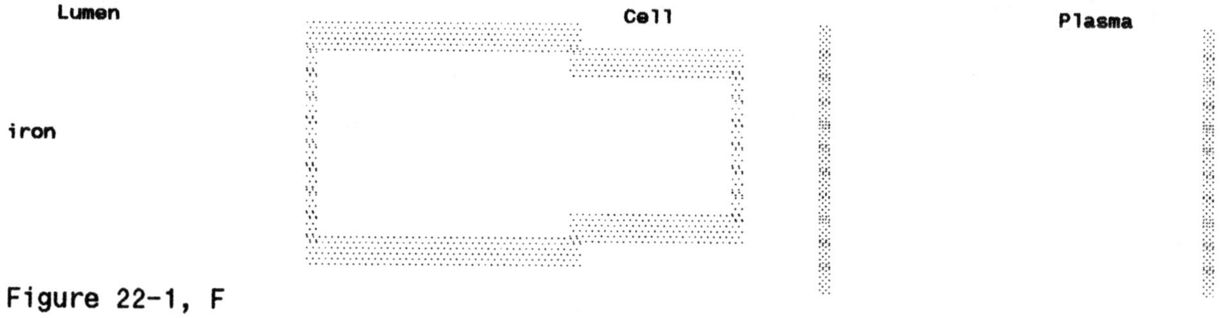

Lumen   Cell   Plasma

iron

Figure 22-1, F

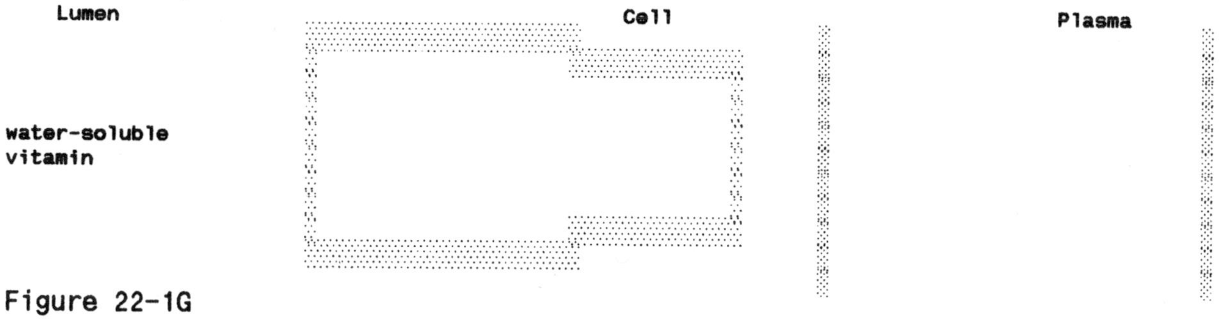

Lumen   Cell   Plasma

water-soluble
vitamin

Figure 22-1G

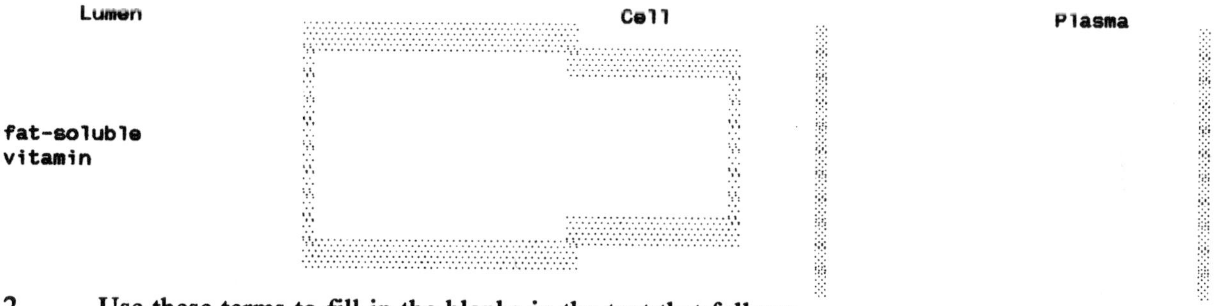

Lumen   Cell   Plasma

fat-soluble
vitamin

2.   Use these terms to fill in the blanks in the text that follows.

CCK	gastrin	long
cephalic	GIP	motilin
digestive enzymes	intestinal	short
gastric		

Digestion can be divided into three phases. The _____ phase begins

before food ingestion, when the idea or sensing of food's presence occurs. The

_____ phase begins as food enters the stomach, and the

_____ phase begins as food enters the duodenum.

283

Stimuli arising from the presence of food in the different GI organs help regulate movement of materials through the tract and the secretion of _____. This regulation involves reflexes that use _____ loops (parasympathetic pathways), _____ (nerve and/or hormone) loops.

Among the best-understood GI hormones are: _____ (from the stomach), which stimulates gastric acid and pepsinogen secretion and gastric motility; _____ (from the intestine), which stimulates gastric and intestinal motility and pepsinogen release; _____ (from the intestine), which stimulates intestinal and pancreatic secretion and inhibits gastric secretion and motility; and _____ (from the intestine), which stimulates gall bladder contraction and inhibits gastric secretion.

3.   Put the name of the proper GI hormone in each blank in the table below.

Hormone	Stimuli	Effects	Role
	amino acids distension pH > 3 parasympathetic activity	increased acid secretion increased antral motility increased pepsinogen secretion	facilitates gastric digestion
	glucose fats hypertonicity	increased intestinal motility decreased gastric secretion and motility	limits gastric emptying; prepares the intestine for substrate
	pH > 4.5	increased gastric motility increased intestinal motility increased pepsinogen secretion	facilitates digestion in intestine
	hypertonicity pH < 4.5 parasympathetic activity	increased pancreatic HCO_3—secretion increased pancreatic zymogen secretion decreased gastric motility decreased gastric secretion	limits gastric emptying; neutralizes chyme leaving the stomach
	fats amino acids	increased pancreatic zymogen secretion increased intestinal secretion increased intestinal motility decreased gastric secretion increased gallbladder contraction	limits gastric emptying; promotes digestion in the intestine

4.	Identify the reflex described in each entry of the table below, which summarizes some of the principal reflexes of the GI tract.

Reflex	Description
Autonomic nervous system reflexes	
	swallowing food relaxes the fundus of the stomach
	acid and hypertonic solutions in the duodenum inhibit gastric emptying
	distension of the stomach and duodenum increase the motility of the ileum, cecum, and colon
	ileocecal sphincter opens when gastric emptying begins
Enteric nervous system reflexes	
	local stimulation of the intestine causes contraction of the muscle immediately above the point of stimulation and relaxation of the muscle below the point of stimulation

5.	Figure 22-2 represents the three phases of digestion. They are staggered to represent their overlap in time (as in Figure 22-14 in the text), with the solid outline representing the actual digestive phase and the shaded outline representing the time just before the phase begins. At the point of each arrow (representing a regulatory agent or process) put a "+" to indicate a stimulating effect or a "-" to indicate an inhibitory effect.

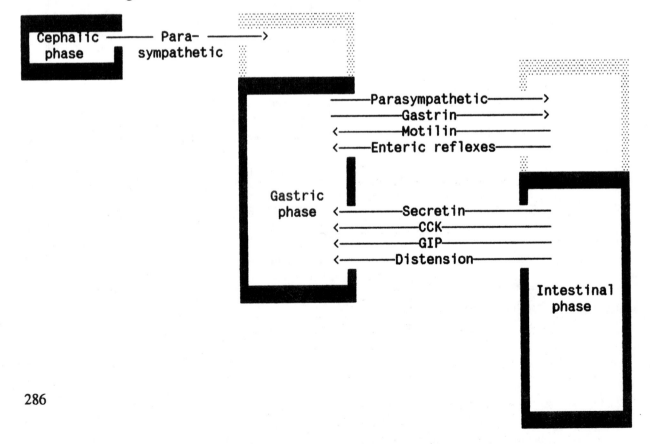

Quick Recall
Review some of the major concepts of this chapter by doing these "quick recall" activities.

1. Tell how and where each of these nutrients is absorbed.

   water

   protein

   carbohydrate

   lipid

   vitamin

2. Give the source and substrate for each enzyme listed.

   amylase

   pepsin

   lipase

   trypsin

   chymotrypsin

   maltase

   sucrase

   lactase

3. List the steps of lipid digestion.

4. List the steps of protein digestion.

5. List the steps of carbohydrate digestion.

6. List the actions of bile (as a digestive agent).

7. Name the three phases of digestion.

Practice Test

Use this practice test to review the topics of this chapter and to prepare for your test on this material.

1. Water is
   a. absorbed actively
   b. absorbed passively
   c. not absorbed in the GI tract
   d. all absorbed by the mouth mucosa
   e. b and d

2. Glucose is absorbed by means of
   a. passive transport
   b. sodium cotransport
   c. amino acid cotransport
   d. bile emulsification
   e. none of the above

3. Which of these releases a substance essential to lipid digestion?
   a. liver
   b. gallbladder
   c. pancreas
   d. a and b
   e. a, b, and c

4. In the colon, chyme
   a. becomes isotonic
   b. becomes hypotonic
   c. becomes hypertonic
   d. remains unchanged
   e. none of the above

5. Galactose competes with _ for its carrier.
   a. maltose
   b. glucose
   c. fructose
   d. aspartame
   e. sucrose

6.   Which of these facilitates lipid digestion?
      a.   intrinsic factor
      b.   bile
      c.   colipase
      d.   pepsin
      e.   b and c

7.   During digestion, lipids may break down to form
      a.   emulsified droplets
      b.   micelles
      c.   chylomicrons
      d.   glycerol
      e.   all of the above

8.   The cephalic phase of digestion
      a.   includes the enterogastric reflex
      b.   may be stimulated by the smell of hot pizza
      c.   begins only when food enters the mouth
      d.   begins only when food enters the stomach
      e.   a and b

9.   Neutral and basic amino acids are
      a.   absorbed by means of the same transport system
      b.   transported by means of separate transport systems
      c.   end products of proteolytic enzyme activity
      d.   b and c
      e.   a and c

10.   Gallbladder contraction is stimulated by
      a.   gastrin
      b.   secretin
      c.   cholecystokinin
      d.   fat in the duodenum
      e.   c and d

11.   The enterogastric reflex involves
      a.   parasympathetic pathways
      b.   distension of the duodenal walls
      c.   inhibition of gastric motility
      d.   a and c
      e.   a, b, and c

12.   The gastroileal reflex involves
      a.   sympathetic pathways
      b.   relaxation of the ileocecal valve
      c.   anticipation of chyme movement out of the stomach
      d.   b and c
      e.   a, b, and c

13. Absorption of vitamin B_{12} requires
    a. binding to a carrier molecule
    b. intrinsic factor
    c. amylase
    d. a and b
    e. b and c

14. Which of these stimulates pancreatic secretion and inhibits gastric activity?
    a. secretin
    b. CCK
    c. pancreatin
    d. gastrin
    e. a and c

15. Lecithin is important in the complete digestion of
    a. carbohydrates
    b. sugars
    c. lipids
    d. proteins
    e. a and b

Answers

Here are answers (or references) to some of the questions presented above.

Word Parts: (your examples may be different) 1-chylomicron/ chymotrypsin, 2-transferrin, 3-hepatic vein, 4-gastrin, 5-cellulose, 6-sinusoid, 7-lobule

Key Terms: Processes: 1. enterogastric reflex 2. gastroileal reflex 3. gastrocolic reflex 4. conjugation 5. lipolysis 6. gastric phase 7. receptive relaxation 8. cephalic phase 9. intestinal phase **Structures/Substances:** 1. gastrin 2. gastric inhibitory peptide [GIP] 3. motilin 4. secretin 5. intrinsic factor 6. chylomicron 7. cholesterol ester 8. cellulose 9. cholecystokinin [CCK] 10. ferritin 11. transferrin 12. hepatocyte 13. mixed micelle 14. sinusoid 15. acidophilus milk 16. amylopectin 17. secretagogue 18. lobule 19. bile canaliculi 20. hepatic vein 21. hepatic portal vein
Enzymes: 1. colipase 2. chymotrypsin 3. phospholipase 4. endopeptidase 5. exopeptidase
Other: 1. anorexia nervosa 2. hypervitaminosis 3. bulimia 4. lactose intolerance

Learning Exercises: 1. (See Figures 22-1 to 22-13 in the text, and Summary items 1,3,4,5 at the end of Chapter 22.) 2. cephalic, gastric, intestinal, digestive enzymes, long, short, gastrin, motilin, GIP, CCK 3. gastrin, GIP, motilin, secretin, cholecystokinin 4. receptive relaxation, enterogastric reflex, gastrocolic reflex, gastroileal reflex, myenteric reflex 5. (Compare your chart to that in Figure 22-15 in the text.)

Quick Recall: (You should be able to answer these questions easily without correction or confirmation by this point in your studies. If you cannot, review your notes, the text chapter, and the previous study activities to find the answers.)

Practice Test: 1-b, 2-b, 3-e, 4-c, 5-b, 6-e, 7-e, 8-b, 9-d, 10-e, 11-e, 12-d, 13-d, 14-a, 15-c

Chapter 23
Endocrine Control of
Organic Metabolism and Growth

Focus
Review this section *first*. It will help you focus on the overall message of this chapter.

Chapter Outline
Read through the outline slowly. This activity will help your mind organize the topics of this chapter.

Characteristics of the absorptive state
      Role of insulin
      Diabetes mellitus: cellular famine in the midst of plenty
      Roles of the liver in the absorptive state
      Transport and storage of lipids
      Protein synthesis
      Somatostatin
Characteristics of the postabsorptive state
      Onset of the postabsorptive state
      Role of glucagon
      Control of glucagon secretion
      Conversion of protein to glucose
      Adrenal hormones
      Metabolic homeostasis in starvation
Regulation of food intake
      Satiety signals and short-term regulation of food intake
      Long-term control of food intake by nutritional state
Growth and metabolism over the life cycle
      Growth and growth hormone
      Effect of aging on body composition
Thyroid hormones and basal metabolic rate
      Regulation of thyroid function
      Thyroid disorders
      Thermoregulation and metabolic adaptation to cold

Learning Objectives

These are the learning goals for this part of the course. After reading the text, attending class, and studying this chapter, you should be able to:

♦ understand how insulin and glucagon regulate blood glucose

♦ distinguish between the absorptive and postabsorptive states

♦ understand the difference between type I and type II diabetes mellitus

♦ describe the adaptive responses of the body to periods of starvation

♦ describe how increases in blood levels of glucose, bulk aspects of ingested food, and neural and hormonal signals produce satiety

♦ understand the factors involved in long-term regulation of body weight

♦ describe how the relative proportions of fat, muscle, and ossified skeleton vary over the life cycle

♦ describe the processes by which thyroid hormones set the body's metabolic rate

♦ describe the adaptive responses of the body to cold

Language of Physiology

Physiology uses its own set of terms, many of which may be unfamiliar to you. This section will help you improve your mastery of key physiological terms.

Word Parts

Here are some combining forms often seen in physiological terms. Give an example of a term that contains each word part listed.

Word Part	Meaning	Example
apo-	from; lack	1
chondro-	cartilage	2
epi-	upon	3
gluc-	glucose, sugar	4
-gon	generate; seed	5
-ism	signifies "condition of"	6
pyro-	heat; fever	7
stat-, stas-	a standing, stopping	8

Key Terms

Read each of the terms in each grouping below aloud, using the pronunciation guide if necessary. This will help you to remember them better than if you read them silently. Then, write out the correct term next to each of the descriptions given.

Terms Related to Processes

absorptive state
basal metabolic rate [BMR]
chondrogenesis (kahn-droh-JEN-es-is)
futile cycle
gluconeogenesis
    (gloo-koh-nee-oh-JEN-es-is)
glucose-sparing
glucostatic hypothesis
    (gloo-koh-STAT-ik)
glycogenesis (gly-koh-JEN-es-is)

glycogenolysis (gly-koh-jen-AHL-is-is)
lipogenesis (lip-oh-JEN-es-is)
lipolysis (lip-AHL-is-is)
lipostatic hypothesis (lip-oh-STAT-ik)
ossification (ahs-sif-ik-AY-shun)
postabsorptive state
proteolysis (proh-tee-AHL-is-is)
thermogenesis (ther-moh-JEN-es-is)
thermostatic hypothesis
    (ther-moh-STAT-ik)

1_____ catabolic process in which a lipid molecule is broken apart to yield its component molecular subunits

2_____ newer hypothesis of long-term regulation of eating, based on the feedback control of eating related to fat deposits in the body

3_____ catabolic process in which glycogen is broken apart to yield separate glucose molecules

4_____ period (of metabolism) during which nutrients are entering the circulation not from outside the body, but from internal stores

5_____ theory of total body weight regulation that states that the heat generated by excess body fat (i.e., an increase in body temperature) serves as a trigger to an automatic reduction in nutrient consumption

6_____ process in the cell involving repeated synthesis and degradation of energy storage molecules, "wasting" energy during the conversions but increasing heat production

7_____ catabolic process in which protein molecules are broken apart to yield smaller polypeptides and/or separate amino acids

8_____ period (of metabolism) during which nutrients are being absorbed into the circulation from the GI lumen

9_____ anabolic process in which a triglyceride is formed from fatty acids and glycerol

10_____ older hypothesis of long-term regulation of eating, based on the feedback control of eating related to the availability of glucose to body cells

11_____ anabolic process in which noncarbohydrates, such as amino acids, are used to form "new" glucose molecules

12_____ anabolic process in which glycogen is formed from separate glucose molecules

13_____ formation of cartilage tissue

14 _____   heat production by the body (to increase overall body temperature); may be the "shivering" (short-term) type resulting from sympathetic stimulation or the "nonshivering" (long-term) type resulting from thyroid responses

15 _____   calcification of soft connective tissue to form hard bone

16 _____   use of fatty acids and ketones as a metabolic energy source, thus saving glucose (the more typical energy source)

17 _____   rate at which the body breaks down stored energy when the person is in an alert (but resting) state and has fasted for 12 hours (often expressed as kcal/kg/day or percentage above or below normal)

Terms related to structures/substances

brown fat
complete protein
epiphyseal plate (ep-ih-FIZ-ee-al)
essential amino acid
high-density lipoprotein (HDL)

ketone (KEE-tohn)
low-density lipoprotein (LDL)
satiety center (sat-EE-et-ee)
very low-density lipoprotein (VLDL)

1 _____   lipoprotein that facilitates lipid uptake into chylomicrons and VLDL

2 _____   reflex center for satiety in the ventromedial region of the hypothalamus

3 _____   dietary protein that contains all essential amino acids (such as meat protein)

4 _____   lipoprotein manufactured in the liver that carries low-molecular-weight lipids to cells

5 _____   special, metabolically active tissue in the human infant (neck, chest, and between the scapulae) that produces heat and channels it to the thorax and vessels that serve the brain

6 _____   lipoprotein formed when a VLDL loses its lighter (lower-molecular-weight) lipid groups to body cells; once formed, it returns to the liver

7 _____   amino acid that is required in the diet, since the human body cannot synthesize it

8 _____   any of several small organic acids (such as acetone) produced by liver cells when excess acetyl-CoA is available

9 _____   cartilaginous "growth region" of a long bone

Terms related to regulatory substances

apoprotein (ap-oh-PROH-teen)
cortisol (KORT-ih-sol)
glucagon (GLOO-kah-gahn)
glycogen synthetase (SIN-thet-ayz)

lipoprotein lipase
proinsulin (proh-IN-soo-lin)
somatomedin (soh-mat-oh-MEE-din)
somatostatin (soh-mat-oh-STAT-in)

1 _____   hormone released by pancreatic delta cells that acts to prevent an overload of the GI system by decreasing GI motility and secretion and pancreatic secretions of enzymes, insulin, and glucagon

2 _____   type of protein needed to activate lipoprotein lipase and to permit chylomicrons and VLDLs to enter the cells lining the intestine

3_____ also called capillary lipase, an enzyme present in capillary endothelium of adipose and some muscular tissue that liberates fatty acids from triglycerides

4_____ insulin-sensitive enzyme that limits the rate of glycogenesis (from glucose-6-phosphate)

5_____ any of a family of insulin-like hormones secreted into the blood by the liver (and perhaps other tissues), promoting mitosis and protein synthesis in target cells

6_____ major postabsorptive, catabolic hormone released from pancreatic alpha cells; it promotes mobilization of glucose from body stores

7_____ steroid hormone secreted by the adrenal cortex (one of the glucocorticoids); it must be present for glucagon to stimulate metabolic pathways

8_____ inactive precursor of insulin, activated within secretory vesicles before release by pancreatic beta cells

Other Key Terms

acromegaly (ak-roh-MEG-al-ee)   hyperglycemia (hy-per-gly-SEE-mee-ah)
core body temperature   hyperthyroidism (hy-per-THY-royd-izm)
dwarfism [pituitary]   hypothyroidism (hy-poh-THY-royd-izm)
gigantism (jy-GANT-izm)   insulin shock
glycouria   osteoporosis (ahs-tee-oh-poh-ROHS-is)
goiter   satiety (sat-EE-et-ee)

1_____ condition of decreased blood glucose concentration caused by an administration of a significant dose of insulin without a concurrent ingestion of sufficient carbohydrates

2_____ condition of net decalcification of the skeleton with advancing age, resulting in the formation of porosities in the bones

3_____ condition of deformity of the hands, feet and face accompanied by skin abnormalities (coarseness); caused by hypersecretion of growth hormone after complete development of the skeleton has occurred

4_____ enlargement of the thyroid gland, causing a bulging of the neck; often results from insufficient dietary intake of iodine (causing a feedback increase of TSH, which stimulates thyroid growth)

5_____ abnormal increase in thyroid hormone secretion, resulting in an increase of the metabolic rate

6_____ abnormal decrease in thyroid hormone secretion, resulting in a decrease in the metabolic rate

7_____ condition of elevated glucose concentration in the blood

8_____ condition of having glucose in the urine

9_____ state of being satiated (feeling "full"; having consumed enough food)

10_____ temperature of the major internal organs (heart, brain, thoracic and abdominal organs), 36° C to 37.6° C in adults

11_____ condition of abnormally insufficient growth of the skeleton, caused by hyposecretion of growth hormone during the developmental years

12_____ condition of abnormally excessive growth of the skeleton, caused by hypersecretion of growth hormone during the developmental years

The Big Picture
Use the activities of this section to help you learn the broader concepts of this chapter.

Learning Exercises

1. For each statement below, write "I" if it applies to insulin or "G" if it applies to glucagon (or "I, G" if it applies to both).

1____ increases glucose uptake from blood by liver, fat, and muscle cells

2____ stimulates enzymes that catalyze glycogenolysis

3____ most important during the absorptive state

4____ most important during the postabsorptive state

5____ stimulates lipoprotein lipase

6____ stimulates hormone-sensitive lipase in the fat cells and release of the products

7____ stimulates gluconeogenesis

8____ increases uptake of some amino acids from blood

9____ regulates blood glucose level

2. Put each of these characteristics into the correct column(s) of the table.

affects about 80% of patients with diabetes
affects about 20% of patients with diabetes
can be treated by altering diet and exercise regimen
can be treated by insulin replacement therapy

insulin-dependent
insulin-independent
results from lack of, or abnormal, insulin receptors
results from inadequate beta-cell secretion

Type I diabetes mellitus	Type II diabetes mellitus

296

3. In each blank in the table below, write "increase" or "decrease."

Factor	Effect on insulin secretion	Effect on glucagon secretion
hyperglycemia		
hypoglycemia		
increased plasma amino acid		
parasympathetic input to pancreas		
sympathetic input to pancreas		
somatostatin		

4. On the graph in Figure 23-1 below, draw a rough line indicating the average percent of body fat from age 20 to age 55.

Figure
23-1

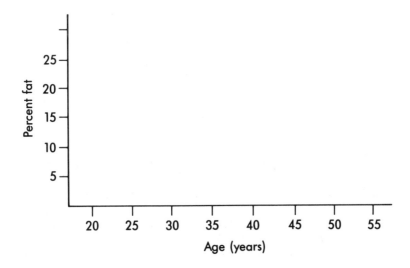

a. How would the shape of a graph of percent body weight of muscle over time compare to the shape of this line?

b. How would the shape of a graph of percent body weight of ossified bone over time compare to the shape of this line?

5. Major thermoregulatory responses are summarized in this table. Fill in the effects, which are missing.

Organ(s)	Response when hypothalamic temperature is below the set point	Explanation of effect on body temperature
cutaneous arterioles	constricted	
sweat glands	no secretion	
pilomotor muscles	contracted	
skeletal muscles	shivering	
adrenal medulla	increased epinephrine secretion	
thyroid	increased TH secretion	

6. Use these terms as labels for Figure 23-2, as indicated.

amino acids
fatty acids

glucose
glycerol
ketones
lactic acid

Figure 23-2

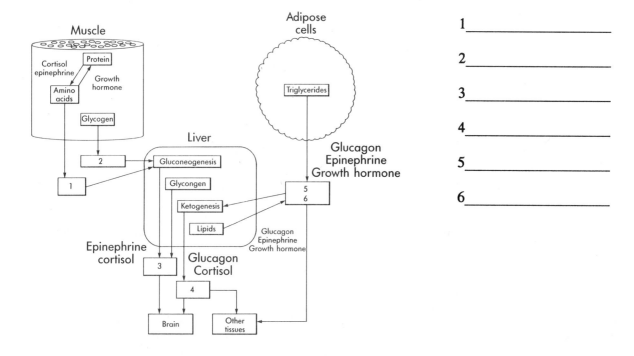

1 _____

2 _____

3 _____

4 _____

5 _____

6 _____

Quick Recall
Review some of the major concepts of this chapter by doing these "quick recall" activities.

1. List the effects of insulin on the blood glucose concentration.

2. List the effects of glucagon on the blood glucose concentration.

3. Name and briefly describe the two major types of diabetes mellitus.

4. List the stimuli that produce satiety.

5. List the factors that may contribute to long-term body weight regulation.

6. List six physiological responses to cold.

Practice Test
Use this practice test to review the topics of this chapter and to prepare for your test on this material.

1. Which of the following statements is correct?
    a. The brain normally uses glucose as an energy source
    b. The brain can metabolize ketones
    c. Skeletal muscle tends to metabolize fatty acids
    d. Skeletal muscle can use internal glycogen
    e. all of the above

2. Which of the following is correct?
    a. The liver can convert protein to glucose
    b. Most protein is stored in skeletal muscle
    c. The brain stores carbohydrates as glycogen
    d. Muscles are always net consumers of energy
    e. a and b

3. Which of these can be said to be a primary hormone of the absorptive state?
    a. glucagon
    b. cortisol
    c. insulin
    d. TSH
    e. a and c

4. Growth hormone
   a. secretion increases during starvation
   b. increases peripheral glucose utilization
   c. increases fatty acid mobilization and use
   d. causes bone length to increase
   e. all are correct

5. Which of the following is correct?
   a. Glucagon elevates plasma glucose by blocking insulin release
   b. Glucagon elevates plasma glucose by blocking insulin receptors
   c. Glucagon elevates plasma glucose by enhancing glycogenolysis
   d. a and b
   e. none of the above

6. Hyperthyroidism would tend to cause
   a. goiter
   b. increased BMR
   c. myxedema
   d. dwarfism
   e. b and c

7. Diabetes mellitus may be caused by
   a. a decrease in number of insulin receptors
   b. an increase in number of insulin receptors
   c. hypersecretion of beta cells
   d. hyposecretion of delta cells
   e. a and c

8. In thyroid follicles, T_3 and T_4 are stored as
   a. thyroxine
   b. thyroglobulin
   c. TSH
   d. iodine
   e. fatty acids

9. Insufficiency of the adrenal cortex may lead to
   a. decreased fluid volume
   b. increased protein catabolism
   c. high blood pressure
   d. decreased plasma K^+
   e. all of the above

10. Somatostatin
    a. decreases beta-cell secretions
    b. decreases alpha-cell secretions
    c. increases glucagon secretion
    d. a and b
    e. a, b, and c

11. Which of these are secreted during starvation?
    a. HGH
    b. glucagon
    c. epinephrine
    d. a and b
    e. a, b, and c

12. Thermoregulation can be accomplished by means of
    a. increased secretion of T_3 and T_4
    b. constriction of cutaneous blood vessels
    c. relaxation of pilomotor muscles
    d. a and b
    e. a, b, and c

13. Which of these produces glucose molecules?
    a. gluconeogenesis
    b. glycogenolysis
    c. glycolysis
    d. ketogenesis
    e. a and b

14. LDLs
    a. are formed when VLDLs lose light lipid groups
    b. are not found in the circulating plasma
    c. return to the liver, once formed
    d. are carbohydrates
    e. a and c

15. Lipoprotein lipase is activated by
    a. trypsin
    b. apoprotein
    c. triglycerides
    d. glucagon
    e. a and b

Answers

Here are answers (or references) to some of the questions presented above.

Word Parts: (your examples may be different) 1-apoprotein, 2-chondrogenesis, 3-epiphyseal, 4-glucagon, 5-glucagon, 6-hyperthyroidism, 7-pyrogen, 8-thermostatic

Key Terms: Processes: 1. lipolysis 2. lipostatic hypothesis 3. glycogenolysis 4. postabsorptive state 5. thermostatic hypothesis 6. futile cycle 7. proteolysis 8. absorptive state 9. lipogenesis 10. glucostatic hypothesis 11. gluconeogenesis 12. glycogenesis 13. chondrogenesis 14. thermogenesis 15. ossification 16. glucose-sparing 17. basal metabolic rate [BMR]
Structures/Substances: 1. high-density lipoproteins [HDL] 2. satiety center 3. complete protein 4. very low-density lipoprotein [VLDL] 5. brown fat 6. low-density lipoprotein [LDL] 7. essential amino acid 8. ketone 9. epiphyseal plate
Regulatory Substances: 1. somatostatin 2. apoprotein 3. lipoprotein lipase 4. glycogen synthetase 5. somatomedin

6. glucagon 7. cortisol 8. proinsulin
Other: 1. insulin shock 2. osteoporosis 3. acromegaly 4. goiter 5. hyperthyroidism 6. hypothyroidism 7. hyperglycemia 8. glycouria 9. satiety 10. core body temperature 11. dwarfism [pituitary] 12. gigantism

Learning Exercises: 1. 1-I, 2-G, 3-I, 4-G, 5-I, 6-G, 7-G, 8-I, 9-I,G 2. Type I: affects about 20% of patients with diabetes, can be treated by insulin replacement therapy, insulin-dependent, results from inadequate beta cell secretion; Type II: affects about 80% of patients with diabetes, can be treated by altering diet and exercise regimen, insulin-independent, results from lack of, or abnormal, insulin receptors 3. (Compare your table with Table 23-3 in the text.) 4. (Compare your graph to Figure 23-20 in the text.) a/b- both muscle and bone would increase slightly until peaking at age 35, then decrease; thus the fat line is a straight upwardly sloped line, whereas fat and muscle lines would resemble flattened bell-shaped lines 5. Arterioles - reduced blood flow to skin, reducing loss of heat to environment; Sweat - reduces evaporative loss of heat to environment; Pilomotor - "fluffs" hair, improving insulation from heat loss; Muscle - produces heat; Adrenal - enhances sympathetic effects listed above; Thyroid - raises BMR, increasing heat production 6. 1-amino acids, 2-lactic acid, 3-glucose, 4-ketones, 5-glycerol, 6-fatty acids

Quick Recall: (You should be able to answer these questions easily without correction or confirmation by this point in your studies. If you cannot, review your notes, the text chapter, and the previous study activities to find the answers.)

Practice Test: 1-e, 2-e, 3-c, 4-e, 5-c, 6-b, 7-a, 8-b, 9-a, 10-d, 11-e, 12-d, 13-e, 14-e, 15-b

Chapter 24
Reproduction and Its Endocrine Control

Focus
Review this section *first*. It will help you focus on the overall message of this chapter.

Chapter Outline
Read through the outline slowly. This activity will help your mind organize the topics of this chapter.

The anatomy of male and female reproductive organs
> Female reproductive system
> Male reproductive system

The genetic basis of reproduction and sex determination
> Meiosis: formation of haploid gametes
> Spermiogenesis
> Oogenesis and follicle development

Determination of genetic sex
Embryonic development of reproductive organs
Hormonal control of sexual maturation
> Role of the hypothalamus and anterior pituitary in puberty
> Gonadal steroids and sexual maturation

Sex hormones and development
Disorders of sexual differentiation
Endocrine regulation of male reproductive function
> Feedback regulation of spermatogenesis and testosterone secretion
> Changes in testicular function with age

Endocrine regulation of female reproductive function
> The ovarian cycle
> Hypothalamic/anterior pituitary stimulation of the ovaries

The uterine or endometrial cycle
> Timeline for the menstrual cycle

Contraception
> Nonhormonal methods of contraception
> Hormonal birth control

The human sexual response
The sexual experience: a whole-body response
Male genital responses
Female genital responses

Learning Objectives

These are the learning goals for this part of the course. After reading the text, attending class, and studying this chapter, you should be able to:

♦ describe the anatomy of male and female reproductive systems

♦ describe how gonadal sex is determined by the sex chromosome complement and how the presence of male or female gonads determines the course of development of male or female internal accessory structures and genital sex

♦ understand the genetic and endocrine causes of representative disorders of sexual development

♦ trace the sequence of events in the formation of male and female gametes and understand the similarities and differences in this process as it occurs in male and female gonads

♦ describe the changes characteristic of male and female puberty and their endocrine basis

♦ describe the endocrine feedback loops that control gonadal function in men and women

♦ trace the events and changes of the menstrual cycle and explain the endocrine roles of the hypothalamus, anterior pituitary, ovarian follicle, and corpus luteum in the control of the cycle

Language of Physiology

Physiology uses its own set of terms, many of which may be unfamiliar to you. This section will help you improve your mastery of key physiological terms.

Word Parts

Here are some combining forms often seen in physiological terms. Give an example of a term that contains each word part listed.

Word Part	Meaning	Example
-arche	beginning; origin	1
-cide	to kill	2
diplo-	twofold, double	3
ejacul-	to throw out	4
haplo-	single	5
liga-	to tie, bind	6
mens- (menstru-)	month (monthly)	7
metr-	uterus	8
ov-, oo-	egg	9
semen-, semin-	seed	10
super-	over, above, excessive	11

Key Terms

Read each of the terms in each grouping below aloud, using the pronunciation guide if necessary. This will help you to remember them better than if you read them silently. Then, write out the correct term next to each of the descriptions given.

Descriptive Terms

bipotential (by-poh-TEN-shal)
gender-dysphoric (dis-FOR-ik)
genetic (sex)
genital (sex)

gonadal (sex) (go-NAD-al)
indifferent (gonads)
secondary (sex characteristics)

1 _____ descriptive term that, when describing sex characteristics, refers to the determination of maleness or femaleness by the presence of appropriate gonads

2 _____ descriptive term that, when describing sex characteristics, refers to determination of maleness or femaleness by the presence of appropriate external genitalia

3 _____ descriptive term that, when describing sex characteristics, refers to the chromosomal code for maleness (Y chromosome) or femaleness (lack of a Y chromosome)

4 _____ term that describes sex-specific body features that develop after puberty

5 _____ in reproductive biology, a term that refers to gonads that have not yet differentiated to become testes or ovaries

6 _____ in reproductive biology, a term that refers to structures that may develop in either of two ways: male or female

7 _____ term that describes someone who is intensely uncomfortable with his or her own genital sex and the sexual identity that should accompany it

Terms related to processes

atresia (a-TREE-jee-ah)
capacitation (kap-as-it-AY-shun)
crossing over
ejaculation (ee-JAK-yoo-lay-shun)
follicular phase (fah-LIK-yoo-ler)
luteal phase (LOO-tee-al)
luteinization (loo-ten-iz-AY-shun)
meiosis (my-OH-sis)
menarche (men-ARK-ee)

menopause
menstrual phase
oogenesis (oh-oh-JEN-es-is)
ovulation (ahv-yoo-LAY-shun)
proliferative phase (proh-LIF-er-ah-tiv)
secretory phase
spermatogenesis (sperm-at-oh-JEN-es-is)
spermiogenesis (sperm-ee-oh-JEN-es-is)

1 _____ term that refers to the process of sperm production (formation of new spermatozoa)

2 _____ process in which homologous bivalents exchange segments of DNA while they are aligned during the first meiotic division, resulting in variation in the daughter cells

3 _____ form of cell (nuclear) division that produces gametes (reproductive cells)

4 _____ term that refers to the entire process of ovum production

5_____ process in which spermatozoa acquire the ability to fuse with an ovum, presumably by means of the action of chemical factors in the female reproductive tract

6_____ also called spermiation — a term that refers to the acquisition of specialized spermatozoan structures (acrosome, flagellum, and so forth) by spermatids

7_____ in the ovary, a process in which some primordial follicles degenerate over time

8_____ one of three major phases of the uterine cycle; characterized by sloughing of the endometrium and flow out of the reproductive tract; it follows the secretory phase if no implantation occurs

9_____ one of three major phases of the uterine cycle; characterized by endometrial development, it begins after menstruation and continues until the beginning of the secretory phase

10_____ one of two phases of the ovarian cycle, lasting from the first day of menstruation to the day of ovulation

11_____ one of three major phases of the uterine cycle; characterized by luteal secretions that intensify the endometrial development begun in the previous proliferative phase

12_____ one of two phases of the ovarian cycle, lasting from the day of ovulation to the first day of menstruation

13_____ process of release of a mature ovum from the ovary

14_____ process of forcefully moving the semen through the urethra and out of the penis

15_____ cessation of ovarian function that typically occurs in the fifth decade of life

16_____ process of forming a corpus luteum (requires LH)

17_____ first menstrual flow in the life of an individual female

Terms related to female structures/substances

cervix (SER-viks)
clitoris (KLIT-or-is)
corpus luteum (LOO-tee-um)
corpus albicans (AL-bik-anz)
endometrium (en-doh-MEE-tree-um)
estradiol (es-trah-DY-ohl)
fallopian tube (fa-LOH-pee-an)
fimbriae (FIM-bree-ay)
graafian follicle (GRAF-ee-an)
labia (LAY-bee-ah)
myometrium (my-oh-MEE-tree-um)

ovary
ovum
polar body
primordial follicle (pry-MOR-dee-al)
progesterone (proh-JEST-er-ohn)
spiral glands
spiral arteries
uterus
vagina
zona pellucida (ZOH-nah pel-OOS-id-ah)

1_____ mature ovarian follicle, the stage of development just before ovulation (release of an ovum)

2_____ progestin, one of two primary reproductive steroids in females; it affects uterine development

3_____ hollow, muscular organ of the female reproductive system, it serves as a passage for sperm (to the ovum) and as the site of development of the embryo/fetus during pregnancy

4_____ term that refers to a cell type formed at each of two different stages of oogenesis; it is not capable of developing into an ovum, but it or its daughter cells eventually degenerate

5_____ layer of viscous material between the ovum and granulosa cells

6_____ female reproductive cell (gamete)

7_____ structure formed on the ovary by a follicle after ovulation; it secretes progesterone and estrogen

8_____ muscular canal between the uterine cervix and the body exterior, it serves to receive the penis (and semen) during intercourse and as the birth canal during labor

9_____ additional blood vessels that develop in the endometrium during the proliferative phase of the menstrual cycle as a result of estrogen stimulation

10_____ also called the oviduct, each (of a pair) is a tube that extends from the uterus to form a loose association with an ovary; it serves to conduct an ovum to the uterus and as a site for fertilization

11_____ erectile external genital organ of the female, it serves as a sensory focus in the sexual response

12_____ exocrine glands that develop in the endometrium during the proliferative phase of the menstrual cycle as a result of estrogen stimulation; they secrete a carbohydrate rich "uterine milk" that can nourish a developing embryo until the placenta is formed

13_____ immature follicles in the ovary consisting of a primary oocyte surrounded by a single layer of granulosa cells, some mature during each reproductive cycle to become primary follicles

14_____ literally "lips," the term refers to two sets of folds that surround and protect the female urethra and vagina (the inner folds are designated "minora," the outer "majora")

15_____ "neck" of the uterus, the narrow portion at the inferior end of the uterus that connects to the vagina

16_____ female gonad, it produces ova on a cyclic basis and secretes hormones — each (of a pair) is located in the pelvic area of the ventral body cavity

17_____ vascular lining of the uterus

18_____ structure left after degeneration of a corpus luteum

19_____ major estrogen, one of two primary reproductive steroids in females; it causes almost all of female-specific changes that occur after puberty

20_____ fingerlike processes at the end of a fallopian tube that surround the ovary and aid an ovum's entry into the tube

21_____ smooth muscle portion of the uterine wall

Terms related to male structures/substances

acrosome (AK-ro-sohm)
bulbourethral gland
  (bul-boh-yoo-REE-thral)
epididymis (ep-ih-DID-im-is)
inhibin (in-HIB-in)
Leydig cell (LAY-dig)
müllerian regression factor (MRF)
  (moo-LAYR-ee-an)
penis
prostate gland (PRAH-stayt)

rete testis (reet TES-tis)
semen (SEE-men)
seminal vesicle (SEM-in-al)
seminiferous tubules (sem-in-IF-er-us)
Sertoli cell (ser-TOH-lee)
spermatogonia (sper-mat-oh-GO-nee-ah)
spermatozoa (sper-mat-oh-ZOH-ah)
testis (TES-tis)
testosterone (tes-TAHS-ter-ohn)
vas deferens (vaz DEF-er-enz)

1 _____ single gland under the bladder and surrounding the upper male urethra, it secretes a large amount of seminal fluid into the reproductive tract

2 _____ male organ supported by three erectile sinuses (two corpora cavernosa, one corpus spongiosum); it serves to introduce semen into the vagina during intercourse and as the focus of sensation in the male sexual response

3 _____ network of tubules that conducts spermatozoa from the seminiferous tubule toward the epididymis (via the efferent ductules)

4 _____ mixture of spermatozoa with fluids secreted by male accessory glands; the fluids nurture the sperm, neutralize acidity, contain prostaglandins that stimulate the female tract, and serve as a medium for sperm transport

5 _____ steroid, it is the primary male sex hormone — it may be converted to estradiol, dihydrotestosterone, or 5α-androstanediol in target cells before it can bind to receptors

6 _____ network of tubules that forms about 80% of the mass of each testis; it possesses cells that give rise to spermatozoa and cells that nurture the developing spermatozoa

7 _____ coiled tubule on the surface of each testis, it serves as a site for the temporary storage (and further development) of spermatozoa

8 _____ body just under the plasma membrane on the anterior aspect of the spermatozoan head; it contains enzymes needed for penetration of an ovum

9 _____ cell of the seminiferous tubule that nurtures developing spermatozoa

10 _____ substance secreted by Sertoli cells of the testis that suppresses development of the müllerian duct structures

11 _____ hormone produced by Sertoli cells that exerts negative feedback control of pituitary secretion, allowing spermatogenesis to be regulated independently of the endocrine function of the testis

12 _____ also called the ductus deferens; it is a tube that conducts spermatozoa from the epididymis through the pelvic cavity and into the unpaired ejaculatory duct (which leads to the urethra)

13 _____ also called an interstitial cell; this type of cell lies outside the seminiferous tubule and secretes testosterone

14 _____ also called Cowper's gland, it is one of a pair of small glands that secrete seminal fluid into the urethra at the base of the penis

15 _____ cells of the seminiferous tubule that give rise to spermatozoa

16 _____ one of a pair of male gonads located within the scrotum (a sack of skin outside the lower pelvic cavity) that produce sperm and hormones

17 _____ one of a pair of male glands that secrete seminal fluid into the vas deferens just before the vas fuses with its mate to become the ejaculatory duct

18 _____ sperm cells, the male reproductive cells (gametes)

Other Terms related to structures/substances

allele (al-EEL)

bivalent (by-VAY-lent)

dehydroepiandrosterone [DHEA]
  (de-hy-droh-ep-ih-an-DRAH-stayr-ohn)

diploid complement (DY-ployd)

gamete (GAM-eet)

genitalia (jen-it-AYL-ee-ah)

gonad (GO-nad)

gonadotropin-releasing hormone [GnRH]

haploid complement (HAP-loyd)

müllerian duct (moo-LAYR-ee-an)

sex chromosome

wolffian duct (WOLF-ee-an)

zygote (ZY-goht)

1 _____ general term referring to primary sex organs (ovaries, testes)

2 _____ term that refers to all reproductive organs (primary organs and accessory organs)

3 _____ hypothalamic secretion that stimulates the anterior pituitary to secrete LH and FSH (LH and FSH are called gonadotropins)

4 _____ chromosome formed by two attached DNA replicates

5 _____ along with androstenedione, one of the major androgens (male hormones) produced by the adrenal cortex

6 _____ general term referring to a reproductive cell (male spermatozoan and/or female ovum) having the haploid complement of chromosomes

7 _____ one of a pair of chromosomes (in the human complement of 23 pairs) that contains information concerning reproductive functions — two types exist: Y and X

8 _____ one of several alternative forms of a gene

9 _____ part of the primitive urogenital tract; this organ may develop to become the male gland/duct system

10 _____ part of the primitive urogenital tract; this organ may develop to become the female internal accessory structures

11 _____ cell that is formed when the male and female gametes fuse to become a single cell with the diploid complement of chromosomes

12 _____ 2n complement of chromosomes, found in most normal body cells (2n = 46 in the human)

13 _____ n complement of chromosomes, found only in the gametes (n = 23 in the human)

Other Key Terms

adrenogenital syndrome
  (ad-ree-no-JEN-it-al)
intrauterine device [IUD]
  (in-trah-YOO-ter-in)
Klinefelter's syndrome (KLYN-fel-terz)
libido (lih-BEE-doh)
spermicide (SPERM-ih-syd)

superfemale
supermale
testicular feminization syndrome
  (tes-TIK-yoo-ler)
tubal ligation (ly-GAY-shun)
Turner's syndrome
vasectomy (vas-EKT-om-ee)

1_____ condition in which genital and gonadal sex are male, but defective androgen receptors result in a failure to masculinize during development

2_____ surgical procedure in which the fallopian tubes are tied shut, then (usually) cut, preventing conception

3_____ condition in which a sex chromosome complement of XYY results in men who appear normal

4_____ condition in which a sex chromosome complement of XXX results in the possibility of reduced fertility; it is accompanied by some degree of mental retardation and/or retarded personality development

5_____ surgical procedure in which the vas deferens (ductus deferens) are tied and cut, preventing sperm from mixing with the semen that is ejaculated

6_____ condition in which an XO (one X only) sex chromosome pattern results in female gonadal sex, but the ovaries do not develop

7_____ condition in which an XXY sex chromosome pattern results in male gonadal sex, but impaired testicular function

8_____ condition of excessive adrenal androgen production, resulting in the masculinization of the external genitals of a female fetus

9_____ device inserted into the uterus that remains there to prevent successful pregnancy

10_____ any substance that tends to kill or incapacitate spermatozoa, used as a contraceptive

11_____ behavioral term that refers to sexual drive

The Big Picture

Use the activities of this section to help you learn the broader concepts of this chapter.

Learning Exercises

1. Identify portions of the female reproductive anatomy as indicated.

cervix   myometrium   uterus body
endometrium   ovary   vagina
fallopian tube

Figure 24-1

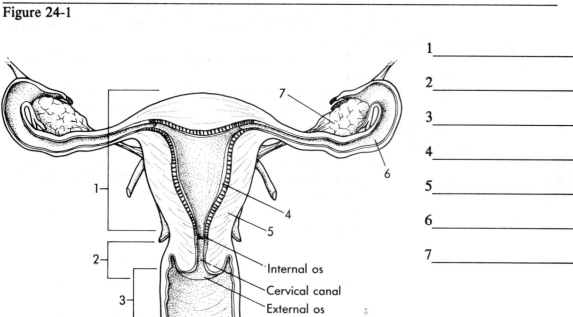

1 _____

2 _____

3 _____

4 _____

5 _____

6 _____

7 _____

Internal os
Cervical canal
External os

2. Use these terms to identify parts of the male reproductive system.

bulbourethral gland   penis   seminal vesicle
ductus deferens   prostate gland   testis
epididymis   scrotum   urethra
glans

Figure 24-2

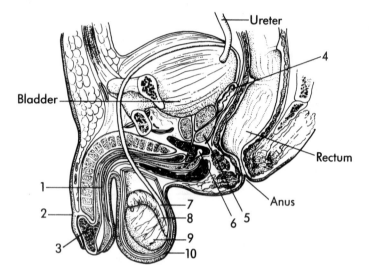

1_____

2_____

3_____

4_____

5_____

6_____

7_____

8_____

9_____

10_____

3. Use these terms to label the appropriate sections of Figure 24-3.

chromosomal sex   genital sex   gonadal sex
gender

Figure 24-3

1. _____

2. _____

Zygote (XX)   Zygote (XY)   3. _____

| No Y | Y present   4. _____

Fetus (with ovaries)   Fetus (with testes)

| Testicular | Testes
  hormones   secrete
  absent   hormones

Fetus (with female   Fetus (with male
external genitals)   genitals)

| Perceived sex | Perceived sex
  and   and
  environment   environment

Adult female identity   Adult male identity

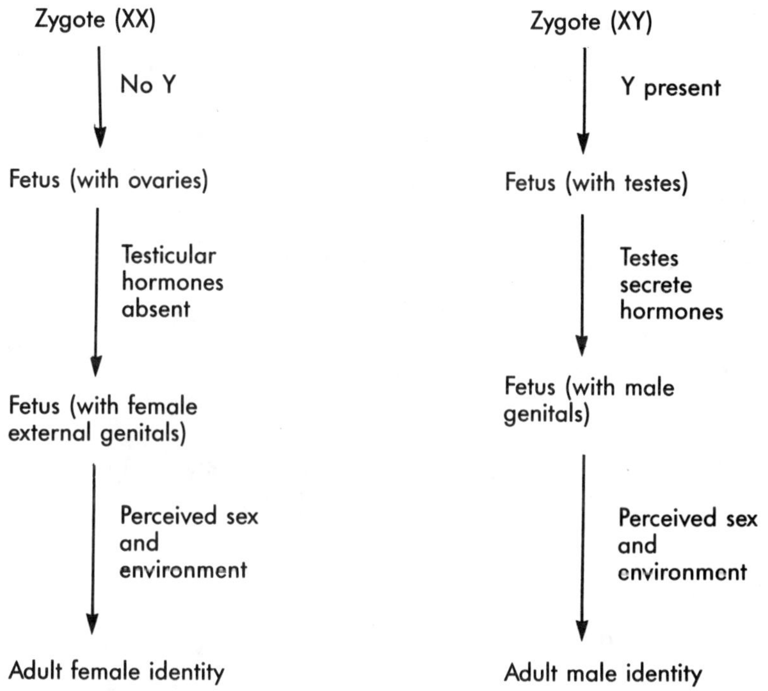

4. Put these phases of sperm development in the order in which they occur.

primary spermatocyte   spermatid   spermatozoan
secondary spermatocyte   spermatogonium

1 _____

2 _____

3 _____

4 _____

5 _____

5. Put these phases of ovum/follicle development in the order in which they occur.

graafian follicle   primary follicle   secondary oocyte
oogonium   primary oocyte   secondary follicle

1_____

2_____

3_____

4_____

5_____

6_____

6. Listed below are effects of endocrine hormones during puberty. Indicate whether the effect is that of estrogen or testosterone.

1_____   stimulates protein synthesis, increasing growth and mature (male pattern) muscle mass

2_____   establishes pattern of fat deposition in breasts, on hips and buttocks, and other areas (also bone growth and female body hair pattern)

3_____   stimulates growth of breast duct system

4_____   stimulates uterine endometrium

5_____   stimulates larynx growth, lowering the voice

6_____   supports spermatogenesis

7_____   significantly increases basal metabolic rate

7. Identify the correct hormones indicated in Figure 24-4.

Figure 24-4

1_____

2_____

3_____

4_____

5_____

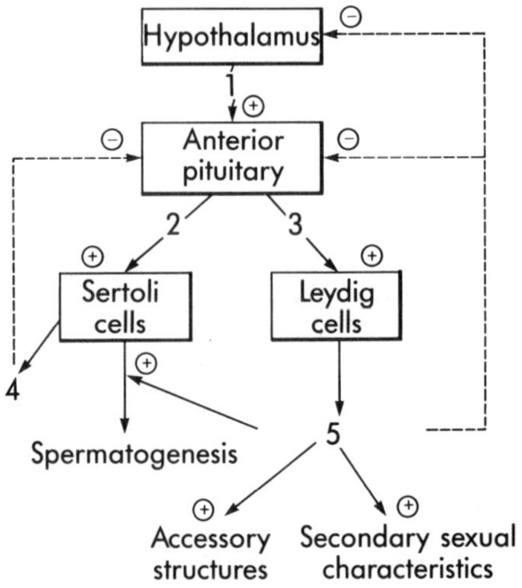

8. Identify these parts of Figure 24-5.

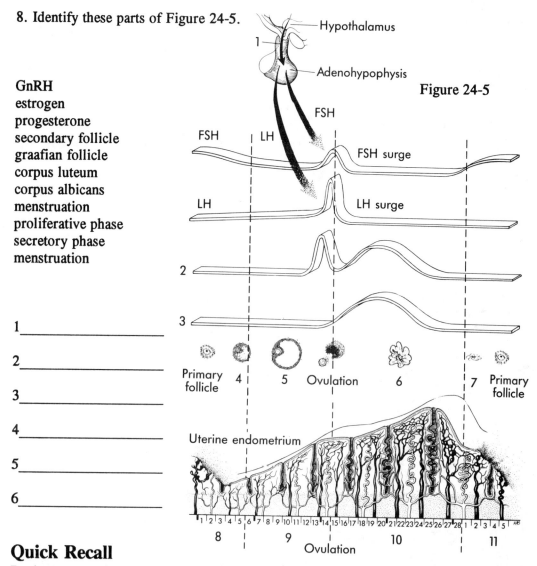

Figure 24-5

GnRH
estrogen
progesterone
secondary follicle
graafian follicle
corpus luteum
corpus albicans
menstruation
proliferative phase
secretory phase
menstruation

1 _____

2 _____

3 _____

4 _____

5 _____

6 _____

Quick Recall

Review some of the major concepts of this chapter by doing these "quick recall" activities.

1. Trace the path of spermatozoa from the site of production to the point of expulsion from the body. (You may want to do this by pencilling in the pathway in Figure 24-2.)

2. List the parts of a mature spermatozoan and each of their functions.

3. List the pathway of an ovum from its production site to a probable point of implantation in the uterus (noting the area in which it is likely to be fertilized). (You may want to do this by pencilling the pathway onto Figure 24-1.)

4. List the steps of sperm development.

5. List the steps of ovum development.

6. Give five effects of estrogens.

7. Give eight effects of testosterone and its metabolites.

8. Name the major phases and events of the female reproductive cycle.

   Uterine:

   Ovarian:

9. Give the general function of GnRH, FSH, and LH in

   males:

   females:

10. List the roles of estrogen and progesterone in the female cycle.

   estrogen:

   progesterone:

Practice Test
Use this practice test to review the topics of this chapter and to prepare for your test on this material.

1.   The müllerian duct differentiates to become
      a.   fallopian tubes
      b.   uterus
      c.   seminiferous tubules
      d.   a and b
      e.   none of the above

2.   In the male fetus
      a.   testosterone prevents degeneration of the wolffian duct
      b.   Sertoli cells secrete müllerian regression factor
      c.   the müllerian duct degenerates
      d.   a and b
      e.   a, b, and c

3.   Which is correct?
        a.   granulosa cells secrete progesterone
        b.   thecal cells secrete estrogen
        c.   androgens are not present in females
        d.   a and b
        e.   a, b and c

4.   Testosterone is secreted by
        a.   Leydig cells
        b.   Sertoli cells
        c.   granulosa cells
        d.   a and b
        e.   none of the above

5.   Which is correct?
        a.   estrogen is trophic to the uterus
        b.   estrogen secretion is high just before ovulation
        c.   estrogen is secreted by the placenta
        d.   a and b
        e.   a, b, and c

6.   Which is correct?
        a.   follicular maturation requires FSH
        b.   follicular maturation requires LH
        c.   rupture of a mature follicle requires LH
        d.   a and c
        e.   a, b, and c

7.   In the luteal phase of the ovarian cycle
        a.   progesterone secretion is low
        b.   LH secretion is maximal
        c.   estrogen secretion increases
        d.   the endometrium becomes secretory
        e.   c and d

8.   Which is correct?
        a.   The endometrium responds only to estrogen
        b.   Menstruation is initiated by vasoconstriction of the spiral arteries
        c.   Menstruation is triggered by a surge in LH
        d.   The endometrium responds to progesterone if primed by estrogen
        e.   a and c

9.   In the male, sperm are formed in the seminiferous tubules in response to
        a.   FSH
        b.   LH
        c.   testosterone
        d.   a and c
        e.   a, b, and c

10. Which is correct?
    a. Sertoli cells secrete testosterone
    b. Sertoli cells provide developing sperm with essential nutrients
    c. Sperm maturation is complete in the seminiferous tubules
    d. Sperm become capacitated in the epididymis
    e. none of the above

11. Components of semen ejaculated from the penis include
    a. fluid from the seminal vesicles
    b. testosterone
    c. fructose
    d. capacitated sperm
    e. both a and c

12. Capacitation of spermatozoa
    a. occurs in the epididymis
    b. occurs in the female tract
    c. is the attachment of a flagellum to the sperm head
    d. is triggered by acrosome enzymes
    e. a and c

13. Fertilization of an ovum is most likely to occur (under standard conditions) in the
    a. fallopian tube
    b. uterus
    c. ovary
    d. cervix
    e. vagina

14. Full expression of male characteristics
    a. never occurs in real life
    b. requires a Y sex chromosome
    c. requires the X sex chromosome
    d. requires two X sex chromosomes
    e. requires adrenal androgens

15. The XXX sex chromosome pattern
    a. is termed "wonderwoman syndrome"
    b. may result in retarded mental development
    c. results in a female with many male characteristics
    d. results in a male with some female characteristics
    e. a and b

Answers

Here are answers (or references) to some of the questions presented above.

Word Parts: (your examples may be different) 1-menarche, 2-spermicide, 3-diploid, 4-ejaculatory duct, 5-haploid, 6-tubal ligation, 7-menstruation, 8-endometrium, 9-oocyte, 10-seminiferous tubule, 11-superfemale

Key Terms: Descriptive: 1. gonadal (sex) 2. genital (sex) 3. genetic (sex) 4. secondary (sex characteristics) 5.

318

indifferent (gonads) 6. bipotential 7. gender-dysphoric

Processes: 1. spermatogenesis 2. crossing over 3. meiosis 4. oogenesis 5. capacitation 6. spermiogenesis 7. atresia 8. menstrual phase 9. proliferative phase 10. follicular phase 11. secretory phase 12. luteal phase 13. ovulation 14. ejaculation 15. menopause 16. luteinization 17. menarche

Female Structures/Substances: 1. graafian follicle 2. progesterone 3. uterus 4. polar body 5. zona pellucida 6. ovum 7. corpus luteum 8. vagina 9. spiral arteries 10. fallopian tube 11. clitoris 12. spiral glands 13. primordial follicle 14. labia 15. cervix 16. ovary 17. endometrium 18. corpus albicans 19. estradiol 20. fimbriae 21. myometrium

Male Structures/Substances: 1. prostate gland 2. penis 3. rete testis 4. semen 5. testosterone 6. seminiferous tubules 7. epididymis 8. acrosome 9. Sertoli cell 10. müllerian regression factor [MRF] 11. inhibin 12. vas deferens 13. Leydig cell 14. bulbourethral gland 15. spermatogonia 16. testis 17. seminal vesicle 18. spermatozoa

Other Structures/Substances: 1. gonad 2. genitalia 3. gonadotropin-releasing hormone [GnRH] 4. bivalent 5. dehydroepiandrosterone [DHEA] 6. gamete 7. sex chromosome 8. allele 9. wolffian duct 10. müllerian duct 11. zygote 12. diploid complement 13. haploid complement

Other Key Terms: 1. testicular feminization syndrome 2. tubal ligation 3. supermale 4. superfemale 5. vasectomy 6. Turner's syndrome 7. Klinefelter's syndrome 8. adrenogenital syndrome 9. intrauterine device [IUD] 10. spermicide 11. libido

Learning Exercises: 1. 1-uterus body, 2-cervix, 3-vagina, 4-endometrium, 5-myometrium, 6-fallopian tube, 7-ovary 2. 1-urethra, 2-penis, 3-glans, 4-seminal vesicle, 5-prostate gland, 6-bulbourethral gland, 7-ductus deferens, 8-epididymis, 9-testis, 10-scrotum 3. 1-chromosomal sex, 2-gonadal sex, 3-genital sex, 4-gender 4. spermatogonium, primary spermatocyte, secondary spermatocyte, spermatid, spermatozoan 5. oogonium, primary oocyte, primary follicle, secondary follicle, graafian follicle, secondary oocyte (See Figure 25-19 in the text for clarification.) 6. Estrogen: 2,3,4; Testosterone: 1,5,6,7 7. 1-GnRH, 2-FSH, 3-LH, 4-inhibin, 5-testosterone 8. 1-GnRH, 2-estrogen, 3-progesterone, 4-secondary follicle, 5-graafian follicle, 6-corpus luteum, 7-corpus albicans, 8-menstruation, 9-proliferative phase, 10-secretory phase, 11-menstruation

Quick Recall: (You should be able to answer these questions easily without correction or confirmation by this point in your studies. If you cannot, review your notes, the text chapter, and the previous study activities to find the answers.)

Practice Test: 1-d, 2-e, 3-d, 4-a, 5-e, 6-e, 7-e, 8-d, 9-d, 10-b, 11-e, 12-b, 13-a, 14-b, 15-b

Chapter 25
Pregnancy, Birth, and Lactation

Focus
Review this section *first*. It will help you focus on the overall message of this chapter.

Chapter Outline
Read through the outline slowly. This activity will help your mind organize the topics of this chapter.

Pregnancy
>   Meeting of the sperm and egg
>   From fertilization to implantation
>   Endocrine functions of the trophoblast and placenta
>   The structure and functions of the placenta
>   The fetal-placental circulation
>   From implantation to birth — the developmental timetable
>   Alteration of maternal physiology by pregnancy

Birth and lactation
>   What determines the length of gestation?
>   The stages of labor
>   Prolactin and lactation
>   Oxytocin and milk letdown
>   The contraceptive effect of lactation
>   Fertility enhancement

Learning Objectives
These are the learning goals for this part of the course. After reading the text, attending class, and studying this chapter, you should be able to:

♦ describe the early development of the human zygote, its implantation in the uterus, and the differentiation of the embryo and chorion

♦ understand the endocrine functions of the corpus luteum and placenta

♦ understand the architecture of the fetal circulation, how it functions in oxygen transport between maternal blood and fetal tissues, and the changes in the circulation that must occur at birth

♦ know the timing of key events of embryonic and fetal development and describe the changes in maternal physiology caused by pregnancy

- describe the stages of labor and the endocrine changes that are hypothesized to initiate labor and increase the strength of uterine contractions as labor progresses

- describe the control of breast development and milk production by prolactin, placental lactogen, progesterone, and estrogen

- trace the hormonal reflex that results in oxytocin secretion and milk letdown when an infant suckles

- describe the treatment for infertility

Language of Physiology
Physiology uses its own set of terms, many of which may be unfamiliar to you. This section will help you improve your mastery of key physiological terms.

Word Parts
Here are some combining forms often seen in physiological terms. Give an example of a term that contains each word part listed.

Word Part	Meaning	Example
-centesis	a piercing	1
chorio-	membrane; skin	2
-cyst	bladder	3
gesta-	to bear, carry	4
miss-	let go; send forth	5
orgasm-	to swell	6

Key Terms
Read each of the terms in each grouping below aloud, using the pronunciation guide if necessary. This will help you to remember them better than if you read them silently. Then, write out the correct term next to each of the descriptions given.

Terms related to processes
effacement (ee-FAYS-ment)
gestation period (jest-AY-shun)
lactation (lak-TAY-shun)
milk letdown

stress-activation
trimester (TRY-mes-ter)

1_____   term that refers to the thinning of the cervix (caused by relaxin) as labor approaches

2_____ process that occurs in the uterine wall during pregnancy, in which the stretching of the muscle increases its contractility (possibly producing uncoordinated contractions — Braxton-Hicks contractions — up to 1 month before labor)

3_____ in reproductive biology, one of three 3-month segments that make up the human gestation period

5_____ period of prenatal development; in humans it lasts 39 weeks (counting from the last menstrual period)

6_____ movement of milk from the alveoli into the duct system of the breast; it involves a reflex in which stimulation of the nipple causes oxytocin release from the posterior pituitary, which in turn causes smooth muscle contraction around the alveoli

7_____ process of milk production and secretion by the mammary glands

Terms related to structures/substances

amnion (AM-nee-ahn)
blastocyst (BLAST-oh-sist)
chorion (KOR-ee-ahn)
colostrum (koh-LAHS-trum)
ductus venosus (DUK-tus ven-OHS-us)
ductus arteriosus
    (DUK-tus ar-teer-ee-OHS-us)
embryo
fetus
foramen ovale (FOR-ah-men oh-VAHL-eh)

human placental lactogen (HPL)
    (plah-SENT-al LAK-toh-jen)
human chorionic gonadotropin (HCG)
    (kor-ee-AHN-ik go-nad-o-TROH-pin)
lactiferous sinus (lak-TIF-er-us)
mammary alveoli (al-VEE-oh-ly)
placenta (plah-SENT-ah)
relaxin (ree-LAKS-in)
umbilical vein
umbilical artery

1_____ stage of human development after implantation (and before the fetal stage) during which most of the organ systems differentiate — the first 8 weeks of gestation

2_____ human at a stage of development after the embryonic stage (i.e., during the last 31 weeks of gestation)

3_____ shunt in the fetal circulation that connects the aorta to the pulmonary artery, bypassing the pulmonary circulation

4_____ chorionic (placental) hormone that prevents the self-destruction of the corpus luteum and stimulates it to maintain its endocrine secretions

5_____ vein that brings blood from the placenta, through the umbilical cord, and to the fetal liver

6_____ hormone produced by the corpus luteum and later by the uterine muscle and placenta; it softens the pelvic girdle's connective tissue and the uterine cervix and may have a role in precipitating labor

7_____ human at a stage of development after the morula stage, characterized by its structure as a hollow ball of cells (the trophoblast), which encloses an inner cell mass (embryoblast)

8_____ fetal blood vessel that shunts the liver circulation to the inferior vena cava

9_____ membrane, derived from the trophoblast, that forms an outer covering of the embryo and later gives rise to the fetal component of the placenta

10_____ thin, yellowish fluid, with a high immunoglobulin content, that is secreted by mammary glands a few days before and a few days after labor

11_____ also called chorionic somatomammotropin, it is a placental hormone that stimulates breast development in preparation for lactation, supports fetal bone growth, and alters the way the mother uses metabolic substrates by substituting lipids for glucose as the cellular energy source

12_____ artery that branches from the fetal descending aorta, then passes through the umbilical cord toward the placenta

13_____ in the mammary glands, the glandular structures that are the sites of milk production

14_____ literally "oval hole," it is a shunt passage in the atrial septum of the atrial heart

15_____ one of a series of widened tubular ducts surrounded by smooth muscle that conduct milk from the mammary alveoli to ducts which empty at the nipple

16_____ inner of two walls that surround the human embryo (the outer wall being the chorion), within which is the embryo floating in amniotic fluid

17_____ organ that mediates transfer of nutrients, gases, and other materials between maternal and fetal blood — and secretes hormones that support the pregnancy

Other Key Terms

amniocentesis (am-nee-oh-sent-EES-is)   ectopic pregnancy
breech birth   patent ductus (PAT-ent DUK-tus)

1_____ diagnostic technique in which amniotic fluid is withdrawn (with a needle and syringe) and floating cells within it are cultured and then karyotyped to determine the genetic character of the developing fetus

2_____ condition in which the ductus arteriosus fails to close after birth, resulting in leakage of blood from the systemic loop into the pulmonary loop

3_____ condition in which a blastocyst implants at a site other than the uterus, thus starting a pregnancy in a nonstandard location

4_____ presentation of the fetus at the time of birth other than the standard head-first presentation

The Big Picture

Use the activities of this section to help you learn the broader concepts of this chapter.

Learning Exercises

1. Use these terms to fill in the blanks found in the text that follows.

blastocyst	fallopian tube	inner cell mass
chorion	fetus	morula
corpus luteum	HCG	placenta

After fertilization in the upper _____, the zygote divides to form first a

_____ of undifferentiated cells and then a _____

consisting of a trophoblast and _____. After implantation, the trophoblast

becomes the _____, which gives rise to the fetal component of the

_____. The _____ becomes an embryo, which after the

eighth week of development is called a _____.

Implantation is followed quickly by secretion of _____, which sustains

the _____ for about the first 4 weeks of pregnancy.

2. Name each hormone described in the items that follow.

estrogen	oxytocin	prolactin
HCG	progesterone	relaxin
HPL		

1 _____ with progesterone, it is secreted by the corpus luteum and placenta — it maintains the endometrium and contributes to breast development

2 _____ with estrogen, it is secreted by the corpus luteum and placenta — it maintains the endometrium, inhibits contraction of the myometrium, and stimulates breast development

3 _____ it is secreted by the placenta in high quantities immediately after implantation — it prevents the self-destruction of the corpus luteum

4 _____ it is secreted by the placenta — it increases fat and carbohydrate metabolism in the mother, making stored nutrients available to the fetus; it also contributes to breast development

5_____ it is secreted by the posterior pituitary — it stimulates uterine contractions and causes milk let-down

6_____ it is secreted by the corpus luteum, placenta, and uterus — it softens the cervix, loosens pelvic ligaments, inhibits uterine contractions, and potentiates the effect of oxytocin

7_____ it is secreted by the anterior pituitary — it maintains milk production after delivery

3. Put these steps in the birth process in the order in which they occur.

oxytocin potentiates strong, coordinated labor contractions, setting up a positive feedback loop
pressure on the cervix triggers increased oxytocin secretion
prostaglandins allow regular uterine contractions that dilate the cervix to 7 to 10 cm
the baby moves through the cervix and vagina
the placenta moves through the birth canal
the number of uterine oxytocin receptors increases
the fetus takes a head-downward position

1_____

2_____

3_____

4_____

5_____

6_____

7_____

4. Identify each of the steps in activity No. 3 as belonging to prelabor, stage one labor, stage two labor, or stage three labor.

1 _____

2 _____

3 _____

4 _____

5 _____

6 _____

7 _____

5. Label the numbered portions of Figure 25-1, then draw arrows to indicate the direction of blood flow throughout the fetal circulatory system. (You may want to color various portions red to indicate the presence of oxygenated blood, blue for deoxygenated blood, and shades of purple to indicate mixing of oxygenated and deoxygenated blood.)

___ductus venosus   ___foramen ovale   ___umbilical arteries
___ductus arteriosus   ___umbilical vein

Figure 25-1

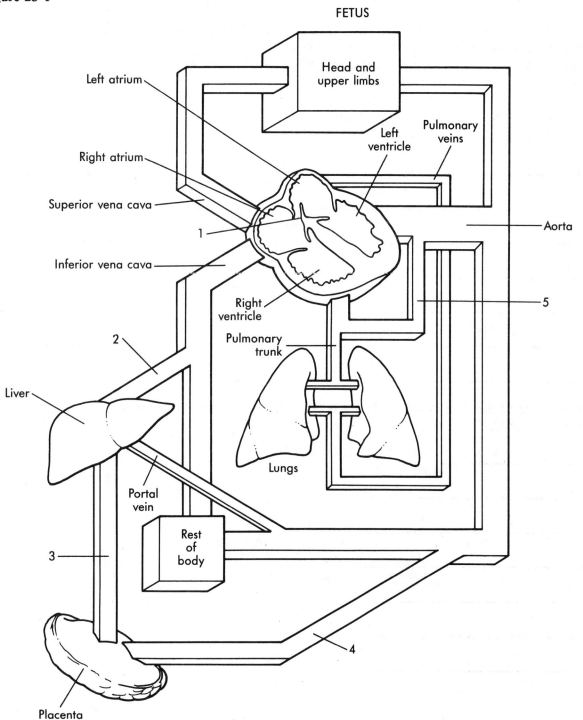

Quick Recall
Review some of the major concepts of this chapter by doing these "quick recall" activities.

1. Name five major stages of human development, beginning with the stage formed at fertilization.

2. List the endocrine functions of the corpus luteum.

3. List the endocrine functions of the placenta.

4. List the changes in fetal circulation that normally occur at birth.

5. List some changes in maternal physiology caused by pregnancy.

6. Name the major events of the three phases of labor.

7. Name five hormones that influence breast development and lactation.

Practice Test
Use this practice test to review the topics of this chapter and to prepare for your test on this material.

1. The chorion is derived from the
   a. embryoblast
   b. trophoblast
   c. placenta
   d. choroid plexus
   e. amnion

2. Immediately after implantation
   a. the corpus luteum self-destructs
   b. the corpus luteum secretes HCG
   c. the chorion secretes HCG
   d. the chorion secretes LH
   e. oxytocin surges

3. The placenta secretes
   a. uterine milk
   b. HCG
   c. oxytocin
   d. progesterone
   e. b and d

4.   A __ implants in the uterine wall.
      a.   zygote
      b.   blastocyst
      c.   morula
      d.   embryo
      e.   fetus

5.   Most differentiation of body systems occurs
      a.   in the first trimester
      b.   in the second trimester
      c.   in the third trimester
      d.   during the embryonic stage
      e.   a and d

6.   Near the end of gestation, progesterone secretion
      a.   has stopped
      b.   is handled by the placenta
      c.   is handled by the corpus luteum
      d.   is handled by the ovaries
      e.   triggers milk letdown

7.   Milk production
      a.   is inhibited by progesterone during pregnancy
      b.   is inhibited by oxytocin
      c.   begins in the first trimester
      d.   is usually termed "milk letdown"
      e.   is inhibited by estrogen during pregnancy

8.   Relaxin
      a.   is secreted by the ovary
      b.   is secreted by the hypothalamus
      c.   promotes softening of the cervix
      d.   a and c
      e.   b and c

9.   Gestation
      a.   is normally four trimesters long
      b.   is normally 39 weeks long
      c.   is normally 42 weeks long
      d.   is normally 360 days long
      e.   a and b

10.   Colostrum
      a.   is secreted by the endometrium
      b.   is also called uterine milk
      c.   is secreted by mammary alveoli
      d.   is secreted until weaning is accomplished
      e.   a and b

11. Passive immunity for a newborn may be imparted by
    a. the placenta
    b. oxytocin injection
    c. colostrum
    d. prostaglandins
    e. passive immunity is not possible in newborns

12. In utero, humans are most susceptible to toxins and drugs
    a. during trimester 1
    b. during trimester 2
    c. during trimester 3
    d. just after birth
    e. while in the birth canal

13. The oxygen dissociation curve of fetal hemoglobin is
    a. the same as for adult Hb
    b. left-shifted compared to the adult curve
    c. right-shifted compared to the adult curve
    d. nonexistent, since fetal lungs are nonfunctional
    e. none of the above

Answers

Here are answers (or references) to some of the questions presented above.

Word Parts: (your examples may be different) 1-amniocentesis, 2-chorionic gonadotropin, 3-blastocyst, 4-gestation, 5-emission, 6-orgasm

Key Terms: Processes: 1. effacement 2. stress-activation 3. trimester 4. gestation period 5. milk let-down 6. lactation **Structures/Substances:** 1. embryo 2. fetus 3. ductus arteriosus 4. human chorionic gonadotropin (HCG) 5. umbilical vein 6. relaxin 7. blastocyst 8. ductus venosus 9. chorion 10. colostrum 11. human placental lactogen (HPL) 12. umbilical artery 13. mammary alveoli 14. foramen ovale 15. lactiferous sinus 16. amnion 17. placenta **Other:** 1. amniocentesis 2. patent ductus 3. ectopic pregnancy 4. breech birth

Learning Exercises: 1. fallopian tube, morula, blastocyst, inner cell mass, chorion, placenta, inner cell mass, fetus, HCG, corpus luteum 2. 1-estrogen, 2-progesterone, 3-HCG, 4-HPL, 5-oxytocin, 6-relaxin, 7-prolactin 3/4. 1-the number of uterine oxytocin receptors increases (prelabor), 2-the fetus takes a head-downward position (prelabor), 3-pressure on the cervix triggers increased oxytocin secretion (prelabor), 4-oxytocin potentiates strong, coordinated labor contractions, setting up a positive feedback loop (stage one), 5-prostaglandins allow regular uterine contractions that dilate the cervix to 7 to 10 cm (stage one), 5-the baby moves through the cervix and vagina (stage two), 7-the placenta moves through the birth canal (stage three) 5. (Compare your figure to Figure 25-12 in the text.) 7. 1-lactiferous sinus, 2-lactiferous ducts, 3-nipple, 4-areola

Quick Recall: (You should be able to answer these questions easily without correction or confirmation by this point in your studies. If you cannot, review your notes, the text chapter, and the previous study activities to find the answers.)

Practice Test: 1-b, 2-c, 3-e, 4-b, 5-e, 6-b, 7-a, 8-d, 9-b, 10-c, 11-c, 12-a, 13-b

Chapter 26
The Immune System

Focus
Review this section *first*. It will help you focus on the overall message of this chapter.

Chapter Outline
Read through the outline slowly. This activity will help your mind organize the topics of this chapter.

Nonspecific components of the immune responses
        Barriers and local cellular defenses
        Inflammation and the complement and kinin-kallikrein systems
        Roles of prostaglandins in inflammation and fever
Specific immune responses
        Distinguishing between self and nonself
        Humoral immunity
        Antibody structure
        Relationship between immunoglobulin structures and actions
        The genetic basis of antibody diversity
        Specific immune system cell types
        Differentiation of the B and T cells
Coordination in the immune system
        Activation of helper T cells
        The kinetics of immune response
Undesirable immune system responses
        Superantigens bypass immune cell specificity
        Transplantation and transfusion reactions
        Hypersensitivity
        Autoimmune diseases

Learning Objectives
These are the learning goals for this part of the course. After reading the text, attending class, and studying this chapter, you should be able to:

♦ describe the nonspecific elements of immune system response

♦ understand the activation and function of complement

♦ know how inflammation develops and promotes immune function

- describe the benefits derived from systemic responses to infection, such as fever and altered blood constituents

- understand the role of the major histocompatibility complex antigens in immune system recognition of self and nonself (antigen presentation complex)

- describe the structure of antibodies and how the structure is related to antigen binding and the biological consequences of binding

- understand the role of antibody-antigen interactions in agglutination, lysis, neutralization, and opsonization

- know the roles in specific immune responses played by helper T cells, cytotoxic T cells, suppressor T cells, and B cells

- be able to describe the development of humoral immunity and the roles of plasma and memory cells

- understand how malfunctions of the immune system lead to hypersensitivity and autoimmune diseases

Language of Physiology

Physiology uses its own set of terms, many of which may be unfamiliar to you. This section will help you improve your mastery of key physiological terms.

Word Parts

Here are some combining forms often seen in physiological terms. Give an example of a term that contains each word part listed.

Word Part	Meaning	Example
anti–	against; resisting	1
glutin–	glue	2
hist–	tissue	3
ops–	appearance; view	4
tax–	to arrange	5
toxi–	poison	6

Key Terms

Read each of the terms in each grouping below aloud, using the pronunciation guide if necessary. This will help you to remember them better than if you read them silently. Then, write out the correct term next to each of the descriptions given.

Descriptive Terms

cytotoxic (syt-oh-TAHKS-ik)   polyclonal (pahl-ee-KLO-nal)
monoclonal (mahn-oh-KLO-nal)

1_____   term that describes something hazardous to cells; this term is sometimes used to name killer T cells

2_____   term that describes a group of antibodies as having been produced by a mixture of B-cell clones

3_____   term that describes a group of antibodies as having been derived from a single B-cell clone

Other Key Terms

ABO system   erythroblastosis fetalis
affinity chromatography   (er-ith-roh-blast-OH-sis fee-TAL-is)
  (kro-mah-TAHG-ra-fee)   Rh system
autoimmune disease (aw-toh-im-YOON)

1_____   blood cell typing system involving an antigen named after rhesus monkeys, in which it was first observed; humans whose cells possess the antigen are identified as "positive" and those without the antigen are identified as "negative"

2_____   method of separation in which antigens are separated from their medium by passing it across surfaces to which monoclonal antibodies (for that antigen) have been attached

3_____   blood cell typing system named for the antigens involved (A, B) and the no-antigen situation (O)

4_____   any of several diseases, such as systemic lupus erythematosus, in which immune responses are improperly directed toward "self antigens" (one's own proteins)

5_____   Rh disease; a condition in which anti-Rh antibodies from a mother enter the bloodstream of an Rh-negative infant and attack its RBCs

Terms related to processes

active immunization
agglutination (ah-gloo-tin-AY-shun)
antigen presentation (ANT-ih-jen)
cell-mediated immunity
chemotaxis (kee-moh-TAKS-is)
complement system
humoral immunity (HYOO-mor-al)
kallikrein-kinin system
  (KAL-ih-kryn KIN-in)

nonspecific immunity
opsonization (ahp-son-iz-AY-shun)
passive immunization
primary immune response
secondary immune response
specific immunity
vaccination

1_____ cascade of enzymatic reactions that is partly responsible for the inflammation reaction (of nonspecific immunity); it results in the formation of kinins, which mediate the inflammation response

2_____ term that refers to general immune response, directed against any and all invaders and injurious stimuli

3_____ process in which a weakened bacterium or virus is injected into a person to stimulate the establishment of permanent immunity

4_____ term that refers to the acquisition of the antibodies from an outside source, such as an antiserum injection, rather than one's own production of antibodies in response to a specific antigen's presence

5_____ process in which antibodies bind to the surface of a foreign cell, tagging it for destruction, and the subsequent recognition of the tagged cell by macrophages

6_____ process in which macrophages ingest foreign antigens, modify them, then display them on the macrophage surface, enhancing the response from corresponding clones of B and T cells

7_____ process in which antibodies link foreign cells together, thus preventing their spread throughout the body

8_____ term that refers to the production of specific antibodies in response to the presence of an antigen (rather than acquisition of antibodies from an outside source, such as an antiserum injection)

9_____ term that refers to immune responses that are directed against specific antigens, rather than injurious stimuli in general

10_____ type of specific immunity conferred by the direct action of T cells (not antibodies)

11_____ process of cell movement in which leukocytes migrate to injured tissues in response to attractants released during the inflammation response

12_____ cascade of enzymatic reactions involving plasma proteins (complement) that can be activated by the specific immune system (classical pathway) or the nonspecific immune system (alternative pathway); the system organizes an attack on bacterial invaders

13_____ specific immune response to a "new" antigen, one that has not previously been presented to the immune system

14_____ specific immune response to an antigen that has already been presented to the immune cells (on a previous occasion)

15_____ type of specific immunity that is conferred by substances (antibodies) present in the plasma of immune individuals

Terms related to structures/substances

antibody (AN-tee-bahd-ee)
antigen (ANT-ih-jen)
antiserum (AN-tee-see-rum)
B cell
bradykinin (brad-ee-KIN-in)
determinant portion
F$_{ab}$ portion (F A B)
hapten
histamine (HIS-tah-meen)
immunoglobulin [Ig]
  (im-yoon-oh-GLOB-yoo-lin)

interferon (in-ter-FEER-ahn)
interleukin-2 (in-ter-LOO-kin two)
lactoferrin (lak-toh-FAYR-in)
lymphokine (LIMF-oh-kyn)
macrophage (MAK-roh-fayj)
major histocompatibility complex
  [MHC] (hist-oh-kom-pat-ih-BIL-it-ee)
perforin (per-FOR-in)
T cell

1_____ substance produced by cells infected by a virus; this substance inhibits replication of some viral DNA and can be passed to uninfected cells (as a form of nonspecific immunity)

2_____ substance secreted by helper T cells; it stimulates T cell multiplication

3_____ family of plasma proteins that act as antibodies, mediating humoral immunity

4_____ toxin secreted by a killer T cell after the cell has bound to its target

5_____ type of histocompatibility antigen found in humans; an antigen that (along with others) helps to identify nucleated cells as belonging to a specific individual

6_____ small molecule that can act as an antigen if it becomes bound to a larger molecule

7_____ substance released by cells that acts to increase capillary permeability

8_____ preparation of serum from an immunized person or animal containing antibodies

9_____ term that signifies the antigen-binding fragment of the Y-shaped antibody molecule, containing the variable region (region with any of several different amino acid sequences)

10_____ term that refers to any macromolecule that produces a specific immune response

11_____ substance (immunoglobulin) secreted by plasma cells that confers humoral immunity

12_____ iron-binding molecule released by neutrophils (WBCs) that reduces the iron available for uptake by bacteria (and thus inhibits bacterial multiplication)

13_____ any of a family of substances released by activated helper T cells that stimulate the action of macrophages and have other immune-stimulating effects

14_____ large phagocytic cells that may also become involved in initiating and controlling specific immune responses

15 _____ one of the products of kallikrein-kinin cascade, it causes vasodilation (which causes the redness and warmth of inflamed areas) and increased capillary permeability (which results in edema and increased lymph production in the affected area)

16 _____ portion of an antigen molecule that binds to the hypervariable segments of the variable region of an antibody

17 _____ type of lymphocyte (WBC) that has antigen-specific receptors on its surface and acts in cell-mediated immunity (name derived from thymus)

18 _____ type of lymphocyte (WBC) that can be activated to differentiate into antibody-secreting plasma cells and mediate humoral immune responses (name derived from bursa of Fabricius in birds)

The Big Picture

Use the activities of this section to help you learn the broader concepts of this chapter.

Learning Exercises

1. Summarize the cellular components of the immune system by giving a brief description of the immune function of each of these cell categories.

Cell	Function
Neutrophil	
Eosinophil	
Basophil	
Monocyte	
B lymphocyte	
T lymphocyte	

2. Identify the subclasses of B cells and T cells by their descriptions below.

cytotoxic (killer) T
  cells
helper T cells

inducer T cells
memory B cells
natural killer T cells

plasma cells
suppressor T cells
virgin B cells

B cells

1_____ differentiate into plasma cells and/or memory cells; they may last for life

2_____ are derived from virgin or memory cells; they respond to a first exposure to an antigen and persist only a few weeks after a primary response

3_____ derived from virgin or memory cells; they respond quickly during a secondary response (by producing plasma and memory cells) and may survive months to years

T cells

4_____ recognize/destroy cells that have been infected with a virus or have been transformed in some way (for example, cancer cells)

5_____ resemble cytotoxic T cells but do not require previous exposure to an antigen

6_____ regulate the immune response; they increase the numbers of cytotoxic T cells, activate B cells, and secrete various lymphokines

7_____ are activated by helper T cells; they stimulate production of new T cells

8_____ inhibit both cell-mediated (T cell) and humoral (B cell) immunity; they limit what might otherwise be an uncontrolled response

3. Identify the parts of Figure 26-1, antibody structure, as indicated.

antigen binding site
light chain

heavy chain
hypervariable region

F_{ab} fragment
F_c fragment

Figure 26-1

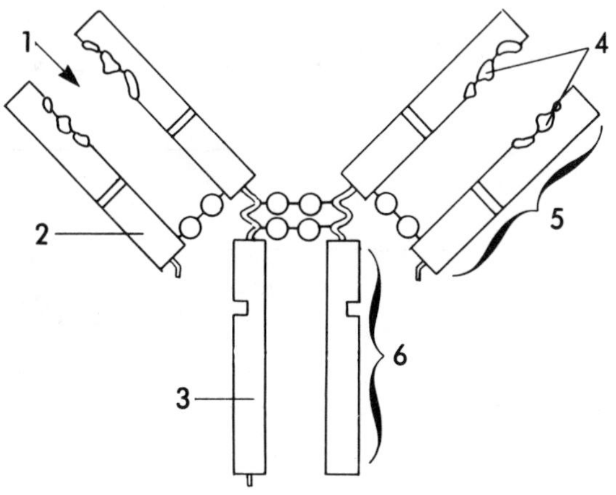

1_____

2_____

3_____

4_____

5_____

6_____

4. Identify these immunoglobulins by matching them with their descriptions.

IgA   IgE   IgM
IgD   IgG

1_____ stimulates phagocytosis and complement reactions (can cross the placenta); identifies microorganisms for engulfment or lysis and provides passive immunity in newborns

2_____ binds to mast cells and basophils; inhibits parasite invasion; stimulates histamine release; involved in allergic reactions

3_____ unknown

4_____ present in saliva, tears, breast milk, and intestinal secretions; agglutinates infectious agents in secretions outside the body

5_____ stimulates phagocytosis and complement reactions; identifies microorganisms for engulfment or lysis

5. Use the terms given to fill in the blanks in the text that follows.

antibody   differentiation   MHC-1
antigen   gene   MHC-2
B cell   histocompatibility   specificity
clone

T cells undergo clonal _____ in the thymus. During this process, various

_____s arise, each with a different receptor _____. The

T-cell receptor resembles an _____ in some respects, but it can bind a foreign

_____ only if the _____ antigen is also present.

_____ antigens are identity tags for the cell-mediated immune system.

They are unique to each individual, arising from the most polymorphic _____ loci

known. _____ antigen is found on all nucleated body cells and directs killer T

lymphocytes to their targets. _____ antigen is found on B cells, macrophages,

and some types of T cell, and it channels interactions between T cells and _____s

that occur in the course of a specific immune response.

6. Fill in the blanks in Figure 26-2 with either "T" or "B."

   Figure 26-2

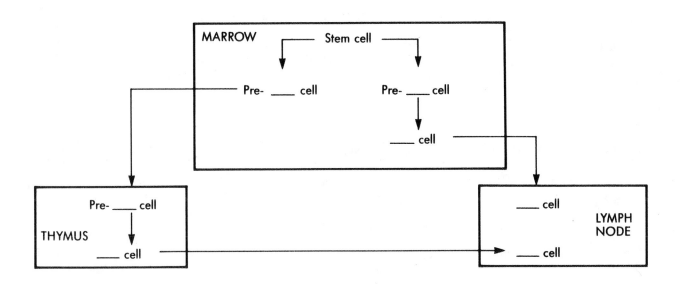

7. Use these terms to fill in the blank portions of the paragraphs below.

cytotoxic   memory   nonself
helper   MHC-1   plasma
inducer   natural killer   suppressor

   Killer, or _____, T cells recognize and attack cells that are

simultaneously displaying _____ antigen and nonself antigen.

_____ cells are not specific but are directed to major classes of

_____ antigens.

   _____ T cells are activated by antigen presented by macrophages,

stimulating _____ T cells to deliver the antigen to activate B-cell clones to

proliferate and give rise to _____ cells and _____ cells.

At the same time, helper T cells stimulate the activity of _____ T cells, which

limit the duration and scope of the immune response.

Quick Recall

Review some of the major concepts of this chapter by doing these "quick recall" activities.

1. Name the two major classes of lymphocytes.

2. List three subclasses of B cells.

3. List five subclasses of T cells.

4. List the major structural components of an antibody molecule.

5. List three factors that contribute to the variability of antibodies.

6. Name five classes of immunoglobulins.

7. Write the two major types of specific immunity.

8. Name two major biochemical systems responsible for the inflammation response.

9. List the two ways in which the complement cascade can be triggered.

10. Compare and contrast specific immunity and nonspecific immunity.

Practice Test

Use this practice test to review the topics of this chapter and to prepare for your test on this material.

1.   Which of the following may be found on the surface of RBCs?
     a.   A antigen
     b.   B antigen
     c.   an Rh factor
     d.   a and b
     e.   a, b, and c

2.   Secretion of antibodies is a function of
     a.   T cells
     b.   B cells
     c.   eosinophils
     d.   a and b
     e.   a, b, and c

3. Humoral immunity involves
    a. antibodies
    b. killer T cells
    c. B lymphocytes
    d. a and b
    e. a and c

4. Macrophages
    a. may be involved in specific immune response
    b. are derived from monocytes
    c. are phagocytic
    d. may exhibit chemotaxis
    e. all of the above

5. T cells undergo clonal differentiation in
    a. the thymus
    b. red bone marrow
    c. lymph nodes
    d. the spleen
    e. a and d

6. Opsonization
    a. requires action by a macrophage
    b. decreases intensity of an immune response
    c. destroys all antigens
    d. is no longer held to be true
    e. all of the above

7. Antibodies are classed as IgG, IgA, and so forth, according to the function of the
    a. F_{ab} portion of the molecule
    b. F_c portion of the molecule
    c. hypervariable region
    d. light chain
    e. antigen

8. MHCs
    a. are antigens
    b. may direct killer T cells to their targets
    c. may regulate interactions between T and B cells during an immune response
    d. is the abbreviation of "macrophage-histamine complexes"
    e. a, b, and c

9. Cytotoxic T cells
    a. may be called natural killer cells
    b. require both an MHC-1 antigen and a "self" antigen
    c. require only a "self" antigen
    d. are involved in cell-mediated immunity
    e. a and d

10. Which of these has a primary function of limiting the immune response?
    a. plasma cell
    b. inducer T cell
    c. suppressor T lymphocyte
    d. cytotoxic T cell
    e. none of the above

11. Functionally, the T-cell receptor is similar to an antibody EXCEPT that the
    a. T cell requires a histocompatibility antigen
    b. antibody requires a histocompatibility antigen
    c. T cell is not alive
    d. antibody is nonspecific
    e. T cell is nonspecific

12. Antibodies may aid in destruction of target cells by means of
    a. opsonization
    b. agglutination
    c. activation of complement cascade
    d. a, b, or c
    e. none of the above

13. The presence of bradykinin may cause
    a. local redness
    b. edema
    c. increased temperature
    d. pain
    e. all of the above

14. Bradykinin is derived from
    a. histamine
    b. antibodies
    c. kallikrein
    d. T lymphocytes
    e. B lymphocytes

15. The complement cascade
    a. may be triggered by a specific immune mechanism
    b. may be triggered by a nonspecific immune mechanism
    c. results in T-cell formation
    d. a and b
    e. a and c

Answers

Here are answers (or references) to some of the questions presented above.

Word Parts: (your examples may be different) 1-antigen, 2-agglutination, 3-histamine, 4-opsonization, 5-chemotaxis, 6-cytotoxic

Key Terms: Descriptive: 1. cytotoxic 2. polyclonal 3. monoclonal **Processes:** 1. kallikrein-kinin system 2.

nonspecific immunity 3. vaccination 4. passive immunization 5. opsonization 6. antigen presentation 7. agglutination 8. active immunization 9. specific immunity 10. cell-mediated immunity 11. chemotaxis 12. complement system 13. primary immune response 14. secondary immune response 15. humoral immunity

Structures/Substances: 1. interferon 2. interleukin-2 3. immunoglobulin (Ig) 4. perforin 5. major histocompatibility complex (MHC) 6. hapten 7. histamine 8. antiserum 9. F_{ab} portion 10. antigen 11. antibody 12. lactoferrin 13. lymphokine 14. macrophage 15. bradykinin 16. determinant portion 17. T cell 18. B cell

Other: 1. Rh system 2. affinity chromatography 3. ABO system 4. autoimmune disease 5. erythroblastosis fetalis

Learning Exercises: 1. neutrophil-immune defenses, eosinophil-defense against parasites, basophil-inflammatory response, monocyte-immune defenses, B lymphocyte-antibody production, T lymphocyte-cellular immune response 2. 1-virgin, 2-plasma, 3-memory, 4-cytotoxic, 5-natural killer, 6-helper T, 7-inducer T, 8-suppressor T 3. 1-antigen binding, site, 2-light chain, 3-heavy chain, 4-hypervariable region, 5-F_{ab} fragment, 6-F_c fragment 4. 1-IgG, 2-IgE, 3-IgD, 4-IgA, 5-IgM 5. differentiation, clone, specificity, antibody, antigen, histocompatibility, histocompatibility, gene, MHC-1, MHC-2, B cell 6. (Compare your figure with Figure 26-14 in the text) 7. cytotoxic, MHC-1, natural killer, nonself, helper, inducer, memory, plasma, suppressor

Quick Recall: (You should be able to answer these questions easily without correction or confirmation by this point in your studies. If you cannot, review your notes, the text chapter, and the previous study activities to find the answers.)

Practice Test: 1-e, 2-b, 3-e, 4-e, 5-a, 6-a, 7-b, 8-e, 9-d, 10-c, 11-a, 12-d, 13-e, 14-c, 15-d